# STATE-OF-THE-ART IMAGING IN STROKE
## VOLUME 2

# STATE-OF-THE-ART IMAGING IN STROKE
## VOLUME 2

BERNHARD SCHALLER
EDITOR

**Nova Biomedical Books**
*New York*

For permission to use material from this book please contact us:
Telephone 631-231-7269; Fax 631-231-8175
Web Site: http://www.novapublishers.com



**Library of Congress Cataloging-in-Publication Data**
*Available upon request*

ISBN 978-1-60021-499-8

*Published by Nova Science Publishers, Inc. ✣ New York*

# Contents

# Introduction

***B. Schaller***
Department of Neuroscience, Karolinska Institute,
Stockholm, Sweden

In the last years, a substantial number of imaging studies hav addressed the neuronal processes underlying recovery after stroke [1]. Although difficult to achieve, several longitudinal studies assessed both clinical recovery and imaging patterns over time and give important inside into the plasticity of the stroked brain. This tendency is supported by the fact that it has become possible to depict biological processes at the cellular and molecular level. These new research methods use magnetic resonance imaging (MRI), positron emission tomography (PET), near-infrared optical imaging, scintigraphy, and autoradiography *in vivo* and *in vitro*. Of primary interest is the development of methods using MRI and PET with which the different kinds of progress of therapy in acute ischemic stroke can be monitored and graphically displayed [2]. Steps to intervene with secondary biochemical, molecular, or inflammatory disturbances were not successful so far. Recent activation studies have provided interesting information about the brain's capacity to reorganize after ischemic stroke and in association with practice and learning. The emerging studies of brain plasticity and its modulation by drugs and other therapies indicate potentially useful approaches to the rehabilitation of adults with brain damage, including damage resulting from cerebral ischaemia.

Recent advances in state-of-the-art imaging techniques make it possible to visualize physiological parameters such as molecular diffusion, tissue perfusion and cortical activation [3]. These techniques greatly contribute to the early detection and to the understanding of the pathophysiological evolution and recovery from ischemic stroke patients. Numerous theories and hypothesis have been forwarded to explain the neurological recovery seen after an acute ischemic stroke [4]. Functional brain imaging has offered an opportunity to visualize cerebral activation associated with recovery from a stroke. Functional MRI, PET, and transcranial magnetic stimulation are now being used to demonstrate activation after stroke associated with specific stimuli or tasks. Relatively stringent criteria can be met to confirm that adaptive functional reorganisation limits disability even in the adult brain: functional brain changes are related to disease burden, can be found in patients with demonstrable pathology but no clinical deficits and can be defined (in motor cortex) even in the absence of volitional recruitment. Initial studies of poststroke responses using fMRI and transcranial magnetic stimulation demonstrate that adaptive reorganisation can be manipulated directly with both pharmacological and behavioural interventions. The combination of strategies based on a strong biological rational with monitoring their effects using highly informative functional brain imaging methods heralds a new era of scientifically-founded post-stroke treatment.

State-of-the-art imaging technology is already being developed to image genes and their impact on cellular function in laboratory animals [5]. Eventually, this may also be possible in humans. One of the paradoxes of advances in diagnostic technology is the neglect of clinical skills. Too often the attitude is to shoot a picture first and ask questions later. Not all that matters can be imaged, and not everything that can be imaged matters—a lesson that some have learned to their patients' sorrow. Ironically, the more advanced the diagnostic technology, the greater the need for refined clinical skills, since the easy diagnoses will be made by the technological aids, leaving the most difficult cases to be resolved by clinical approaches and judgment. For this reason, the ethical aspects of our doing are of utmost importance, so that the excellent new state-of-the-art imaging methods are of advantage and not of handicap to our patients. But let us open to window to an interesting area in which the state-of-the-art imaging will be in the center of our handling. However, stroke is only one, but an important example of this process.

In the second part of this book, the main attention is on imaging the poststroke phase and their implication on treatment. This part of the book will give important insight in the future of imaging in stroke and their interaction with clinical aspects. Stroke care has become a specialised field, requiring input from different subspecialists forming a multidisciplinary team.

## References


[1] Schaller B, Jacobs AH, Graf R. Hemispheric dominance for the cortical control of swallowing in humans: a contribution to better understand cortical organization? *Eur. J. Radiol.* 2004; 51:290-1.

[2] Schaller B, Graf R, Sanada Y, et al. Hemodynamic changes after occlusion of the posterior sagittal sinus: an experimental PET study in cats. *Am. J. Neuroradiol.* 2003; 24:1876-80.

[3] Schellinger PD; Fiebach JB, Hacke W. Imaging-based decision making in thrombolytic therapy for ischemic stroke: present status. *Stroke* 2003; 34:575-83.

[4] Ward NS, Brown MM, Thompson AJ, et al. The influence of time after stroke on brain activations during a motor task. *Ann. Neurol.* 2004; 55:829-34.

[5] Hoehn M, Kustermann E, Blunk J, et al. Monitoring of implanted stem cell migration in vivo: a highly resolved in vivo magnetic resonance imaging investigation of experimental stroke in rat. *Proc. Natl. Acad. Sci. USA* 2002; 99:16267-16272.

In: State-of-the-Art Imaging in Stroke, Volume 2
Editor: Bernhard Schaller, pp. 1-39
ISBN 978-1-60021-499-8


*Chapter I*

# Cell Transplantation after Stroke: The Role of *In Vivo* Imaging

*Michel Modo[1, 3], Jack Price[2,3] and Steve C. R. Williams[1]*
[1]Neuroimaging Research Group – Neurology
[2]Department of Neurosciences
[3]Center for Cellular and Integrative Biology, Institute of Psychiatry,
King's College London, London, UK

## A. Introduction

Stroke is the leading cause of adult disability in the Western world and the second leading cause of death in the world [1]. To date, pharmacological interventions have shown some promise in improving outcome of ischaemic stroke if treatment is administered during the acute phase (<6 hours after onset) [2]. Initiation of treatment during the acute phase of a stroke remains a challenge, but can be greatly aided by the use of neuroimaging techniques, such as magnetic resonance imaging [3]. The development of inclusion and exclusion criteria based on physiological markers of ischaemic damage, such as the presence of a penumbra, rather than reported time of symptom onset are also likely to improve the efficacy and utility of these treatments [4]. However, despite some therapeutic successes, these approaches still, in the main, aim to limit the inflicted damage and currently are not addressing the potential to replace lost cells or to support brain plasticity. Consequently, many patients remain disabled and suffer from a persistent loss of quality of life.

Neural transplantation provides an alternative therapeutic strategy based on neurobiological principles that can rescue damaged neurons by means of trophic factor support whilst sustaining the re-organization of existing pathways, and, ultimately, providing novel functional cells which can integrate into the damaged circuitry [5,6]. Pioneering studies with omental tissue gained from a free fold of the peritoneum suggested that tissue transplantation can improve the functional outcome after a stroke [7-9]. These studies presented a rationale for more extensive studies using fetal brain tissue during the 1990s that resulted in a more robust and extensive functional recovery [10-17]. Refinement of the transplant material to contain exclusively an homogenous source of stem cells has further provided the proof-of-principle that transplantation of 'immature' cells can alleviate ischaemia-induced impairments [18,19]. Similar pre-clinical successes have been reported by means of pre-differentiated neuroteratocarcinoma cells [20,21], Sertoli cells [22], and bone marrow cells [23,24]. Nonetheless, some of the studies have disappointed showing, for instance, only a few cells surviving [25] or differentiation into a low number of neurons derived from bone marrow cells [23;26]. Thus, raising doubts about whether cell transplantation exerts a beneficial effect through integration of new cells into existing circuitry.

In global ischaemia, only fetal tissue from the CA1 subfield region of the hippocampus, but not from the CA3 cell region recovered behavioural impairments due to the selective CA1 damage [27] suggesting that not any type of cell can functionally replace cells lost within a neural circuit. In this case, specific cell replacement is necessary to produce a behavioural effect. Still, transplantation of astrocytes or microglia can also improve behavioural functions [28,29] implying that neuronal replacement might not always be a necessary condition. Recovery after a stroke might not be as clearly dependent on a point-to-point reconnection of neural circuitry as is the case in global ischaemic brain damage. Spontaneous recovery in stroke, for instance, is often observed and thought to be a consequence of re-organization of neural networks remote from the lesion site (diaschisis)[30], re-organization or unmasking of transcallosal connectivity allowing homologous areas in the contralateral hemisphere to take over lost functions [31], areas neighbouring the infarct taking over functions [32] or the use of different behavioural strategies to solve the same task [33]. In addition to re-construction or reinnervation of neural circuitry, cell transplantation could support these various processes of endogenous recovery and promote improvements in lost functions. Additionally, the ability of transplanted cells to deliver or stimulate secretion of trophic factors can potentially prevent apoptotic cells from dying [34] and reduce secondary (Wallerian) degeneration [17] leading to an improved outcome in long-term assessments. Upregulation of neurodevelopmental proteins after stroke [35,36] and transplantation [37] further indicate that transplants might exert beneficial effects by various mechanisms in addition to integration into local neuronal cell assemblies. Cell transplantation might therefore provide additional support to the existing response of endogenous stem cells to the infarction [38]. This would also explain why non-neuronal cells, such as bone marrow cells, exert beneficial effects despite only a small proportion of transplanted cells transdifferentiating into neurons (i.e. from cells typically producing a different organ system). Consequently, the combination of several mechanisms could be responsible for transplantation-induced recovery after a stroke (Table 1).

It has also emerged that various aspects of the transplantation procedure itself can influence the recovery after a stroke (Table 2). Notably, the number of cells transplanted can affect recovery, as it is generally presumed that there is a direct positive correlation between the quantity of administered "therapeutic entities" and the degree of recovery.

**Table 1. based on (Dunnett and Björklund, 1994)**

| Mechanisms | Description | Example |
|---|---|---|
| Non-specific | • side-effects of surgery | • caudate lesions alleviate Parkinson's disease |
| | • placebo effect | • Placebo effect observed in double blind clinical trial (Freeman et al., 1999) |
| | • enriched environment | • use of impaired forelimb after lesion improves forelimb's function (Humm et al., 1998) |
| Pharmacological | • secretion of missing neurotransmitters | • dopamine transplants for Parkinson's disease (Chen et al., 1999) |
| Trophic | • release of trophic factors | • adrenal grafts secrete trophic factors that stimulate sprouting in brain (Hansen et al., 1995) |
| | • stimulation of host release of trophic factors | • sham injection results in sprouting of axons (Batchelor et al., 2002) |
| Host Response | • upregulation of developmental proteins | • upregulation of ApoE levels after transplantation (Modo et al., 2003b) |
| | • upregulation of endogenous stem cell response | • subventricular zone sproliferate and migrate to stroke lesion (Arvidsson et al., 2002) |
| | • host inflammatory response | • rejection response promotes recovery (Brejanac et al., 1996) |
| | • support endogenous plasticity | • diaschisis |
| Reconstruction | • grafted cells restore missing/damaged connections | • grafts integrate into tri-synaptic pathway in hippocampus after global ischemia (Hodges et al., 1996) |
| | • grafts re-grow tissue | |
| Reinnervation | • grafts integrate into existing neural circuitry | • striatal grafts restore cortico-striato-pallidal circuits (Wictorin, 1992) |
| Bridge Graft | • grafts provide substrate for regeneration of damaged axons | • axonal re-growth in spinal cord dissection (Xu et al., 1997) |

It is, however, unclear how many cells will be needed to achieve a maximal or minimal therapeutic effect. Although Borlongan et al. [20] have demonstrated that viability and survival of transplanted cells determine the degree of recovery, to date, no clear dose-response relationship has been reported between number of transplanted cells or surviving cells that would allow a calculation of a dose-response curve. Moreover, the level of viability of the transplanted cells (i.e. what proportion of cells are alive in the transplant) has been poorly addressed and there is currently no indication as to what level of viability should be used as a cut-off to exclude transplant material. All preparations of cells *in vitro* will result in some cell death and transplantation of a certain number of dead cells. Transplantation of only dead cells into an ischaemic lesion results in a substantial worsening of the lesion and behavioral impairment [39], but transplantation of dead cells into other brain regions did not affect outcome. The placement of cells in relation to the ischaemic injury might therefore be a crucial factor influencing recovery. Modo et al. [40], for instance, demonstrated that transplantation of cells into both the ischaemic and non-ischaemic hemisphere resulted in recovery of somatosensory functioning, whereas intracerebroventricular transplants allowed control-like spatial learning. We may therefore conclude that despite the seemingly ubiquitous properties of stem cells, the site of implantation is undoubtedly critical [37]. However, it is also possible that recovery processes are localized and that implantation of cells in a particular area might promote recovery processes preferentially in one area rather than in another resulting in different functions being restored.

Apart for the site of implantation, the timing of implantation might also be an important determinant in functional recovery. Transplants into acute lesions appear to survive less well than those implanted more than one week after ischaemia [14]. An inhospitable lesion environment characterized by cell death and macrophage infiltration is likely to also be detrimental to transplanted cells. On the other hand, the upregulation of trophic factors involved in brain plasticity, acting to recover the damage after the acute effects of ischaemia have cleared, might provide a more supportive environment for cell implantation. The best results of transplants have therefore been reported with implantation times between 8-21 days after lesioning [14,41-44].

**Table 2. How imaging can address the factors influencing graft-mediated recovery**

| Influencing factors | The role of *in vivo* imaging |
|---|---|
| Site of lesion | Stereotactic coordinates of location can be determined |
| Severity of lesion | Measurement of lesion volume |
| Graft survival | Contrast agent-labeling prior to transplantation allows cellular tracking |
| Number of grafted cells | Change in signal due to contrast agent-labeled cells potentially can determine how many cells are contained within an area |
| Sites of Implantation | Injection tract visible on $T_2$*-weighted images |
| Effect on host re-organization | fMRI can probe how functional activity changes as the brain re-organizes |
| Inflammatory/immunological response | *In vivo* labeling of macrophages with contrast agent |

It also still remains unclear if the extent of ischaemic brain damage should determine the number of transplanted cells needed to achieve a therapeutic effect. In a clinical setting, it can be assumed that depending on particular lesion characteristics, such as lesion size or the presence of a penumbra, the number of cells to be transplanted would need to be adjusted to account for individual differences between patients. Clearly, many factors influence transplant-mediated behavioural recovery and in order to provide a robust implementation of cell transplantation in a clinical environment, it will be important to determine all the salient factors for the most effective treatment strategy.

Until recently, immunohistochemical analysis of grafted cells has been the sole line of investigation to determine the characteristics of transplanted cells and their anatomical and functional integration *in situ*. However, the 'snapshot' results acquired *ex vivo* by histopathology at one particular time point are limited in their ability to capture the dynamic nature of the evolution of a lesion and processes of recovery. The advent of neuroimaging systems for small animals has therefore opened up a new opportunity to study, in a preclinical setting, stroke lesions and therapeutic interventions prior to their clinical implementation. Neuroimaging, such as positron emission tomography (PET) and magnetic resonance imaging (MRI), have been instrumental in improving the diagnosis of ischaemic lesions and gaining a better understanding of the processes involved in lesion formation [45]. Gaining an understanding of how transplants affect damage leads to a better appreciation of the mechanisms involved in graft-mediated repair. *In vivo* monitoring by means of neuroimaging therefore offers the prospect to determine how cell transplants affect the lesion and its progression over time [46]. Not only can MRI identify and trace the evolution of the lesion, but labeling of cells *in vitro* prior to implantation with a contrast agent also allows the tracking of these transplanted cells in the living brain opening new vistas to understanding why these cells migrate to areas of damage whilst promoting functional improvements [46,47]. The introduction of contrast agents with the potential for molecular imaging will permit the repeated *in vivo* assessment of molecular aspects of the lesion environment [48,49] and help to identify the molecular underpinnings of transplant-induced brain plasticity. Molecular imaging will therefore in the future provide a new tool in our understanding of how cell transplants facilitate functional recovery after a stroke. Advances in the imaging of cell transplants in stroke, to date have mainly focused on experimental studies in animal models of stroke.

## B. Experimental Knowledge

Fetal tissue transplants can be detected on MR images as they form a mass that is distinct from the rest of the brain [50-52]. The vascular properties of the graft are also distinct from the rest of the brain and can also be distinguished from brain tumours based on the characteristics of contrast agent influx [53]. However, cell transplants will generally not form a distinct mass, but will migrate and ideally integrate seamlessly within the host parenchyma. By virtue of these properties and a lack of graft-derived vasculature, it is not possible to identify cell transplants by conventional structural MRI [54]. However, the introduction of contrast agents to label cells prior to transplantation was pioneered in the early 1990s [55,56] and has recently initiated a new avenue to *in vivo* investigations.

## *In Vitro* Preparations for *In Vivo* Cell Tracking

The development of contrast agents, such as ultra small particles of iron oxide (USPIO), generate enough contrast due to the 'blooming effect' in $T_2$*-weighted MR images [57] that they allow detection at very low concentrations [58]. Incorporation of these particles into cells therefore allows the imaging of a small number of cells in the brain and may even lead to *in vivo* single-cell imaging [59,60]. Phagocytic cells, such as macrophages, will ingest USPIO *in vitro* [61] and *in vivo* in the blood stream [62], whereas neural cells do not appear to readily take-up these larger molecules. Hoehn et al. [63] have shown that the combination of iron oxide particles with a transfection agent, usually used to transfer DNA into cells, improves cellular uptake to allow efficient incorporation of contrast agents into the cells for *in vitro* and *in vivo* imaging. Similarly, modification of the contrast agent's surface can render them more amenable to cell labeling [64,65]. For instance, Bulte et al. [66] designed a novel contrast agent based on dendrimers that are readily chaperoned into the cell. These magnetodendrimers label a variety of cells within a reasonable time frame (i.e. hours rather than days) whilst affording a robust *in vivo* detection of transplanted cells. Smaller contrast agents based on Gadolinium (Gd) are more readily taken-up into cells [54], but their inherent lower signal enhancement demands a greater load of the contrast agent to be incorporated into the cells to be detected *in vivo*. To this end, Daldrup-Link et al. [67] also recently suggested that Gd-based agents are more amenable to the development of multimodal agents which incorporate a fluorescent dye to afford *in vivo* optical imaging and corroboration by fluorescent histology. As Crich et al. [68] indicated the potential of Gd-based contrast agents to provide a positive contrast (hyperintense signal) in $T_1$-weighted MR images is considered more reliable since a negative contrast (hypointense signal) on $T_2$- or $T_2$*-weighted MR images can be a consequence of injection tract damage or blood from the meninges bleeding into the implantation site. To circumvent these issues, the design of novel pulse sequences which can produce a positive signal on $T_2$-weighted MR images whilst nulling the signal from the surrounding tissue or blood [69] will constitute useful developments to provide a sensitive and specific imaging approach to cellular tracking. The higher susceptibility of iron-based contrast agents and their ease of detection currently make them a more popular choice for cellular imaging.

As contrast agents consist of a metal particle as an inner sphere, the potential exposure of the cell to this metal particle in high concentrations can impact on cellular viability. It is therefore paramount to investigate if the concentration of contrast agent to be used will affect the viability of the labeled cells. Although it can generally be presumed that cell labeling will reduce the cell viability, Hoehn et al. [63], for instance, reported that cell viability was even superior in labeled than in non-labeled cells. Nonetheless, determining the effect of cell labeling on cell viability is crucial as transplantation of compromised cells might ultimately lead to a poor survival of transplanted cells.

Not only is cell viability an important issue to be tested *in vitro* prior to transplantation, but it is also important to understand the effect of the contrast agent on cellular functions. The most basic function that can be affected by labeling of cells with a contrast agent is proliferation. Proliferation is an essential step in the differentiation of neural precursor cells. Compromising cellular division can therefore limit the cells' ability to differentiate, integrate to detect the transplanted cell compared to the same cell being contained within a larger voxel (as the signal arising from each voxel constitutes a signal average for all cells in that volume). Some reports suggest that with conventional USPIOs, it is possible to detect as few as 40 labelled cells per voxel *in vitro* and 500 labelled cells *in vivo* [63]. The use of micron sized particles of iron oxides (MPIOs) even allows detection of a single cell *in vivo* [60]. *In vivo* detection after transplantation into stroke-damaged brains is complicated by the proliferation of the transplanted cells. As the cells proliferate, the amount of contrast agent contained within each daughter cell is halved. It is therefore more difficult to detect these cells after cell division. Modo et al. [54] reported that after 7 days of cell proliferation cells were no longer detectable based on the fluorescent signal of a bimodal contrast agent *in vitro* suggesting that if cells are permitted to proliferate, they will become undetectable by MRI. In contrast, Hoehn et al. [63] indicated that cells labelled with USPIOs were still detectable after 10 cell divisions *in vitro*.

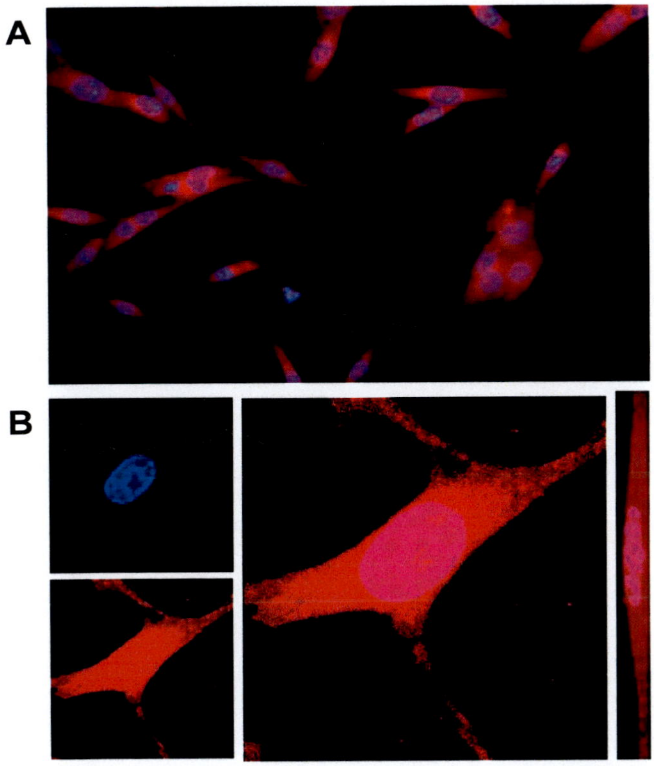


Figure 1. *In vitro* labeling of stem cells with a bimodal contrast agent. A. Conditionally immortalized neural stem cells from the MHP36 cell line grow *in vitro* and by incubation with the bimodal contrast agent GRID, these cells will incorporate the contrast agent and allow detection of cells by both MRI and fluorescent microscopy. Incorporation of this bimodal agent into cells does not appear to alter the cells phenotype in vitro or in vivo. However, it is still unclear if contrast agents might exert an effect on the cells ability to promote behavioural improvements. B. Thousands of molecules of GRID are taken up by stem cells into their cytoplasm rendering the whole cell red. In a co-culture experiment, it has been shown that leakage and re-uptake does not appear to pose a significant problem with this contrast agent (Modo et al., 2002c).

and subsequently promote functional recovery *in vivo*. Moreover, some division/differentiation of stem cells is required before the cellular programs involved in migration can be initiated [70]. In order to guarantee a similar mechanism of recovery a transplantation of stem cells, it is therefore essential that proliferation of cells is larg unaffected by incorporation of a contrast agent. Modo et al. [54] have demonstrated MHP36 cells which are conditionally immortalized retain their ability to proliferate *in v* after cell labeling and that these transplanted cells differentiated into both neurons and g cells in global ischemic brains. Although in general contrast agent labeling does not seem affect the cells ability to proliferate and differentiate [71,72], Kostura et al. [73] rece reported that labeling of mesenchymal stem cells with Feridex (an iron-based clinica approved contrast agent) specifically affects the cells' potential to differentiate i chondrocytes *in vitro* and *in vivo*, but not their adipogenic or osteogenic potential. Th results imply that there might be subtle effects of cell labeling that will only become appa after more extensive investigations into their effects on cellular functioning.

The localization of contrast agents inside the cell might influence the effect th compounds exert on cellular functioning. Hoehn et al. [63] demonstrated that the USI combined with a transfection agent localized the contrast agent to the lysosomes. Howe reports of incorporation of USPIOs within cells after prolonged exposure [74,75] raise question as to which approach might be more desirable, faster labeling or omission of transfection agent? It is thought that localization to the endosomes will improve the reten of the contrast agent within the cell and not interfere with any crucial functioning of the c Although the cytoplasm provides a larger space within the cell, localization of the cont agent to the cytoplasm is less desirable as it might interfere with cellular functi Especially, the use of Gd-based contrast agents that necessitate a larger number of molec to be incorporated might only find the necessary space within the cytoplasm. By attach specific 'guidance' molecules to contrast agents, it is also possible to preferentially l particular cellular compartments [76]. It is still unclear how contrast agents interact with cellular functions and if these interactions could be detrimental.

Although, contrast agents might not interfere with cellular functioning during the b periods of *in vitro* observation, it is less clear how the metal particles forming the i sphere of contrast agents will affect cell functioning over time after they have lost t protective outer sphere. Currently, it is not known if and over what time period the o sphere of contrast agents might disintegrate. Depending on the type of metal particle concentration, and its localization, the effect on cellular functioning might be negligib might lead to cell death. At present, there are no indications if this is indeed a problem t considered prior to potential clinical applications. Although metabolizing of iron-b contrast agents with transplanted cells is a possibility (as part of the normal iron metaboli and some cells can even be engineered to draw iron from the endogenous pool [77], it is unlikely that this will be the case for Gd-based contrast agents.

The type of metal particle and its concentration within a transplanted cell will determine its detection limit *in vivo*, but also depend on the pulse sequences and hardwa be used. For instance, a higher magnetic field strength in the main, intensifies the effect o contrast agent [78]. Moreover, the possibility to have a higher spatial resolution for the s time of imaging reduces partial volume effects. The smaller voxel size makes it more li

A final check before venturing to *in vivo* imaging is to determine if the contrast agent might leak from the transplanted cell and inadvertently label host cells yielding a false positive response. The use of the bimodal contrast agent GRID, detectable by both MRI and fluorescent microscopy, has allowed Modo et al. [54] to demonstrate in a co-culture system, in which cells labeled with the red fluorescent GRID and the green fluorescent dye PKH67 were grown together for 2 weeks, that there was no crossing over of labels between cells. This implies that leakage and re-uptake does not constitute a significant problem.

However, it is still unclear if these *in vitro* experiments can reliably predict what happens *in vivo*. The presence of macrophages, microglia and astrocytes *in vivo* might promote leakage and re-uptake. A cell-autologuous markers, such as green fluorescent protein (GFP), might, for example, allow a more robust corroboration of cellular tracking by MRI.

## Tracking the Migration of Transplanted Cells in the Living Brain

In vivo detection of contrast agent-loaded cells is contingent on a sufficient signal change induced by the (super-) paramagnetic properties of the agents inside the cells. The limitations of in vivo detection are also dependent on the concentration of contrast agent (the less signal attenuation caused by an agent, the more needs to be incorporated inside the cell), the number of cells to be detected and the voxel volume.

As mentioned above, the magnitude of signal change expected based on a paramagnetic effect (i.e. weakly attracted to magnetic field, such as gadolinium-based agents on a $T_1$-weighted MR image), will be more difficult to detect in vivo compared to superparamagnetic effects (i.e. magnetic moments align within individual particles and produce a very strong paramagnetic effect, such as an iron oxide-based agent on $T_2$*-weighted images). Nonetheless, the potential to detect the cells as a hyperintensity (bright signal) on a $T_1$-weighted MR scan is advantageous as a hypointensity (dark signal) on $T_2$-weighted MR images is not unequivocally attributable the contrast agent-labeled cells [54,68,69]. Still, '$T_1$'-agents generally also exert a signal change on $T_2$-weighted MR images that is often easier to detect due its superparamagnetic properties [54]. Interpretation of $T_2$-weighted MR images in vivo is complicated by the fact that air bubbles, injection tract damage, and small bleeds, can also produce hypointense contrasts that could be mistaken for transplanted cells. An additional issue with superparamagnetic effects is that a high concentration of molecules within cells or a large number of cells within a voxel will cause a 'blooming effect' that will occupy an area larger than occupied by the cells. This potentially occludes important information regarding anatomy or the presence of damage. The 'blooming effect' can, nevertheless, be exploited if the aim is to detect only a few cells in vivo. Unfortunately, no formula has been reported in the literature to calculate how much contrast agent needs to be contained within a cell to allow a reliable detection. At present, no ideal contrast agent exists that would allow the detection of only a few cells by means of a quantifiable hyperintense (positive) signal enhancement without occluding potential damage or anatomical detail.

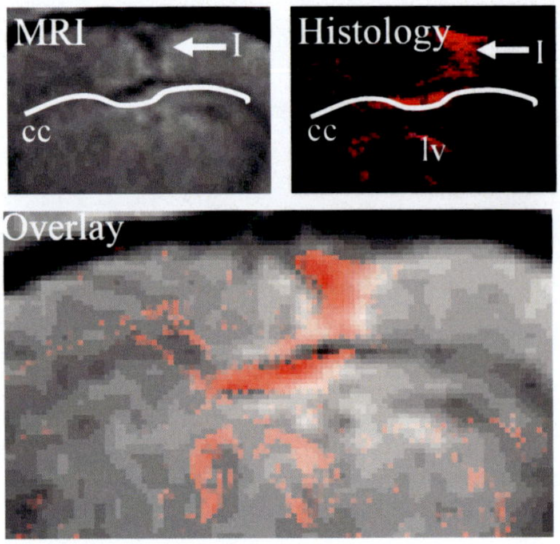


Figure 2. Detecting stem cells labeled with a bimodal contrast agent by MRI and fluorescent histology. In vitro labeling of neural stem cells with the bimodal contrast agent GRID allows their detection in the damaged brain by both MRI and fluorescent histology. The bimodality of this agent allows a direct corroboration of the cells detected by either modality (Modo et al., 2002c). The negative signal (dark spots) on the MRI scan to trace transplanted cells in the damaged brain could also be caused by other phenomena, such as an air bubble or a small bleed. Being able to therefore corroborate by histology that this reduced MRI signal intensity is indeed due to the transplanted cells corroborates the MRI detection of transplanted cells. (I = injection tract; cc = corpus callosum; lv lateral ventricles).

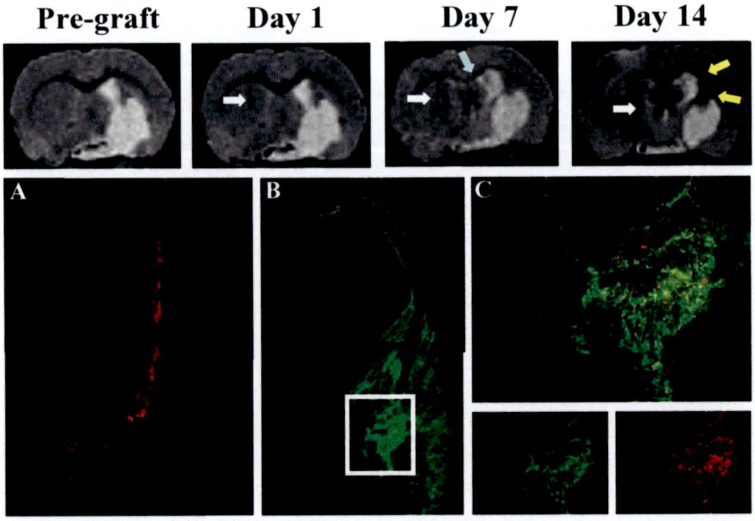


Figure 3. Serial *in vivo* tracking of the migration of transplanted stem cells by MRI. Being able to visualize the area of damage prior to transplantation also ensures that any changes observed following transplantation are indeed due to the implantation procedures of contrast agent-labeled cells. The serial scanning of the same subject over time by MRI offers a dynamic representation of cell migration *in vivo* that could not be gained by traditional histological methods. Post-mortem analyses at the final time point can be used to corroborate in vivo detection of, for instance, the initial injection tract (A), but can also be used to probe the cells integration into the damaged tissue (B) and its differentiation into site-appropriate phenotypes (C) (Red indicates GRID-labeled transplanted cells, Green indicates GFAP-positive astrocytes). This approach gives us the technology to probe how cell migration and integration into damaged tissues lead to behavioural improvements (Modo et al., 2004b).

To date, most studies have mainly focused on the proof-of-principle that detection of transplanted cells is feasible in vivo, but applications of this approach are now emerging for ischaemia-damaged brains. Once cells can be visualized in vivo, it is possible to study the significance of cell survival, migration and functional integration to behavioural performance. However, so far, the focus has been mainly to locate the transplanted cells (54) and to visualize their migration [63,74,75,79,80]. These studies demonstrate that it is possible to locate cells on the day after transplantation to the injection tract. A popular choice has been to locate the injection tract in the contralateral hemisphere and to observe how cells migrate along the corpus callosum to the site of injury [63,74,75,79] where they will differentiate into site-appropriate phenotypes and participate in processes of repair [37,40,79].

Kim et al. [81] demonstrated the same phenomenon by in vivo bioluminescence, although the poorer in vivo spatial resolution of this technique did not provide sufficient detail to implicate a particular structure in migration. Migration of cells has also been observed after intracisternal implantation, although migration did not appear to involve the corpus callosum [80]. The speed of migration of these bone marrow cells was calculated as 65μm/hr by measuring their distance from the injection site. The lack of migration along the corpus callosum after intracisternal injection might suggest that transcallosal migration is specific to contralateral injections. The migration towards the lesion, however, seems to be a common phenomenon among embryonic, neural and bone marrow stem cells.

To ensure that these in vivo observations are indeed due to transplanted cells, control injections of cells not labeled with a contrast agent are essential to exclude injection tract damage as a possible cause of the hypointense signal delineating the injection tract [54]. Furthermore, to avoid the potential misidentification of macrophages which have taken-up contrast agent from dead transplanted cells, transplantation of dead cells labeled with a contrast agent is recommended [80]. Generally, the hypointense circular area denoting the deposit disappears over time suggesting that the contrast agent is not readily taken up in a significant number of host cells apart of macrophages. The presence of contrast agent within macrophages at these time points indicates that these cells clear the contrast agent from the brain. In animals with a stroke, caution is demanded when transplanting dead cells into the infarct area as it can increase lesion volume by ~30% [39] and therefore should not be considered a viable control condition for studies investigating the effect of transplanted cells on lesion volume or behavioural recovery.

Although, Zhang et al. [80] reported behavioural improvements in animals with contrast agent-loaded bone marrow cells, it is unclear if this would indeed also be the case for neural stem cell transplants which might act through different mechanisms of recovery. Also, the inhibition of mesenchymal stem cells by iron oxide particle incorporation to differentiate into chondrogenesis [73] implies that some effects might be subtle and hence might not be observed immediately. Consequently, it will be important to determine if contrast agent-loading of cells will affect their potential to promote brain repair over protracted (>6 months) time periods. So far, most reports have only focused on the first month following transplantation and did not observe any deleterious effects. To determine the long-term viability of this approach more chronic time points will need to be addressed to test if the contrast agent will disappear or exert a delayed deleterious effect on transplanted cells.

The reliable detection of transplanted cells in vivo is only the preliminary step towards the use of MRI as a means to study how transplanted cells exert their beneficial effects on behaviour. It is only of limited clinical use to know that cells will migrate and survive, unless they will promote behavioural recovery. It therefore remains to be evaluated if speed or distance of migration and graft survival as determined by contrast agent-enhanced MRI will be important indices that can inform us about the influence of transplanted stem cells on behavioural improvements after a stroke.

## Effect of Transplanted Cells on Lesion Progression

Labeling of cells with contrast agents allows tracing of cells *in vivo*, but does not address the issue of how transplanted cells alter the damaged brain in order to provide functional and behavioural recovery. Serial MRI can capture the ischaemic lesion prior to transplantation and follow the progression of this lesion over time to investigate if grafting of cells will halt lesion progression or might even reverse the size of the lesion. Roberts et al. [82] have demonstrated the potential of this approach by transplanting neural stem cells in rats with bilateral 3-NPA-induced damage of the striatum. Comparison of lesion volumes pre- and post-transplantation in addition to other anatomical measures, such as striatal atrophy, revealed that grafting did not significantly reduce the volume of the lesion, but halted the progression of striatal atrophy. A correlational analysis with behavioural observations indicated that this striatal preservation was linked to preservation of motor function. These results also revealed that deficits in behaviour do not necessarily correlate with lesion volume, but relate to anatomical measures that are directly involved in the neural substrate responsible for a particular task.

Depending on the severity of a stroke, many different neuroanatomical structures can be affected and contribute to behavioural impairments. Identifying which neural substrate is responsible for a particular behaviour and/or recovery is important as cells could be directly implanted in this locale. The use of contrast agents, however, might inadvertently complicate the assessment of damage as the hypointense (dark) MR signal indicating transplanted cells might interfere with the hyperintense (bright) 'lesion-signal'. Determining that transplanted cells rescue damaged tissue would be difficult to ascertain as changes in the signal in this neuroanatomical structure could be due to the contrast agent inside transplanted cells rather than a change in the tissue properties. Thus, it would be difficult to determine the relationship between changes in the neural substrate and behaviour. The continued monitoring of lesion progression and the potential to assess recurrent strokes needs to be warranted in a clinical setting. So far, it is therefore unclear to what degree contrast agent-loaded cells would impact on the serial chronic assessment of ischaemic lesions.

Ideally, a $T_1$-attenuating agent should be developed to allow the reliable detection of cells *in vivo*. The use of $T_1$-weighed MR scans to detect transplanted cells would have only minimal impact on the ability of mainly $T_2$-based measurements to evaluate the progression or recurrence of an ischaemic insult.

## Integrating Cellular Imaging with Stroke Imaging

MRI currently affords the most versatile *in vivo* assessment of stroke [3]. Perfusion and diffusion imaging allow an early detection of ischaemic damage, possibly even the detection of a penumbra [83], whereas $T_2$-weighted MR images permit a robust assessment of chronic damage. Functional MRI (fMRI) further probes the functional significance of damage [84] and can help us to determine the neural substrates of behavioural dysfunctions [85]. Furthermore, excitement about fMRI as a translational technique relates to its ability to study functional reorganization in the brain of both animal and human subjects [86,87].

Considering that little is known about how cell transplants exert their beneficial effects, the integration of fMRI and cellular tracking will indicate if there is a relationship between degree of functional re-organization and infiltration of transplanted cells. The analytical potential lies in determining to what degree transplanted cells are "attracted" by damage (66), if there is a correlation between speed or extent of migration and stroke damage, and more importantly if the rate of migration and functional re-organization of the damaged brain have any significance for behavioural recovery. The next step would then be to optimize these mechanisms with an aim to further improve the efficacy of cell therapy. A distinction should be made here in that functional recovery refers to changes in the functional architecture of the brain (i.e. the pathways or regions that are elicited during a particular task), whereas behavioural recovery is indicated by changes in the performance of a given task.

Combining imaging techniques, such as PET and MRI, into a single device [88] can further enhance our abilities to study the fundamental processes of how ischaemic episodes progress to chronic lesion. The higher specificity and sensitivity of radioligands for PET imaging can complement the higher spatial resolution of MRI, hence supplying highly specific molecular and very detailed anatomical images of disease pathology. Studying how transplanted cells interact with the host brain and result in upregulation of specific neurodevelopmental proteins could lead to a molecular understanding of cell-mediated brain repair. Studying plasticity events, such as diaschis [89,90], in preclinical models in relation to cell transplantation will help to disentangle whether transplanted cells support host re-organization by supplementing host-processes or whether they provide a novel mechanism by which functional plasticity is achieved.

Likewise, further experimental knowledge can also be gained from integrating MRI with optical imaging methods. The use of bimodal agents could, for instance, afford the localization of transplanted cells *in vivo* by MRI and report on gene expression inside these cells by means of a fluorescent signal being produced by proteins binding to the contrast agent. Likewise, bioluminescent imaging of transgenic animals expressing GFP (or any other fluorescent signal) linked to a particular gene could help to illuminate the particular expression patterns of, for instance, neurodevelopmental genes in the process of differentiation of transplanted precursor cells. Further development of this technology may allow investigations into the expression of genes at particular locations of the transplanted cells and the response of the gene expression of the host (by means of GFP-bioluminescence). A greater understanding of the developmental changes that transplanted cells are undergoing *in vivo* (e.g. differentiation or transdifferentiation) and the response of the host to grafted cells could be gained from the integration of these *in vivo* imaging techniques. Nonetheless, the technical challenges of this multimodal imaging are enormous.

Thorough preclinical testing involving neuroimaging will therefore address the potential of cell transplantation to promote behavioural improvements in patients suffering from stroke damage. Unlike the development of pharmaceutical compounds, no clear guidelines exist as to what should be considered sufficient pre-clinical evidence that cell transplants should progress to clinical trials. Mere cell survival, migration or differentiation in the absence of behavioural improvements cannot, in isolation, justify exposing patients to the risk of surgery. Therefore the ability to promote behavioural change would be a *conditio sine qua non* to consider a particular approach a viable treatment.

## C. Clinical Knowledge

Based on pre-clinical evidence proving the behavioural efficacy of predifferentiated human neuroteratocarcinoma (NT2) cells in animal models [21], Kondziolka et al. [91] conducted a small clinical trial probing safety and efficacy of this procedure in 12 patients with stroke. Either 2 or 6 million cells were transplanted into the infracted basal ganglia. In 4 patients, large areas of the regional cortex also showed signs of infarction. Arterial supply to the area of infarction was, however, not evaluated prior to transplantation. During frequent subsequent visits to assess the safety and efficacy of the procedure over 52 weeks, patients were assessed on both the National Institute of Health Stroke Scale (NIHSS) and the European Stroke Scale (ESS). Additionally, at baseline and 6 months after implantation, patients were rated on the Barthel Index (BI). No significant side-effect of the surgery or tumour formation were observed in any of the patients indicating that the grafting procedure can be considered safe. In a patient that died at 27 months post-transplantation, cells with a typical polyploidy caryotype of hNT cells were found in the periphery of the infarct area [92]. These transplanted cells expressed neurofilament markers indicative of neuronal differentiation. However, the extent of graft survival or its relevance to clinical outcome are unclear from the report. At 24 weeks post-implantation, 50% of the patients showed some improvements on the assessment scales, whereas 25% of patients showed a decline in performance. Kondziolka et al. [91] indicated that improvements were not consistent and that the means of efficacy assessment were not optimized in this study. The assessment of long-term recovery in stroke patients poses a major challenge, especially due to the heterogeneity of the lesion size and location. No integrated balanced scale (including motor, cognitive, and emotional factors) currently exists that would allow an adequate long-term follow-up of this group of patients.

A follow-up phase II trial further elaborated on the efficacy testing by incorporating an extensive neuropsychological battery of tests [93] that encompassed a wider variety of assessment factors and included appropriate control groups. However, no data validating this test battery on stroke patients for long-term assessment has been published. In this phase II trial, a larger sample of patients was implanted with either 5 or 10 million cells in the area of infarction confined to the basal ganglia. Few improvements were observed after cell transplantation, with the exception of marked improvements on the Rey Complex Figure test in patients that suffered a stroke in the non-dominant hemisphere. In patients with a stroke in the dominant hemisphere, no similar improvements were observed on any of the assessed functions. Alongside news of a phase I trial using porcine fetal neural cells being stopped due to adverse side-effects in two patients [94], these studies predict that the translation of pre-clinical efficacy into therapeutic success is not straightforward. However, the specific improvement of a sub-group of patients on a particular task implies that the benefits of cell transplantation might crucially, at least in the first phase of development, depend on patient selection and elaborate psychometric testing to establish a proof-of-efficacy.

## How Does the Lesion Affect Graft Efficacy?

The type (ischaemic or haemorrhagic) and location of a stroke are likely to impact on the potential success of cell therapy. Most pre-clinical studies have focused on ischaemic stroke and consequently little is known about the efficacy of cell therapy in, for instance, haemorrhagic stroke. Although a few investigations have been conducted in pre-clinical haemorrhagic stroke models [95], the scarce evidence and current lack of comparison with ischaemic stroke models does not warrant the inclusion of haemorrhagic stroke patients in clinical trials at this time.

Likewise, to date, most pre-clinical stroke studies have focused on a fairly acute implantation period (up to about 3 weeks following the ischaemic insult), whereas inclusion in clinical trials has mainly be conducted on patients with stroke damage that has been stable for several months. The variability of the time of transplantation from 7 to 55 months [91] could also contribute to the difference in efficacy observed between pre-clinical and clinical studies. As mentioned above, the time of transplantation might be crucial to harness the maximal regenerative power of cell therapy. The burden here is on pre-clinical studies to provide more thorough assessments of the therapeutic window for cell therapy.

A stroke in the basal ganglia results in a completely different behavioural impairment compared to a stroke confined to the cortex. Depending on the lesion location, different types of recovery mechanisms might be more important than others. To recover a particular type of damage, it might therefore be necessary to induce transplanted cells to mainly act, for instance, through support of diaschisis, rather than to replace whole connections. Replacing interneurons with their local connections might be easier to accomplish than re-wiring connections between distinct regions (such as getting dopaminergic cells to re-connect the substantia nigra and caudate putamen in Parkinson's disease). So far, pharmacological agents have, in the main, shown efficacy limiting the progression of ischaemic damage in the cortex, but have shown less success in reducing striatal damage. The differential vulnerability of striatal and cortical cells [96] might account for some of these differences and might indicate that repair of this damage by cell transplantation might rely, at least in part, on different mechanisms. Again, no pre-clinical studies have addressed this issue to suggest clear guidelines to define inclusion/exclusion criteria for initial clinical studies.

Not only does the location of the stroke matter, but also the type of behaviour to be recovered. Some behaviours depend on specific connections being formed, whereas others, such as motor tasks, are more dependent on, for instance, the level of dopamine-transmission in the caudate putamen. It is therefore conceivable that grafts mainly exerting a pharmacological effect, such as secretion of dopamine, are more likely to affect an aspect of behaviour that is less dependent on a point-to-point connection.

Moreover, impairment on a behavioural task is not an isolated entity being damaged that needs repairing. Behaviour consists of the orchestrated sequences of different basic processes, some of which may have been compromised by the area of damage. For instance, if the neural substrate for attention has been damaged, it is likely that all behavioural tasks involving attention will show an impairment. Recovery on these tasks can therefore be expected if the neural substrates of attention have been 'repaired'. Understanding both the impaired behaviour and underlying damage will increase our ability to successfully reverse the behavioural impairments by means of cell therapy. As mentioned above, it is therefore important to thoroughly assess patients for the type of impairment that is to be recovered with an extensive test battery to cover a variety of basic processes. The more consistent the lesion, the more likely a similar behavioural impairment profile can be expected. Consistency among patients to be included in an efficacy study will be paramount to determine a clear treatment effect.

Also, irrespective of location and type of damage, if efficacy is linked to a particular mechanism that these cells exert, a relationship between the quantity of cells and recovery should be observed [97]. It is therefore also conceivable that a larger lesion (or more severe behavioural deficits) might need more cells than a smaller lesion. Although Kondziolka et al. [91] reported that clinical outcome, size of infarction or time since infarction did not correlate in their sample of 12 patients, only a larger sample would provide the analytical power to generalize these findings. A carefully designed dose-response study factoring in lesion volume by means of a pre-transplant MRI scan might help to address this important issue in order to optimize therapeutic efficacy.

## Immunosuppressed or Immunocompetent Hosts?

The need for immunosuppression also remains to be addressed appropriately. Kondziolka et al. [91] administered cyclosporine A (6 mg/kg body weight per day orally for 1 week prior and 8 weeks post-grafting) and methylprednisolone (40 mg intravenously during implantation) in their phase I trial. There are conflicting reports regarding the necessity of immunosuppression for fetal transplantation experiments in patients with Parkinson's disease. Some authors profess that it is a necessary condition at least in the short-term to guarantee satisfactory graft survival [98], whereas others argue that graft survival is similar even without immunosuppression [99,100]. Although it might still be unclear if immunosuppression is a necessary element in transplantation for stroke, it is, however, important to investigate this issue since graft rejection or the inflammatory response to grafted cells can improve behavioural function [101] and therefore inadvertently provide an alternative non-specific mechanism to facilitate recovery.

Although great insight can be gained from pre-clinical studies regarding the use of a xenogenic, allogenic or syngenic cell or tissue sources, the immune system of rodents is not as sensitive as that of human patients and it is therefore difficult to predict if immunosuppression is required. Some studies in rodents suggest that no immunosuppression is required for neural stem cells as their MHC expression is fairly low [48] and the blood-brain barrier might prevent immune detection allowing concordant xenografts to survive [102]. Even in primate models long-term survival of mouse xenografts or allografts have been observed with minimal or no immunosuppression [103,104]. Still, other studies demonstrate clearly improved survival of grafted cells with extensive immunosuppression regimes [105]. Although these studies predominantly employed fetal transplants that contain immunogenic microglia and endothelial cells, they reveal that the immune privilege of the brain is not absolute. Being able to administer cell therapy without the need for immunosuppression, however, would be greatly beneficial to the patient in order to reduce side-effects, such as renal failure. Immunosuppression in acute stroke can also affect the inflammatory response to the damage [106]. It is unclear if this influence is beneficial or detrimental, since microglia and macrophages have been implicated in the process of brain repair [107], and immunosuppressants, such as cyclosporine A, are also known to reduce lesion volume in pre-clinical models [106]. Carefully designed pre-clinical studies should address these issues.

## Neuroimaging as a Core Clinical Assessment

The use of $^{11}$C-PK-11195 as a PET-ligand can reveal the microglia response to transplanted cells and provide a fairly non-invasive approach to visualize the inflammatory reaction in both animals and humans (108,109). Although, clinical studies of cell grafts in stroke patients did not visualize the microglia response to transplanted cells, Meltzer et al. [110] imaged patients with both serial MRI and PET. Transplanted cells improved the glucose metabolism in the infarcted area and correlated with enhanced performance on clinical tests. An increased metabolism at 6 months following grafting was suggested as evidence that inflammation could not account for these results. However, at present little is known about the clinical time course of a graft rejection response and it must be assumed that it is possible that an inflammatory or rejection response to grafted cells could persist for extended time periods. The presence of macrophages at the site of implantation/infarction has been reported by Nelson et al. [92] even 27 months after transplantation. Future imaging with more specific PET ligands [111] or contrast agent-mediated tracking of macrophages [112] could help to address these issues.

Serial MRI measurements should allow a quantitative assessment of the effects of grafted cells on the host tissue [113] and provide an indication as to the anatomical substrates that could lead to behavioural improvements. The recent development of voxel based morphometry (VBM) has provided exciting new insights into the progression of neurological disorders, such as Alzheimer's disease [114], by identifying minute changes taking place over years of pathology. Similar approaches could reveal insights into subtle graft mechanisms, such as prevention of secondary atrophy, which cannot easily be detected by immunohistochemical methods due to intra-subject variability. Likewise, the implementation of robust functional MRI (fMRI) paradigms [84,115] sensitive to, for instance, ischaemic lesions confined to the non-dominant basal ganglia, could provide evidence as to the effect of grafted cells on host plasticity, whereas diffusion tensor imaging (DTI) Jones et al. [116] could complement these observations to reveal if there is any sparing or reconstruction of damaged fibers. The application of these technologies in a serial fashion at frequent intervals will increase the ability of clinical investigators to determine the relevant mechanisms of recovery and optimize transplantation procedures.

Although these approaches will provide evidence of the effect of transplanted cells in the host brain, they do not provide any direct information as to the survival or location of the transplanted cells. As mentioned above, the development of cellular tracking by MRI and PET are promising new developments to allow a 'direct' assessment of grafted cells. Being able to visualize the survival of grafted cells will allow us to determine if graft-mediated recovery is truly dependent on graft survival and if there is a relationship between the number of surviving cells and the extent of recovery. Furthermore, distinguishing whether grafted cells slowly die over time or disappear due to an immune reaction will need to be considered for the long-term management of stroke as it might become necessary for these patients to undergo further repeated implantations of cells to prevent subsequent degeneration.

Not only is the survival of grafted cells relevant to recovery, but also placement or location of the grafted cells can affect behavioural function. It is conceivable that graft placement within the ischaemic penumbra might support damaged cells in addition to providing new cells that will 're-wire' the area. The location of cells within this region might therefore afford a more efficacious intervention than if cells merely integrate into a peri-infarct area where cells remained intact. Still, at present there is limited scientific evidence for either scenario. The use of cellular tracking by means of contrast agents allowing the specific visualization of transplanted cells will contribute to the resolution of these issues. The current and future developments of cellular and molecular imaging techniques will greatly benefit our ability to address these questions *in vivo* in both pre-clinical and clinical settings.

## D. Aspects for the Future

The development and design of contrast agents that afford visualization of cells and molecules *in vivo* will be of great benefit to the investigation of the development, degeneration and regeneration of the brain [117]. At present, mainly radioligands for PET imaging have the ability to visualize particular molecules *in vivo* in human patients. However, the development of smart contrast agents that only change the MR signal upon binding to a molecule of interest [118] and magnetic relaxation switches that use particular molecules or proteins as catalysts to dose-dependently change the $T_2$ signal on an MR scan [119], hold great promise for future applications of MR to visualize molecular aspects of disease and regeneration serially *in vivo*.

These developments in 'molecular medicine' will lead to a greater understanding of disease processes by providing us with a refined toolbox to help identify different sub-groups of patients that is based on the molecular characterization of pathological processes rather than upon presentation of symptoms. It will also allow us to recognize the molecular events which precipitate degeneration and regeneration. However, these advances are dependent on the engineering of contrast agents that will target specific molecules. Although it is currently possible to attach antibodies to contrast particles [120], these constructs are often too large to cross the blood-brain barrier or they provide a background that is too noisy to afford specific imaging of a molecule of interest. It is unrealistic to believe that 'smart' contrast agents will be developed to all types of molecules. Instead, it is more likely that contrast agent design will specifically address a need to image the more important molecules that could be used as hallmarks for particular biological events.

Finding hallmarks of molecular processes is largely guided by genetics and the neuropathological assessment of diseased brains. However, there is an increasing need to develop *in vivo* markers of these 'hallmark' processes. Although the development of molecular imaging markers will aim to fulfill this role and complement the *ex vivo* analyses of molecular aberrations, an interdisciplinary approach is necessary to develop *in vivo* surrogate markers of disease progression and repair.

## Developing Surrogate Imaging Markers

Surrogate markers of behavioural recovery can consist of imaging indices that allow an independent and objective measurement of disease progression and reversal. Imaging indices are therefore also increasingly used in clinical trials as inclusion/exclusion criteria or to stratify patients into experimental groups. As pathological assessment of tissue is, in the main, only possible upon death of the patient, limited information as to the process or state of the disease at onset can be gained. However, it is pathological information at the onset of the disease that will be the most helpful clinically for diagnosis and treatment. Neuroimaging is often the only tool that clinicians can use to gain an insight into the early pathological processes in a patient's brain.

Based on pre-clinical models, it is therefore possible to devise imaging strategies that will allow the assessment of these early hallmarks of disease. For instance, combined diffusion and perfusion imaging of stroke has largely been the consequence of extensive pre-clinical studies assessing the potential of these imaging strategies to visualize early ischaemic events that can serve as surrogate markers of pathology. These indices inform the clinician about the potential to intervene based on the physiological state of the cerebrovascular event rather than based on symptom-onset [121].

The physiological state of the damage will also determine the ability of cells contained within this tissue to respond to, for instance, a pharmacological challenge that would normally lead to a signal transmission within this area detectable on MRI scans. This pharmacological MRI (phMRI), currently used in animal and human research [122,123], might provide a new means to assess the functional status of the penumbra. In chronic patients that might undergo neural transplantation, phMRI might also help to identify which particular type of cell has been lost by ischaemia and would need to be replaced. It would then be possible to pre-differentiate cells *in vitro* along a particular pathway that would allow the appropriate phenotype to arise after implantation. PhMRI could then again be used to assess if indeed cell replacement has occurred to a sufficient level that will allow adequate signal transmission. Similar studies in rodent models of Parkinson's disease have already shown the promise of this approach and corroborated these findings in relation to PET and autoradiography [124]. Upon transplantation of dopamine-secreting cells into the previously dopamine-depleted striatum, behavioural functions and striatal activity were restored. Restoration of the BOLD response in the striatum to amphetamine-administration can therefore serve as a surrogate marker of the functional effectiveness of the grafted cells [124]. Nonetheless, the potential of pharmacological MR in pre-clinical models of stroke is unclear as no well-designed studies have so far been reported that could highlight its potential as a surrogate marker of functional damage.

Currently, one of the main foci of functional imaging in stroke is the use of fMRI of somatosensory impairments. These can be observed in both pre-clinical and clinical settings. Although fMRI is currently used to study the ability of the damaged somatosensory cortex to re-organize [84], it is less clear at present how this information could be harnessed to guide intervention or provide a surrogate marker of treatment efficacy. Would a successful treatment be expected to have more of the traditional somatotopic map being preserved because the treatment will have preserved more of the structural integrity of the region or would it result in greater change in the region reflecting greater plasticity? Clearly, fMRI of somatosensory processing is paramount to our understanding of how patients recover after a stroke, but it is less well understood how these changes can be used to guide or validate therapeutic interventions. Controlled pre-clinical studies will help to gain a better understanding of how somatosensory plasticity could be used as an imaging index of behavioural recovery that is dependent upon treatment intervention. The use of neural transplantation will require novel approaches to probe the potential integration of grafted cells into existing neural networks or to ascertain if new cell assemblies consisting of grafted cells are developed. The use of contrast agents to label cells prior to transplantation to study their arrival in the somatosensory cortex and the consequent change in functional processing of somatosensory information will improve our understanding about how transplanted cells promote functional change leading to behavioural recovery.

Currently, the main imaging surrogate marker employed in stroke studies consists of a measurement of lesion volume as detected from $T_2$-weighted MR images. Consequently, pre-clinical studies investigating the efficacy of pharmacological agents often use lesion volume as a sole surrogate marker of treatment success without recourse to behavioural assessment. Although, it has often been reported that there is a good corroboration between the extent of damage and behavioural impairment [125], observations that other measures, such as leukocyte infiltration, can show better correlations with improvements in behavioural function [126,127] imply that lesion volume *per se* might not always be the most appropriate surrogate marker. Behavioural measures are often deemed to be rather crude and show spontaneous recovery which can complicate the long-term interpretation of these results. However, long-term imaging follow-up with extensive concomitant behavioural testing in rodents can potentially provide a more robust assessment of the consequences of stroke [128]. These circumstances might, for instance, inform us as to why lesion progression does not necessarily translate into a worsening of function. It is therefore likely that it will be the long-term functional benefits that will be a significant determinant if a therapy will successfully translate to the clinic.

The use of extensive behavioural testing in addition to serial MRI will indicate which imaging index will be a good predictor of treatment success as assessed by behavioural recovery [129]. Neuroanatomical substrates might be better predictors of performance on particular tasks and reveal novel insights as to the mechanisms by which grafted cells had an effect in, for instance, preserving striatal, but not cortical tissue. To translate these tasks into the clinical setting would then require the assessment of behavioural function heavily reliant on striatal function to ensure the assessment of striatal tissue integrity. It is therefore imperative that stroke patients undergo a comprehensive testing battery in addition to serial imaging. This will be the central theme of a *C*ore *A*ssessment *P*rogram for *I*ntracerebral *T*ransplantation in *Stroke* (CAPIT-Stroke).

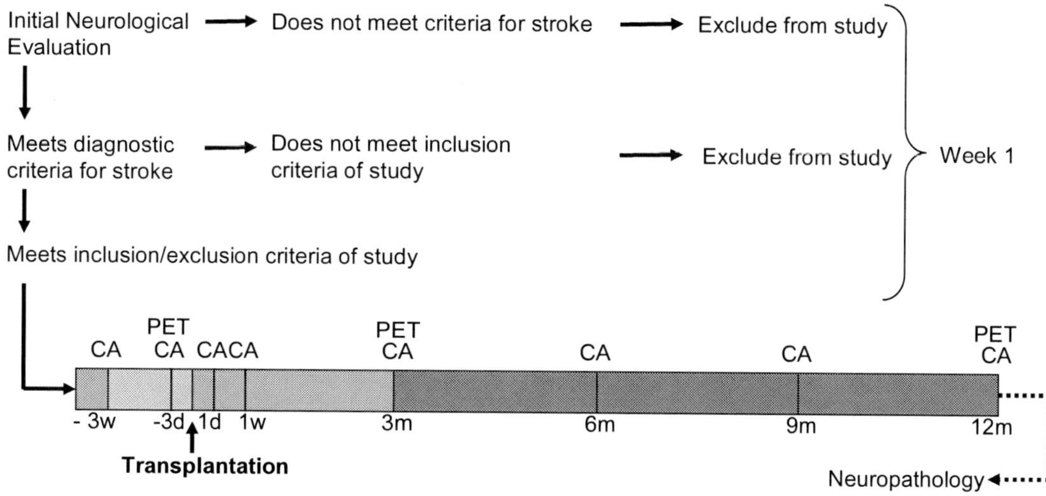


Figure 4. A Core Assessment Program for Intracerebral Transplantation (CAPIT) in stroke. Based on the original CAPIT (Lanston et al., 1992), a similar protocol can be suggested for stroke. On presentation at the acute stroke ward, a neurological and neuroimaging examination will be needed to determine if the patient indeed fulfills the criteria for a stroke and if the presentation falls within the inclusion/exclusion criteria of the clinical trial. However, contrary to Parkinson's disease, transplantation after a stroke should be within a month or so after symptom presentation since pre-clinical studies suggest that later implantation limits the efficacy of the grafted cells. A thorough core assessment (CA) of these patients should be undertaken that includes very extensive neuropsychological testing and at least a T2-weighted MRI scan at all relevant time points. The more data that can be gained from these patients, the more we can understand why these patients improve or which factors are relevant to their recovery. Ideally, PET scanning would also be undertaken to ensure that grafted cells are not undergoing rejection or that the inflammatory/immunological response to the injection tract is related to behaviour. Patients should also receive two complete check-ups every year following the 1st year of assessment to ensure that no deleterious effects appear later in life. This data will also be extremely important to determine in the future if these patients might benefit from further transplants. Every effort should be made to ensure that the brains of these patients will be available for neuropathological examination upon their death to investigate if cells survived and if an immunological response to grafted cells was mounted by the host.

## Developing a Comprehensive Assessment Battery for Cell Therapy

Akin to the CAPIT assessments devised for Parkinson's and Huntington's disease [130-132], imaging-dependent patient classification and follow-up will be crucial to compare results from mulitcenter stroke trials (Figure 4). However, it will be difficult to strike a balance between clearly defined core elements of the trials that allow direct comparisons, whilst also providing sufficient flexibility to researchers to specifically design experiments that address a particular problem. The main difference to the design of pre-clinical studies is the lack of a finite time point at which transplanted brains could be assessed. For this reason, it is not possible to conceive of a trial that would only assess the safety of the procedure, but it would demand long-term follow-up of these patients akin to efficacy assessment. Depending on the design of these initial 'safety' studies, it is possible that these patients will also be included in a more robust efficacy study. Having a consistent general assessment procedure in place would ensure that meta-analyses of the data across trials could be performed with fewer patients as data from different studies could be pooled.

The core assessment should consist of clearly defined inclusion/exclusion criteria that are based on clinical diagnosis, neuropsychological testing and neuroimaging. In the first instance, it would be desirable that very narrow inclusion criteria should be set to include only ischaemic strokes of a particular size range and restricted location that afford a consistent neuropsychological profile. In line with pre-clinical results the time for transplantation should be around 1 month following the stroke as this has been shown to the be the time-frame within which transplantation appears to be most effective. However, further pre-clinical testing is desirable to provide further guidance as to the practical aspects of the transplantation procedure. Neuroimaging should play a central role in these assessments. The absolute minimal requirement should be $T_2$-weighted MR images at various time points that would allow a serial assessment of changes in the brain. Not only can $T_2$-weighted MR images provide an unequivocal identification of the evolution of damage within a few days following a stroke, but they also afford a distinction between ischaemic and haemorhagic infarction [133] providing the basis to include/exclude patients that could not easily be distinguished based on acute clinical symptoms. Identifying a penumbral region might also be desirable, as it is generally presumed that preservation of damaged cells and tissues will have a greater effect on behavioural recovery than cell replacement [134]. The use of PET imaging to visualize the penumbra by $^{18}$F-fluoromisonidazole [135] and the microglia response by $^{11}$C-PK-11195 [136] is desirable at crucial time points, but due to the low dissemination of PET scanners, it cannot be assumed that all groups would have adequate access to the facilities that it should be considered a core analytical technique. The use of molecular or cellular imaging approaches should also be treated with caution at this stage. Although, it is invaluable to gain information about the location and survival of the transplanted cells, the labeling of cells with contrast agents is currently not proven to be safe for long-term assessment. A similar cautionary note needs to be raised regarding the current development of molecular MR contrast agents. Thorough pre-clinical testing is needed to ensure that these additional manipulations of cells do not impact on the transplanted cells. Nonetheless, in the future, it would be desirable to integrate these exciting novel imaging methods into clinical trials to gain further information about how these cells behave in the human brain. The more extensive the imaging component of the pre-surgical planning and follow-up, the more information can be gained as to the mechanisms involved in the observed behavioural improvements.

Every effort should also be made to ensure that at post-mortem the brains of patients participating in these trials are available for neuropathological examinations. Detecting transplanted human cells in a human brain will pose a challenge. However, in some cases, such as neuroteratocarcinoma cells, it will be possible to use alternative markers that can unequivocally lead to the identification of the cells. For instance, transplantation of male cells into a female brain would allow identification of grafted cells based on 'staining' techniques that reveal the Y chromosome present in all male, but not in female cells. Autologous transplants, however, might need specific labeling before transplantation to allow identification of cells post-mortem. A neuropathological assessment should ideally comprise the identification (and stereological counting) of transplanted cells in addition to phenotypic characterization of cells, assessment of an inflammatory/immunological response, and the expression of neurodegenerative/developmental proteins. It is also important that neuropathological assessment of human specimens will parallel pre-clinical analyses to ensure that future pre-clinical studies aimed at the refinement of the transplantation approach will address issues raised in these clinical studies. The greater control over experimental conditions in pre-clinical studies compared to clinical studies allows a more robust assessment of cause and effect relationships. In clinical studies, it is often difficult to ascertain if behavioural improvements are indeed due to a novel treatment since other factors will undoubtedly contribute to the final outcome.

## Integration with Existing Treatments

Unlike in pre-clinical studies, clinical studies are not merely interested in determining if there is a therapeutic effect of a particular intervention, but the aim should be to provide the best possible patient care. During the acute phase of stroke, the main aim of the clinical team must be to stabilize the patient, in case of blockage of an artery to reperfuse the compromised tissue and ideally provide support to dying cells upon reperfusion. At present, the best approach to achieve this end is by means of pharmacological intervention. Although these interventions might only show modest success in some cases, currently they are the best proven interventions and therefore constitute the first line of treatment. Although it is conceivable that 'off-the-shelf' cell transplants will be available in the future, at present clinical trials should aim to first establish the efficacy of cell therapy as a complementary treatment rather than a primary intervention.

Hence, it is likely that, as in the clinical trials conducted to date, cell implantation will be primarily aimed at the more chronic timeframe of stroke impairment. So far, the only therapeutic intervention that has gained wide-spread clinical appeal during this chronic phase of stroke recovery is rehabilitation therapy. Although pre-clinical studies imply that cell therapy can provide substantial benefits to patients, combining cell therapy with rehabilitation therapy has been demonstrated to further improve the effectiveness of the grafts and in some cases has even been reported to be an essential feature of graft-mediated recovery [138,139]. However, it is important that appropriate assessment will be performed on patients which did not receive a transplant, but the same rehabilitation program to ensure that the observed improved recovery is indeed due to a combination of cell therapy and rehabilitation and not merely due to more attention and rehabilitation training in the treated group.

Recent clinical trials using sham-surgery [139-141] highlighted the need for more robust clinical designs and assessments to be considered for future trials to provide an unequivocal answer to the question of graft efficacy. Concerns regarding the inflammatory response to an injection tract (i.e. the potential effect of sham-surgery) being the source of the observed improvements [142,143] can be adequately addressed by means of PET imaging of the microglia response and its relation to behaviour. Ultimately, one would hope that pre-clinical and clinical trials will determine the effectiveness of grafts to remedy behavioural dysfunction and determine the conditions which need to be considered to ensure the success of cell transplants.

## What Determines the Clinical Success of Cell Transplantation?

An extensive pre-clinical development program that assesses the efficacy of cell therapy in combination with practical factors that will impact upon the efficacy of the treatment is an essential step in the preparation for clinical trials (Figure 5). The phase II trial reported by Stilley et al. [144] implies that some patients might benefit more than others from transplant therapy. In the first instance, it will be important to clearly identify this cohort of patients and gain a better understanding of why these patients showed a more marked improvement. Initial pre-clinical studies can only provide a proof-of-concept and merely solicit an indication as to which patients might benefit most, or not at all, from this intervention.

If clinical trials lead to hypotheses about potential mechanisms or factors that might influence recovery, these should be addressed further in pre-clinical trials that can then re-formulate clinical interventions to optimize transplant therapy.

Existing and novel neuroimaging techniques are playing an increasing role in informing scientists and clinicians about the effects of transplanted cells and improve our understanding of the anatomical and functional effects these cells produce. By further improving the imaging assessment of transplanted cells by, for instance, the use of contrast agents to visualize cells directly in the brain (as in pre-clinical studies), it will become possible to control and manipulate the factors that lead to treatment success. The combination of the state-of-the-art imaging with state-of-the-art regenerative biology will hopefully lead to the development of a successful therapy that will alleviate patient suffering and decrease the number of patients facing life-long impairment due to the damage inflicted by a stroke.

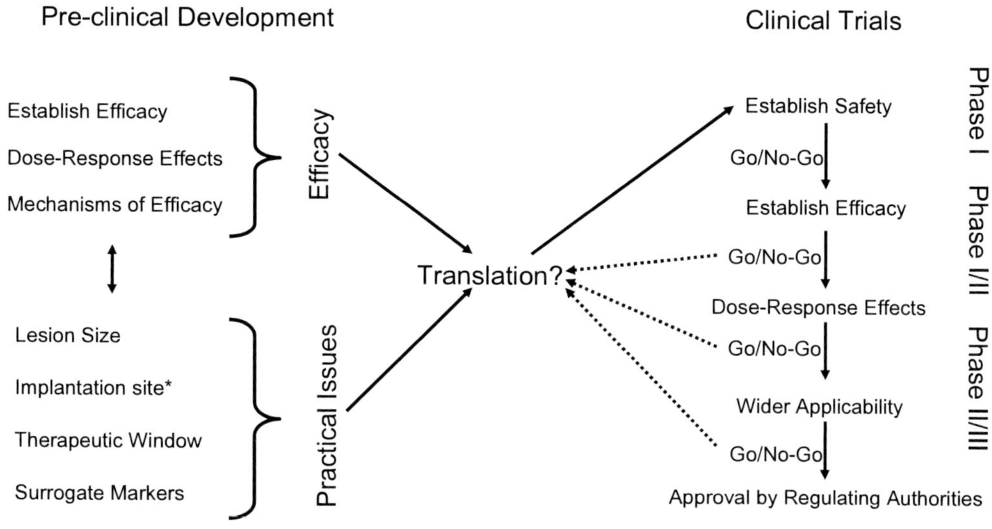


Figure 5. Basic steps in the development of cell transplantation as a routine treatment. A thorough pre-clinical development needs to be in place to ensure that the efficacy of transplanted cells provides an indication as to their potential success in remedying behavioural dysfunctions in human patients. Ideally some of this efficacy testing will be performed on non-human primates to ensure that a complex immune system and highly-specialized gyrencephalic brain do not limit the applicability of the approach developed in rodent models. Establishing a dose-response relationship that could provide indications as to the number of cells to be transplanted in human patients would also improve the understanding of how these cells exert beneficial effects. Additionally, practical issues, such as where these cells should be implanted (*or administered intravenously) or if the number of cells to be administered should be dictated by lesion size, will need to be addressed in pre-clinical models to ensure that patient studies have the best possible chance of a positive outcome. Pre-clinical models should also address the issue of a therapeutic window. The clinical trials reported to date, largely used patients that had a stroke at least 7 months before transplantation, whereas pre-clinical models suggest that the most effective time period of administration consists of ~2 weeks following the infarction. Pre-clinical models will be essential in addressing these issues before clinical trials will establish efficacy. Based on these pre-clinical results, decisions will need to be made as to the adequacy and completeness of these results to guide clinical trials. As clinical trials progress, go/no-go decisions will have to be made at each step depending on safety, efficacy or side-effects of cell therapy. However, issues arising from these clinical trials should be addressed again in pre-clinical studies to optimize therapeutic success and ensure maximum efficacy of cell transplantation before it will become available as an approved 'routine' treatment.

# E. Take-Home-Message

Cell transplantation for stroke is in the process of becoming a therapeutic entity in the clinical arena. At present, however, many questions remain to be answered. Pre-clinical studies provide invaluable information as to the efficacy and the optimal conditions for the administration of cell therapy. Nonetheless, some questions can only be addressed in carefully designed and conducted clinical trials. It is neuroimaging, encompassing PET and MRI, that will be essential in the preclinical development of these therapies by providing potentially objective surrogate markers of graft efficacy for clinical assessment. The use of neuroimaging will also characterize the suitability of patients for transplantation. Especially in the initial phases of clinical development, the use of a well-defined clinical population based on imaging and neuropsychological parameters will be extremely helpful to determine the efficacy of cell transplantation. The development of a general protocol for the conduct of clinical trials of cell therapy in stroke is highly desirable to allow comparison of studies. Neuroimaging should play a central role in this assessment and the development of novel imaging approaches should be implemented to allow maximal information to be extracted from each trial. It is hoped that these considerations will bring a safe and long-lasting relief to patients suffering from stroke impairments.

## References

[1] Ingall T. Stroke - incidence, mortality, mobidity and risk. *Journal of Insurance Medicine* 2004; 36:143-152.

[2] Wagner KR, Jauch EC. Extending the window for acute stroke treatment: thrombolytics plus CNS protective therapies. *Experimental Neurology* 2004; 188:195-199.

[3] Modo M, Hopkins K, Virley D, et al. Transplantation of neural stem cells modulates apolipoprotein E expression in a rat model of stroke. *Experimental Neurology* 2003; 183:320-329.

[4] Derdeyn CP. Physiological neuroimaging: Emerging clinical applications. *Journal of the American Medical Association 2001*; 285:3065-3068.

[5] Björklund A, Lindvall O. Cell replacement therapies for central nervous system disorders. *Nature Neuroscience* 2000; 3:537-544.

[6] Szentirmai O, Carter BS. Genetic and cellular therapies for cerebral infarction. *Neurosurgery* 2004; 55:283-297.

[7] Goldsmith HS, Duckett S, Chen W-F. Prevention of cerebral infarction in the monkey by omental transposition to the brain. *Stroke* 1978; 9:224-229.

[8] Goldsmith HS. Omental transplantation for stroke and TIA's. *Journal of Neurosurgery* 1987; 66:152-153.

[9] Goldsmith HS, Sax DS. Omental transposition for cerebral infarction: A 13-year follow-up study. *Surgical Neurology* 1999; 51:342-346.

[10] Grabowski M, Brundin P, Johansson BB. Fetal neocortical grafts implanted in adult hypertensive rats with cortical infarcts following a middle cerebral artery occlusion: Ingrowth of afferent fibers from the host brain. *Experimental Neurology* 1992;116:105-121.

[11] Grabowski M, Christofferson RH, Brundin P, et al. Vascularization of fetal neocortical grafts implanted in brain infarcts in spontaneously hypertensive rats. *Neuroscience* 1992; 51:673-682.

[12] Grabowski M, Brundin P, Johansson BB. Functional integration of cortical grafts placed in brain infarcts of rats. *Annals of Neurol*ogy 1993; 34:362-368.

[13] Nishino H, Koide K, Aihara N, et al. Striatal grafts in the ischemic striatum improve pallidal GABA release and passive avoidance. *Brain Research Bulletin* 1993; 32:517-520.
[14] Grabowski M, Johansson BB, Brundin P. Survival of fetal neocortical grafts implanted in brain infarcts of adult rats: The influence of postlesion time and ago of donor tissue. Experimental *Neurology* 1994; 127:126-136.
[15] Grabowski M, Johansson BB, Brundin P. Neocortical grafts placed in the infarcted brain of adult rats: Few or no efferent fibers grow from transplant to host. *Experimental Neurology* 1995; 134:273-276.
[16] Grabowski M, Sorensen JC, Mattsson B, et al. Influence of an enriched environment and cortical grafting on functional outcome in brain infarcts of adult rats. *Experimental Neurology* 1995; 133:96-102.
[17] Mattson B, Sorensen JC, Zimmer J, et al. Neural grafting to experimental neocortical infarcts improves behavioral outcome and reduces thalamic atrophy in rats housed in enriched but not in standard environments. *Stroke* 1997; 28:1225-1232.
[18] Sinden JD, Rashid-Doubell F, Kershaw TR, et al. Recovery of spatial learning by grafts of a conditionally immortalized hippocampal neuroepithelial cell line into the ischaemia-lesioned hippocampus. *Neuroscience* 1997; 81:599-608.
[19] Gray JA, Hodges H, Sinden J. *Prospects for the clinical application of neural transplantation with the use of conditionally immortalized neuroepithelial stem cells.* Philosophical Transactions of the Royal Society of London B 1999; 354:1407-1421.
[20] Borlongan CV, Saporta S, Poulos SG, et al. Viability and survival of hNT neurons determine degree of functional recovery in grafted ischemic rats. *NeuroReport* 1998; 9:2837-2842.
[21] Borlongan CV, Tajima Y, Trojanowski JQ, et al. Transplantation of cryopreserved human embryonal carcinoma-derived neurons (NT2N cells) promotes functional recovery in ischaemic rats. *Experimental Neurology* 1998; 149:310-321.
[22] Saporta S, Cameron DF, Borlongan CV, et al. Survival of rat and porcine sertoli cell transplants in the rat striatum without cyclosporine-A immunosuppression. *Experimental Neurology* 1997; 146:299-304.
[23] Li Y, Chen J, Chen XG, et al. Human marrow stromal cell therapy for stroke in rat: neurotrophins and functional recovery. *Neurology* 2002; 59:514-523.
[24] Iihoshi S, Honmou O, Houkin K, et al. A therapeutic window for intravenous administration of autologous bone marrow after cerebral ischemia in adult rats. *Brain Research* 2004; 1007:1-9.
[25] Saporta S, Borlongan CV, Sanberg PR. Neural transplantation of human neurotreratocarcinoma (hNT) neurons into ischemic rats. Quantitative dose-response analysis of cell survival and behavioral recovery. *Neuroscience* 1999; 91:519-525.
[26] Zhao LR, Duan WM, Reyes M, et al. Human bone marrow stem cells exhibit neural phenotypes and ameliorate neurological deficits after grafting into the ischemic brain of rats. *Exp. Neurol.* 2002; 174:11-20.
[27] Hodges H, Sownski P, Fleming P, et al. Contrasting effects of foetal CA1 and CA3 hippocampal grafts on deficits on spatial learning and working memory induced by global ischaemia in the rat. *Neuroscience* 1996; 72:959-988.

[28] Bradbury EJ, Kershaw TR, Marchbanks RM, et al. Astrocyte transplants alleviate lesion induced memory deficits independently of cholinergic recovery. *Neuroscience* 1995; 65:955-972.

[29] Kitamura Y, Takata K, Inden M, et al. Intracerebroventricular injection of microglia protects against focal brain ischemia. *J. Pharmacol. Sci.* 2004; 94:203-206.

[30] Seitz RJ, Azari NP, Knorr U, et al. The role of diaschisis in stroke recovery. *Stroke* 1999; 30:1844-1850.

[31] Reinecke S, Lutzenburg M, Hagemann G, et al. Electrophysiological transcortical diaschisis after middle cerebral artery occlusion (MCAO) in rats. *Neuroscience Letters* 1999; 261:85-88.

[32] Bach-y-Rita P. Brain plasticity as a basis for recovery of function in humans. *Neuropsychologia* 1990; 28:547-554.

[33] Dobkin BH. Strategies for stroke rehabilitation. *Lancet Neurol.* 2004; 3:528-536.

[34] Ourednik J, Ourednik V, Lynch WP, et al. Neural stem cells display an inherent mechanism for rescuing dysfunctional neurons. *Nat. Biotechnol.* 2002; 20:1103-1110.

[35] Pennypacker KR, Hernandez H, Benkovic S, et al. Induction of presenilins in the rat brain after middle cerebral arterial occlusion. *Brain Res. Bull.* 1999; 48:539-543.

[36] Cramer SC, Chopp M. Recovery recapitulates ontogeny. *Trends in Neuroscience* 2000; 23:265-271.

[37] Modo M, Stroemer RP, Tang E, Patel S, Hodges H (2003c) Effects of implantation site of dead stem cells in rats with stroke damage. *NeuroReport* 14:39-42.

[38] Arvidsson A, Collin T, Kirik D, et al. Neuronal replacement from endogenous precursors in the adult brain after stroke. *Nat. Med.* 2002; 8:963-970.

[39] Modo M, Mellodew K, Rezaie P. In vitro expression of major histocompatibility class I and class II antigens by conditionally immortalized murine neural stem cells. *Neuroscience Letters* 2003; 337:85-88.

[40] Modo M, Stroemer RP, Tang E, et al. Effects of implantation site of stem cell grafts on behavioral recovery from stroke damage. *Stroke* 2002; 33:2270-2278.

[41] Nieto-Sampedro M, Manthrope M, Barbin G, et al. Injury-induced neuronotrophic activity in adult rat brain: Correlation with survival of delayed implants in the wound cavity. *Journal of Neuroscience* 1983; 3:2219-2229.

[42] Gibbs RB, Cotman CW. Factors affecting survival and outgrowth from transplants of entorhinal cortex. *Neuroscience* 1987; 21:699-706.

[43] Zhou FC, Auerbach S, Azmitia E. Denervation of serotenergic fibers in the hippocampus induced a trophic factor which enhances the maturation of transplanted serotenergic neurons but not norepinepherine neurons. *Journal of Neuroscience Research* 1987; 17:235-246.

[44] Okano H, Ogawa Y, Nakamura M, et al. Transplantation of neural stem cells into the spinal cord after injury. *Semin. Cell Dev. Biol.* 2003; 14:191-198.

[45] Hoehn M, Nicolay K, Franke C, et al. Application of magnetic resonance to animal models of cerebral ischemia. *J. Magn. Reson. Imaging* 2001; 14:491-509.

[46] Modo M, Roberts TJ, Sandhu JK, et al. In vivo monitoring of cellular transplants by magnetic resonance imaging and positron emission tomography. *Expert Opinion on Biological Therapy* 2004; 4:145-155.

[47] Bulte JWM, Duncan ID, Frank JA. In vivo magnetic resonance tracking of magnetically labelled cells after transplantation. *Journal of Cerebral Blood Flow and Metabolism* 2002; 22:899-907.

[48] Modo M, Williams SCR. MRI and novel contrast agents for molecular imaging. In: *Biomedical imaging in experimental neuroscience*. (van Bruggen N, Roberts T, eds), pp 293-322. Boca Raton, FL: CRC Press. 2003.

[49] Modo M, Williams SCR. Molecular imaging by magnetic resonance imaging. *Rivista di Neuroradiologia* 2003; 16:23-27.

[50] Norman AB, Thomas SR, Pratt RG, et al. Magnetic resonance imaging of rat brain following kainic acid-induced lesions and fetal striatal tissue transplants. *Brain Research* 1989; 483:188-191.

[51] Norman AB, Thomas SR, Pratt RG, et al. (1990) T1 and T2 weighted magnetic resonance imaging of excitotoxin lesions and neural transplants in rat brain in vivo. *Experimental Neurology* 1990; 109:164-170.

[52] Guzman R, Meyer M, Lovbald KO, et al. Striatal grafts in a rat model of Huntington's disease: Time course comparison of MRI and histology. *Experimental Neurology* 1999; 156:180-190.

[53] Norman AB, Thomas SR, Pratt RG, et al. A magnetic resonance imaging contrast agent differentiates between the vascular properties of fetal striatal tissue transplants and gliomas in rat brain in vivo. *Brain Research* 1989; 503:156-159.

[54] Modo M, Rezaie P, Heuschling P, et al. Transplantation of neural stem cells in a rat model of stroke: assessment of short-term graft survival and acute host immunological response. *Brain Res*. 2002; 958:70-82.

[55] Norman AB, Thomas SR, Pratt RG, et al. Magnetic resonance imaging of neural transplants in rat brain using a supraparamagnetic contrast agent. *Brain Research* 1992; 594:279-283.

[56] Hawrylak N, Ghosh P, Broadus J, et al. Nuclear magnetic resonance (NMR) imaging of iron-oxide-labeled neural transplants. *Experimental Neurology* 1993; 21:181-192.

[57] Kim JK, Kucharczyk W, Kenkelman RM. Cavernous hemangiomas: Dipolar susceptibility artifacts at imaging. *Radiology* 1993; 187:735-741.

[58] Bulte JW, Kraitchman DL. Iron oxide MR contrast agents for molecular and cellular imaging. *NMR Biomed*. 2004; 17:484-499.

[59] Dodd SJ, Williams M, Suhan JP, et al. Detection of single mammalian cells by high-resolution magnetic resonance imaging. *Biophysical Journal* 1999; 76:103-109.

[60] Shapiro EM, Skrtic S, Sharer K, et al. (2004) MRI detection of single particles for cellular imaging. *Proceedings of the National Academy of Science* 2004; 101:10901-10906.

[61] Raynal I, Prigent P, Peyramaure S, et al. Macrophage endocytosis of superparamagnetic iron oxide nanoparticles: mechanisms and comparison of ferumoxides and ferumoxtran-10. *Invest. Radiol*. 2004; 39:56-63.

[62] Schroeter M, Saleh A, Wiedermann D, et al. Histochemical detection of ultrasmall superparamagnetic iron oxide (USPIO) contrast medium uptake in epxerimental brain ischemia. *Magnetic Resonance in Medicine* 2004; 52:403-406.

[63] Hoehn M, Kustermann E, Blunk J, et al. Monitoring of implanted stem cell migration in vivo: A highly resolved in vivo magnetic resonance imaging investigation of experimental stroke in rat. *Proceedings of the National Academy of Science* 2002; 99:16267-16272.

[64] Lewin M, Carlesso N, Tung C-H, et al. Tat peptide-derivatized magnetic nanoparticles allow in vivo tracking and recovery of progenitor cells. *Nature Biotechnology* 2000; 18:410-414.

[65] Allen MJ, MacRenaris KW, Venkatasubramanian PN, et al. Cellular delivery of MRI contrast agents. *Chemistry and Biology* 2004; 11:301-307.

[66] Bulte JWM, Ben-Hur T, Miller BR, et al. MR microscopy of magnetically labeled neurospheres transplanted into the Lewis EAE rat brain. *Magnetic Resonance in Medicine* 2003; 50:201-205.

[67] Daldrup-Link HE, Rudelius M, Metz S, et al. Cell tracking with gadophrin-2: A bifunctional contrast agent for MR imaging, optical imaging, and fluorescence microscopy. *European Journal of Nuclear Medicine and Molecular Imaging* 2004; 31:1312-1321.

[68] Crich SG, Biancone L, Cantaluppi V, et al. Improved route for the visualization of stem cells labeled with a Gd-/Eu-chelate as dual (MRI and fluorescence) agent. *Magn. Reson. Med.* 2004; 51:938-944.

[69] Coristine AJ, Foster P, Deoni SC, et al. Positive contrast labeling of SPIO loaded cells in cell samples and spinal cord. In: *International Society for Magnetic Resonance in Medicine*, p 163. Kyoto, Japan; 2004.

[70] Englund U, Bjorklund A, Wictorin K. Migration patterns and phenotypic differentiation of long-term expanded human neural progenitor cells after transplantation into the adult rat brain. *Brain Res. Dev. Brain Res.* 2002; 134:123-141.

[71] Arbab AS, Bashaw LA, Miller BR, et al. Intracytoplasmic tagging of cells with ferumoxides and transfection agent for cellular magnetic resonance imaging after cell transplantation: Methods and techniques. *Transplantation* 2002; 76:1123-1130.

[72] Arbab AS, Bashaw LA, Miller BR, et al. Characterization of biophysical and metabolic properties of cells labeled with superparamagnetic iron oxide nanoparticles and transfection agent for cellular MR imaging. *Radiology* 2003; 229:838-846.

[73] Kostura L, Kraitchman DL, Mackay AM, et al. (2004) Feridex labeling of mesenchymal stem cells inhibits chondrogenesis but not adipogenesis or osteogenesis. *NMR Biomed* 2004;17:513-517.

[74] Jendelovà P, Herynek V, DeCroos J, et al. Imaging the fate of implanted bone marrow stromal cells labeled with superparamagnetic nanoparticles. *Magnetic Resonance in Medicine* 2003; 50:767-776.

[75] Jendelovà P, Herynek V, Urdzkovà L, et al. Magnetic resonance tracking of transplanted bone marrow and embryonic stem cells labeled by iron oxide nanoparticles in rat brain and spinal cord. *Journal of Neuroscience Research* 2004; 76:232-243.

[76] Heckl S, Debus J, Jenne J, et al. CNN-Gd3+ enables cell nucleus molecular imaging of prostate cancer cells: The last 600 nm. *Cancer Research* 2002; 62:7018-7024.

[77] Cohen B, Dafni H, Meir G, et al. Ferritin as novel MR-reporter for molecular imaging of gene expression. *Proceedings of the International Society for Magnetic Resonance in Medicine* 2004; 11:1707.

[78] Rinck PA, Muller RN. Field strength and dose dependence of contrast enhancement by gadolinium-based MR contrast agents. *Eur. Radiol.* 1999; 9:998-1004.

[79] Modo M, Mellodew K, Cash D, et al. Mapping transplanted stem cell migration after a stroke: A serial, in vivo magnetic resonance imaging study. *Neuroimage* 2004; 21:311-317.

[80] Zhang ZG, Jiang Q, Zhang R, et al. Magnetic resonance imaging and neurosphere therapy of stroke in rat. *Annals of Neurology* 2003; 53:259-263.

[81] Kim D-E, Schellingerhout D, Ishii K, et al. Imaging of stem cell recruitment to ischemic infarcts in a murine model. *Stroke* 2004; 35:952-957.

[82] Roberts TP, Rourkey HA. Diffusion weighted magnetic resonance imaging in stroke. *Eur. J. Radiol.* 2003; 45:185-94.

[83] Guadagno JV, Donnan GA, Markus R, et al. Imaging of the ischaemic penumbra. *Current Opinion in Neurology* 2004; 17 61-67.

[84] Rijntes M, Weiller C. Recovery of motor and language abilities after stroke: The contribution of functional imaging. *Progress in Neurobiology* 2002; 66:109-122.

[85] Sauter A, Reese T, P¢rszàsz R, et al. Recovery of function in cryoprotected cerebral cortex in rat stroke model assessed by functional MRI. *Magnetic Resonance in Medicine* 2002; 47:759-765.

[86] Dijkhuizen RM, Ren J, Mandeville JB, et al. Functional magnetic resonance imaging of reorganization in rat brain after stroke. *Proceedings of the National Academy of Science* 2001; 98:12766-12771.

[87] Dijkhuizen RM, Singhal AB, Mandeville JB, et al. Correlation between brain reorganization, ischemic damage, and neurologic status after transient focal cerebral ischemia in rats: A functional magnetic resonance imaging study. *Journal of Neuroscience* 2003; 23:510-517.

[88] Marsden PK, Strul D, Keevil SF, et al. Simultaneous PET and NMR. *Br. J. Radiol.* 2002; 75 Spec No:S53-59.

[89] Carmichael ST, Tatsukawa K, Katsman D, et al. Evolution of diaschisis in a focal stroke model. *Stroke* 2004; 35:758-763.

[90] Mir HM, Tatsukawa KJ, Carmichael ST, et al. Metabolic correlates of lesion-specific plasticity: an in vivo imaging study. *Brain Res.* 2004; 1002:28-34.

[91] Kondziolka D, Wechsler L, Goldstein S, et al. Transplantation of cultured human neuronal cells for patients with stroke. *Neurology* 2000; 55:565-569.

[92] Nelson PT, Kondziolka D, Wechsler L, et al. Clonal human (hNT) neuron grafts for stroke therapy: Neuropathology in a patient 27 months after implantation. *American Journal of Pathology* 2002; 160:1201-1206.

[93] Stilley CS, Ryan CM, Kondziolka D, et al. Changes in cognitive function after neuronal cell transplantation for basal ganglia stroke. *Neurology* 2004; 63:1320-1322.

[94] Savitz SI, Rosenbaum DM, Dinsmore JH, et al. Cell transplantation for stroke. *Ann. Neurol.* 2002; 52:266-275.

[95] Jeong SW, Chu K, Jung KH, et al. Human neural stem cell transplantation promotes functional recovery in rats with experimental intracerebral hemorrhage. *Stroke* 2003; 34:2258-2263.

[96] Bernaudin M, Nouvelot A, MacKenzie ET, et al. Selective neuronal vulnerability and specific glial reactions in hippocampal and neocortical organotypic cultures submitted to ischaemia. *Experimental Neurology* 1998; 150:30-39.

[97] Vendrame M, Cassady J, Newcomb J, et al. Infusion of human umbilical cord blood cells in a rat model of stroke dose-dependently rescues behavioral deficits and reduces inarct volume. *Stroke* 2004; 35:2390-2395.

[98] Hauser RA, Sandberg PR, Freeman TB, et al. (2002) Bilateral human fetal striatal transplantation in Huntington's disease. *Neurology* 2002; 58:1704; author reply 1704.

[99] Henderson BT, Clough CG, Hughes RC, et al. Implantation of human fetal ventral mesencephalon to the right caudate nucleus in advanced Parkinson's disease. *Arch. Neurol.* 1991; 48:822-827.

[100] Freed CR, Greene PE, Breeze RE, et al. Transplantation of embryonic dopamine neurons for severe Parkinson's disease. *N. Engl. J. Med.* 2001; 344:710-719.

[101] Bresjanac M, Sagen J, Seigel G, et al. (1997) Xenogeneic adrenal medulla graft rejection rather than survival leads to increased rat striatal tyrosine hydroxylase immunoreactivity. *J. Neuropathol. Exp. Neurol.* 1997; 56:490-498.

[102] Modo M, Cash D, Mellodew K, et al. Tracking transplanted stem cell migration using bifunctional, contrast agent-enhanced, magnetic resonance imaging. *Neuroimage* 2002; 17:803-811.

[103] Bakay RA, Boyer KL, Freed CR, et al. Immunological responses to injury and grafting in the central nervous system of nonhuman primates. *Cell Transplant* 1998; 7:109-120.

[104] Virley D, Ridley RM, Sinden J, et al. Primary CA1 and conditionally immortal MHP36 cell grafts restore conditional discrimination learning and recall in marmosets after excitotoxic lesions of the hippocampal CA1 field. *Brain* 1999; 122:2321-2335.

[105] Cicchetti F, Fodor W, Deacon TW, et al. Immune parameters relevant to neural xenograft survival in the primate brain. *Xenotransplantation* 2003; 10:41-49.

[106] Yu G, Hess DC, Borlongan CV. Combined cyclosporine-A and methylprednisolone treatment exerts partial and transient neuroprotection against ischemic stroke. *Brain Res.* 2004; 1018:32-37.

[107] Rabchevsky AG, Streit WJ. Grafting of cultured microglial cells into the lesioned spinal cord of adult rats enhances neurite outgrowth. *J. Neurosci. Res.* 1997; 47:34-48.

[108] Puschban Z, Waldner R, Seppi K, et al. Failure of neuroprotection by embryonic striatal grafts in a double lesion rat model of striatonigral degeneration (multiple system atrophy). *Exp. Neurol.* 2000; 164:166-175.

[109] Cicchetti F, Brownell AL, Williams K, et al. Neuroinflammation of the nigrostriatal pathway during progressive 6-OHDA dopamine degeneration in rats monitored by immunohistochemistry and PET imaging. *Eur. J. Neurosci.* 2002; 15:991-998.

[110] Meltzer CC, Kondziolka D, Villemagne VL, et al. Serial [18F] fluorodeoxyglucose positron emission tomography after human neuronal implantation for stroke. *Neurosurgery* 2001; 49:586-591; discussion 591-582.

[111] Venneti S, Lopresti BJ, Wang G, et al. PET imaging of brain macrophages using the peripheral benzodiazepine receptor in a macaque model of neuroAIDS. *J. Clin. Invest*. 2004; 113:981-989.

[112] Saleh A, Schroeter M, Jonkmanns C, et al. In vivo MRI of brain inflammation in human ischaemic stroke. *Brain* 2004; 127:1670-1677.

[113] Dunnett SB, Björklund A. Mechanisms of function of neural grafts in the injured brain. In: *Functional Neural Transplantation* (Dunnett SB, Bjorklund A, eds), pp 531-567. New Yrok, NY: Raven Press, 1994.

[114] Chan D, Fox NC, Jenkins R, et al. Rates of global and regional cerebral atrophy in AD and frontotemporal dementia. *Neurology* 2001; 57:1756-1763.

[115] Feydy A, Carlier R, Roby-Brami A, et al. Longitudinal study of motor recovery after stroke: Recruitment and focusing of brain activation. *Stroke* 2002; 33:1610-1617.

[116] Jones DK, Lythgoe D, Horsfield MA, et al. Characterization of white matter damage in ischemic leukoaraiosis with diffusion tensor MRI. *Stroke* 1999; 30:393-397.

[117] Jacobs AH, Winkler A, Dittmar C, et al. Prospects of molecular imaging in neurology. *Journal of Cellular Biochemistry* 2002; 39:98-109.

[118] Louie AY, Meade TJ. Recent advances in MRI: Novel contrast agents shed light on in vivo biochemistry. *Trends in Biochemical Sciences* 2000; :7-11.

[119] Perez JM, O'Loughin T, Simeone J, et al. DNA-based magnetic nanoparticle assembly acts as a magnetic relaxation nanoswitch allowing screening of DNA-cleaving agents. *Journal of the American Chemical Society* 2002; 124:2856-2857.

[120] Sipkins DA, Gjibels K, Tropper FD, et al. (2000) ICAM-1 expression in autoimmune encephalitis visualized using magnetic resonance imaging. *Journal of Neuroimmunology* 2000; 104:1-9.

[121] Warach S. New imaging strategies for patient selection for thrombolytic and neuroprotective therapies. *Neurology* 2001; 57 S48-S52.

[122] Leslie RA, James MF. Pharmacological magnetic resonance imaging: A new application for functional MRI. *Trends in Pharmacolgical Science* 2000; 21:314-318.

[123] Honey G, Bullmore ET. Human pharmacological MRI. Trends in Pharmacolgical *Science* 2004; 25:366-374.

[124] Chen YI, Brownell A-L, Galpern W, et al. Detection of dopaminergic cell loss and neural transplantation using pharmacological MRI, PET, and behavioral assessment. *NeuroReport* 1999; 10:2881-2886.

[125] Belayev L, Busto R, Zhao W, et al. Effect of delayed albumin hemodilution on infarction volume and brain edema after transient middle cerebral artery occlusion in rats. *J. Neurosurg*. 1997; 87:595-601.

[126] Miljkovic-Lolic M, Silbergleit R, Fiskum G, et al. Neuroprotective effects of hyperbaric oxygen treatment in experimental focal cerebral ischemia are associated with reduced brain leukocyte myeloperoxidase activity. *Brain Res*. 2003; 971:90-94.

[127] Schabitz WR, Berger C, Kollmar R, et al. Effect of brain-derived neurotrophic factor treatment and forced arm use on functional motor recovery after small cortical ischemia. *Stroke* 2004; 35:992-997.

[128] Virley D, Beech JS, Smart SC, et al. A temporal MRI assessment of neuropathology after transient middle cerebral artery occlusion in the rat: Correlations with behavior. *Journal of Cerebral Blood Flow and Metabolism* 2000; 20:563-582.

[129] Duncan PW. Measuring recovery of function after stroke: Clinical and measurement issues in selecting stroke outcome measures in clinical trials. In: *Restorative Neurology: Advances on Pharmacotherapy for Recovery after Stroke*. (Goldstein LB, ed), pp 225-239. Armonk, NY: Futura Publishing; 1998.

[130] Lanston W, Widner H, Goetz CG, et al. Core assessment program for intracerebral transplantations (CAPIT). *Movement Disorder*s 1992; 7:2-13.

[131] Quinn N, Brown R, Craufurd D, et al. Core Assessment Program for Intracerebral Transplantation in Huntington's Disease (CAPIT-HD). *Mov. Disord.* 1996; 11:143-150.

[132] Widner H, Defer GL. Dyskinesias assessment: from CAPIT to CAPSIT. Core Assessment Program for Intracerebral Transplantations. Core Assessment Program for Surgical Interventional Therapies. *Mov. Disord.* 1999; 14 Suppl 1:60-66.

[133] Stadnik TW, Osteauz M. Actual trends in diagnosis/thrombolytic therapy of acute cerebral stroke. *European Journal of Radiology* 2001; 38:28-40.

[134] Lindvall O, Kokaia, Z. Recovery and rehabilitation in stroke: Stem Cells. *Stroke* 2004; 35:2691-2694.

[135] Markus R, Donnan GA, Kazui S, et al. Statistical parametric mapping of hypoxic tissue indetified by [18F]fluoromisonidazole and positron emission tomography following acute ischemic stroke. *Neuroimage* 2002; 16:425-433.

[136] Wictorin K Anatomy and connectivity of intrastriatal striatal transplants. Progress in Neurobiology 1992; 38:611-639.

[137] Polgar S, Borlongan CV, Koutouzis TK, et al. Implications of neurological rehabilitation for advancing intracerebral transplantation. *Brain Reseach Bulletin* 1997; 44:229-232.

[138] Döbrössy M, Dunnett SB. Motor training effects on recovery of function after striatal lesions and striatal grafts. *Experimental Neurology* 2003; 184:274-284.

[139] Freeman TB, Vawter DE, Leaverton PE, et al. Use of placebo surgery in controlled trials of a cellular-based therapy for Parkinson's disease. *N. Engl. J. Med.* 1999; 341:988-992.

[140] Dekkers W, Boer G. Sham neurosurgery in patients with Parkinson's disease: is it morally acceptable? *J. Med. Ethics* 2001; 27:151-156.

[141] Boer GJ, Widner H. Clinical neurotransplantation: core assessment protocol rather than sham surgery as control. *Brain Res. Bull.* 2002; 58:547-553.

[142] Chen YC, Galpern WR, Brownell AL, et al. Detection of dopaminergic neurotransmitter activity using pharmacologic MRI: Correlation with PET, microdialysis, and behavioral data. *Magnetic Resonance in Medicine* 1997; 38:389-398.

[143] Batchelor PE, Porritt MJ, Martinello P, et al. Macrophages and Microglia Produce Local Trophic Gradients That Stimulate Axonal Sprouting Toward but Not beyond the Wound Edge. *Mol. Cell Neurosci.* 2002; 21:436-453.

[144] Humm JL, Kozlowski DA, James DC, et al. Use-dependent exacerbation of brain damage occurs during an early post-lesion vulnerable period. *Brain Research* 1998; 783:286-292.

[145] Allen MJ, MacRenaris KW, Venkatasubramanian PN, et al. Cellular delivery of MRI contrast agents. *Chemistry and Biology* 2004; 11:301-307.

[146] Bulte JWM, Ben-Hur T, Miller BR, et al. MR microscopy of magnetically labeled neurospheres transplanted into the Lewis EAE rat brain. *Magnetic Resonance in Medicine* 2003; 50:201-205.

[147] Daldrup-Link HE, Rudelius M, Metz S, et al. Cell tracking with gadophrin-2: A bifunctional contrast agent for MR imaging, optical imaging, and fluorescence microscopy. *European Journal of Nuclear Medicine and Molecular Imaging* 2004; 31:1312-1321.

[148] Crich SG, Biancone L, Cantaluppi V, et al. Improved route for the visualization of stem cells labeled with a Gd-/Eu-chelate as dual (MRI and fluorescence) agent. *Magn. Reson. Med.* 2004; 51:938-944.

[149] Coristine AJ, Foster P, Deoni SC, et al. Positive contrast labeling of SPIO loaded cells in cell samples and spinal cord. In: *International Society for Magnetic Resonance in Medicine*, p 163. Kyoto, Japan; 2004.

[150] Englund U, Bjorklund A, Wictorin K. Migration patterns and phenotypic differentiation of long-term expanded human neural progenitor cells after transplantation into the adult rat brain. *Brain Res. Dev. Brain Res.* 2002; 134:123-141.

[151] Arbab AS, Bashaw LA, Miller BR, et al. Intracytoplasmic tagging of cells with ferumoxides and transfection agent for cellular magnetic resonance imaging after cell transplantation: Methods and techniques. *Transplantation* 2002; 76:1123-1130.

[152] Arbab AS, Bashaw LA, Miller BR, et al. Characterization of biophysical and metabolic properties of cells labeled with superparamagnetic iron oxide nanoparticles and transfection agent for cellular MR imaging. *Radiology* 2003; 229:838-846.

[153] Kostura L, Kraitchman DL, Mackay AM, et al. (2004) Feridex labeling of mesenchymal stem cells inhibits chondrogenesis but not adipogenesis or osteogenesis. *NMR Biomed* 2004;17:513-517.

[154] Jendelovà P, Herynek V, DeCroos J, et al. Imaging the fate of implanted bone marrow stromal cells labeled with superparamagnetic nanoparticles. *Magnetic Resonance in Medicine* 2003; 50:767-776.

[155] Jendelovà P, Herynek V, Urdzkovà L, et al. Magnetic resonance tracking of transplanted bone marrow and embryonic stem cells labeled by iron oxide nanoparticles in rat brain and spinal cord. *Journal of Neuroscience Research* 2004; 76:232-243.

[156] Heckl S, Debus J, Jenne J, et al. CNN-Gd3+ enables cell nucleus molecular imaging of prostate cancer cells: The last 600 nm. *Cancer Research* 2002; 62:7018-7024.

[157] Cohen B, Dafni H, Meir G, et al. Ferritin as novel MR-reporter for molecular imaging of gene expression. *Proceedings of the International Society for Magnetic Resonance in Medicine* 2004; 11:1707.

[158] Rinck PA, Muller RN. Field strength and dose dependence of contrast enhancement by gadolinium-based MR contrast agents. *Eur. Radiol.* 1999; 9:998-1004.

[159] Modo M, Mellodew K, Cash D, et al. Mapping transplanted stem cell migration after a stroke: A serial, in vivo magnetic resonance imaging study. *Neuroimage* 2004; 21:311-317.

[160] Zhang ZG, Jiang Q, Zhang R, et al. Magnetic resonance imaging and neurosphere therapy of stroke in rat. *Annals of Neurology* 2003; 53:259-263.

[161] Kim D-E, Schellingerhout D, Ishii K, et al. Imaging of stem cell recruitment to ischemic infarcts in a murine model. *Stroke* 2004; 35:952-957.

[162] Roberts TP, Rourkey HA. Diffusion weighted magnetic resonance imaging in stroke. *Eur. J. Radiol.* 2003; 45:185-94.

[163] Guadagno JV, Donnan GA, Markus R, et al. Imaging of the ischaemic penumbra. *Current Opinion in Neurology* 2004; 17 61-67.

[164] Rijntes M, Weiller C. Recovery of motor and language abilities after stroke: The contribution of functional imaging. *Progress in Neurobiology* 2002; 66:109-122.

[165] Sauter A, Reese T, P¢rszàsz R, et al. Recovery of function in cryoprotected cerebral cortex in rat stroke model assessed by functional MRI. *Magnetic Resonance in Medicine* 2002; 47:759-765.

[166] Dijkhuizen RM, Ren J, Mandeville JB, et al. Functional magnetic resonance imaging of reorganization in rat brain after stroke. *Proceedings of the National Academy of Science* 2001; 98:12766-12771.

[167] Dijkhuizen RM, Singhal AB, Mandeville JB, et al. Correlation between brain reorganization, ischemic damage, and neurologic status after transient focal cerebral ischemia in rats: A functional magnetic resonance imaging study. *Journal of Neuroscience* 2003; 23:510-517.

[168] Marsden PK, Strul D, Keevil SF, et al. Simultaneous PET and NMR. *Br. J. Radiol.* 2002; 75 Spec No:S53-59.

[169] Carmichael ST, Tatsukawa K, Katsman D, et al. Evolution of diaschisis in a focal stroke model. *Stroke* 2004; 35:758-763.

[170] Mir HM, Tatsukawa KJ, Carmichael ST, et al. Metabolic correlates of lesion-specific plasticity: an in vivo imaging study. *Brain Res.* 2004; 1002:28-34.

[171] Kondziolka D, Wechsler L, Goldstein S, et al. Transplantation of cultured human neuronal cells for patients with stroke. *Neurology* 2000; 55:565-569.

[172] Nelson PT, Kondziolka D, Wechsler L, et al. Clonal human (hNT) neuron grafts for stroke therapy: Neuropathology in a patient 27 months after implantation. *American Journal of Pathology* 2002; 160:1201-1206.

[173] Stilley CS, Ryan CM, Kondziolka D, et al. Changes in cognitive function after neuronal cell transplantation for basal ganglia stroke. *Neurology* 2004; 63:1320-1322.

[174] Savitz SI, Rosenbaum DM, Dinsmore JH, et al. Cell transplantation for stroke. *Ann. Neurol.* 2002; 52:266-275.

[175] Jeong SW, Chu K, Jung KH, et al. Human neural stem cell transplantation promotes functional recovery in rats with experimental intracerebral hemorrhage. *Stroke* 2003; 34:2258-2263.

[176] Bernaudin M, Nouvelot A, MacKenzie ET, et al. Selective neuronal vulnerability and specific glial reactions in hippocampal and neocortical organotypic cultures submitted to ischaemia. *Experimental Neurology* 1998; 150:30-39.

[177] Vendrame M, Cassady J, Newcomb J, et al. Infusion of human umbilical cord blood cells in a rat model of stroke dose-dependently rescues behavioral deficits and reduces inarct volume. *Stroke* 2004; 35:2390-2395.

[178] Hauser RA, Sandberg PR, Freeman TB, et al. (2002) Bilateral human fetal striatal transplantation in Huntington's disease. *Neurology* 2002; 58:1704; author reply 1704.

[179] Henderson BT, Clough CG, Hughes RC, et al. Implantation of human fetal ventral mesencephalon to the right caudate nucleus in advanced Parkinson's disease. *Arch. Neurol.* 1991; 48:822-827.

[180] Freed CR, Greene PE, Breeze RE, et al. Transplantation of embryonic dopamine neurons for severe Parkinson's disease. *N. Engl. J. Med.* 2001; 344:710-719.

[181] Bresjanac M, Sagen J, Seigel G, et al. (1997) Xenogeneic adrenal medulla graft rejection rather than survival leads to increased rat striatal tyrosine hydroxylase immunoreactivity. *J. Neuropathol. Exp. Neurol.* 1997; 56:490-498.

[182] Modo M, Cash D, Mellodew K, et al. Tracking transplanted stem cell migration using bifunctional, contrast agent-enhanced, magnetic resonance imaging. *Neuroimage* 2002; 17:803-811.

[183] Bakay RA, Boyer KL, Freed CR, et al. Immunological responses to injury and grafting in the central nervous system of nonhuman primates. *Cell Transplant* 1998; 7:109-120.

[184] Virley D, Ridley RM, Sinden J, et al. Primary CA1 and conditionally immortal MHP36 cell grafts restore conditional discrimination learning and recall in marmosets after excitotoxic lesions of the hippocampal CA1 field. *Brain* 1999; 122:2321-2335.

[185] Cicchetti F, Fodor W, Deacon TW, et al. Immune parameters relevant to neural xenograft survival in the primate brain. *Xenotransplantation* 2003; 10:41-49.

[186] Yu G, Hess DC, Borlongan CV. Combined cyclosporine-A and methylprednisolone treatment exerts partial and transient neuroprotection against ischemic stroke. *Brain Res.* 2004; 1018:32-37.

[187] Rabchevsky AG, Streit WJ. Grafting of cultured microglial cells into the lesioned spinal cord of adult rats enhances neurite outgrowth. *J. Neurosci. Res.* 1997; 47:34-48.

[188] Puschban Z, Waldner R, Seppi K, et al. Failure of neuroprotection by embryonic striatal grafts in a double lesion rat model of striatonigral degeneration (multiple system atrophy). *Exp. Neurol.* 2000; 164:166-175.

[189] Cicchetti F, Brownell AL, Williams K, et al. Neuroinflammation of the nigrostriatal pathway during progressive 6-OHDA dopamine degeneration in rats monitored by immunohistochemistry and PET imaging. *Eur. J. Neurosci.* 2002; 15:991-998.

[190] Meltzer CC, Kondziolka D, Villemagne VL, et al. Serial [18F] fluorodeoxyglucose positron emission tomography after human neuronal implantation for stroke. *Neurosurgery* 2001; 49:586-591; discussion 591-582.

[191] Venneti S, Lopresti BJ, Wang G, et al. PET imaging of brain macrophages using the peripheral benzodiazepine receptor in a macaque model of neuroAIDS. *J. Clin. Invest*. 2004; 113:981-989.

[192] Saleh A, Schroeter M, Jonkmanns C, et al. In vivo MRI of brain inflammation in human ischaemic stroke. *Brain* 2004; 127:1670-1677.

[193] Dunnett SB, Björklund A. Mechanisms of function of neural grafts in the injured brain. In: *Functional Neural Transplantation* (Dunnett SB, Bjorklund A, eds), pp 531-567. New Yrok, NY: Raven Press, 1994.

[194] Chan D, Fox NC, Jenkins R, et al. Rates of global and regional cerebral atrophy in AD and frontotemporal dementia. *Neurology* 2001; 57:1756-1763.

[195] Feydy A, Carlier R, Roby-Brami A, et al. Longitudinal study of motor recovery after stroke: Recruitment and focusing of brain activation. *Stroke* 2002; 33:1610-1617.

[196] Jones DK, Lythgoe D, Horsfield MA, et al. Characterization of white matter damage in ischemic leukoaraiosis with diffusion tensor MRI. *Stroke* 1999; 30:393-397.

[197] Jacobs AH, Winkler A, Dittmar C, et al. Prospects of molecular imaging in neurology. *Journal of Cellular Biochemistry* 2002; 39:98-109.

[198] Louie AY, Meade TJ. Recent advances in MRI: Novel contrast agents shed light on in vivo biochemistry. *Trends in Biochemical Sciences* 2000; :7-11.

[199] Perez JM, O'Loughin T, Simeone J, et al. DNA-based magnetic nanoparticle assembly acts as a magnetic relaxation nanoswitch allowing screening of DNA-cleaving agents. *Journal of the American Chemical Society* 2002; 124:2856-2857.

[200] Sipkins DA, Gjibels K, Tropper FD, et al. (2000) ICAM-1 expression in autoimmune encephalitis visualized using magnetic resonance imaging. *Journal of Neuroimmunology* 2000; 104:1-9.

[201] Warach S. New imaging strategies for patient selection for thrombolytic and neuroprotective therapies. *Neurology* 2001; 57 S48-S52.

[202] Leslie RA, James MF. Pharmacological magnetic resonance imaging: A new application for functional MRI. *Trends in Pharmacolgical Science* 2000; 21:314-318.

[203] Honey G, Bullmore ET. Human pharmacological MRI. Trends in Pharmacolgical *Science* 2004; 25:366-374.

[204] Chen YI, Brownell A-L, Galpern W, et al. Detection of dopaminergic cell loss and neural transplantation using pharmacological MRI, PET, and behavioral assessment. *NeuroReport* 1999; 10:2881-2886.

[205] Belayev L, Busto R, Zhao W, et al. Effect of delayed albumin hemodilution on infarction volume and brain edema after transient middle cerebral artery occlusion in rats. *J. Neurosurg*. 1997; 87:595-601.

[206] Miljkovic-Lolic M, Silbergleit R, Fiskum G, et al. Neuroprotective effects of hyperbaric oxygen treatment in experimental focal cerebral ischemia are associated with reduced brain leukocyte myeloperoxidase activity. *Brain Res*. 2003; 971:90-94.

[207] Schabitz WR, Berger C, Kollmar R, et al. Effect of brain-derived neurotrophic factor treatment and forced arm use on functional motor recovery after small cortical ischemia. *Stroke* 2004; 35:992-997.

[208] Virley D, Beech JS, Smart SC, et al. A temporal MRI assessment of neuropathology after transient middle cerebral artery occlusion in the rat: Correlations with behavior. *Journal of Cerebral Blood Flow and Metabolism* 2000; 20:563-582.

[209] Duncan PW. Measuring recovery of function after stroke: Clinical and measurement issues in selecting stroke outcome measures in clinical trials. In: *Restorative Neurology: Advances on Pharmacotherapy for Recovery after Stroke*. (Goldstein LB, ed), pp 225-239. Armonk, NY: Futura Publishing; 1998.

[210] Lanston W, Widner H, Goetz CG, et al. Core assessment program for intracerebral transplantations (CAPIT). *Movement Disorders* 1992; 7:2-13.

[211] Quinn N, Brown R, Craufurd D, et al. Core Assessment Program for Intracerebral Transplantation in Huntington's Disease (CAPIT-HD). *Mov. Disord.* 1996; 11:143-150.

[212] Widner H, Defer GL. Dyskinesias assessment: from CAPIT to CAPSIT. Core Assessment Program for Intracerebral Transplantations. Core Assessment Program for Surgical Interventional Therapies. *Mov. Disord.* 1999; 14 Suppl 1:60-66.

[213] Stadnik TW, Osteauz M. Actual trends in diagnosis/thrombolytic therapy of acute cerebral stroke. *European Journal of Radiology* 2001; 38:28-40.

[214] Lindvall O, Kokaia, Z. Recovery and rehabilitation in stroke: Stem Cells. *Stroke* 2004; 35:2691-2694.

[215] Markus R, Donnan GA, Kazui S, et al. Statistical parametric mapping of hypoxic tissue indetified by [18F]fluoromisonidazole and positron emission tomography following acute ischemic stroke. *Neuroimage* 2002; 16:425-433.

[216] Wictorin K Anatomy and connectivity of intrastriatal striatal transplants. Progress in Neurobiology 1992; 38:611-639.

[217] Polgar S, Borlongan CV, Koutouzis TK, et al. Implications of neurological rehabilitation for advancing intracerebral transplantation. *Brain Reseach Bulletin* 1997; 44:229-232.

[218] Döbrössy M, Dunnett SB. Motor training effects on recovery of function after striatal lesions and striatal grafts. *Experimental Neurology* 2003; 184:274-284.

[219] Freeman TB, Vawter DE, Leaverton PE, et al. Use of placebo surgery in controlled trials of a cellular-based therapy for Parkinson's disease. *N. Engl. J. Med.* 1999; 341:988-992.

[220] Dekkers W, Boer G. Sham neurosurgery in patients with Parkinson's disease: is it morally acceptable? *J. Med. Ethics* 2001; 27:151-156.

[221] Boer GJ, Widner H. Clinical neurotransplantation: core assessment protocol rather than sham surgery as control. *Brain Res. Bull.* 2002; 58:547-553.

[222] Chen YC, Galpern WR, Brownell AL, et al. Detection of dopaminergic neurotransmitter activity using pharmacologic MRI: Correlation with PET, microdialysis, and behavioral data. *Magnetic Resonance in Medicine* 1997; 38:389-398.

[223] Batchelor PE, Porritt MJ, Martinello P, et al. Macrophages and Microglia Produce Local Trophic Gradients That Stimulate Axonal Sprouting Toward but Not beyond the Wound Edge. *Mol. Cell Neurosci.* 2002; 21:436-453.

[224] Humm JL, Kozlowski DA, James DC, et al. Use-dependent exacerbation of brain damage occurs during an early post-lesion vulnerable period. *Brain Research* 1998; 783:286-292.

In: State-of-the-Art Imaging in Stroke, Volume 2
Editor: Bernhard Schaller, pp. 41-74
ISBN 978-1-60021-499-8


*Chapter II*

# Longitudinal Optical Imaging Study for Locomotor Recovery after Stroke

***Ichiro Miyai***
Neurorehabilitation Research Institute, Bobath Memorial Hospital,
Osaka, 536-0023, Japan

## Abstract

To investigate neural mechanisms underlying locomotor recovery, optical imaging technique using near-infrared spectroscopy is suitable because of its flexibility, portability, and excellent time resolution. The technique is based on the idea that absorption of near-infrared light are mainly caused by chromophores including oxygenated hemoglobin and deoxygenated hemoglobin in human tissue. Cortical activation can be assessed as changes levels of regional hemoglobin oxygenation. Typically activation can be assessed by increased levels of oxygenated hemoglobin and decreased levels of deoxygenated hemoglobin. In locomotor tasks the former marker appear to be much more sensitive. In healthy subjects, walking at 1km/hr was associated by cortical activation that centered in the medial sensorimotor cortices and supplementary motor areas. Walking or running at higher speed does not necessarily increase activation in the sensorimotor cortices but enhance activation in other cortical regions such as the premotor cortex and prefrontal cortex. This observation might be associated with hierarchical structures of locomotor control in human including the cerebral cortex, basal ganglia, brainstem, cerebellum, and spinal cord. In patients with stroke, cortical activation patterns during hemiparetic gait were characterized by asymmetrical activation in the sensorimotor cortex and recruitment of the premotor cortex and the prefrontal regions. Recruitment of multiple cortical areas appears to depend of size of lesion and severity of motor impairment. Importantly activation patterns could be modified by rehabilitative intervention. For instance, facilitation technique, by which therapists assisted patients to walk by pressing the hip forward and backward to ensure the stability of the stance and swing phase of the paretic leg, induced enhanced activation in the motor related areas, particularly in the premotor area. Partial body weight support during gait training on the treadmill tended to decrease sensorimotor activation in patients with stroke but not in controls. A longitudinal optical imaging study revealed that locomotor recovery was associated with improvement of asymmetrical activations in the sensorimotor cortex as well as enhanced activation in the premotor cortex. Because of its excellent time resolution, real-time monitoring of neurorehabilitation might be possible to evaluate immediate effects of rehabilitative interventions on cortical activation. Thus optical imaging technique might not only provide a powerful tool for human studies for cerebral mechanisms underlying functional recovery after brain damage but also contribute to establishment of brain-based as well as evidence-based strategies for neurorehabilitation.

**Keywords:** locomotion, near-infrared spectroscopy (NIRS), optical imaging, stroke, hemiparesis, gait, functional recovery, and neurorehabilitation.

## Introduction

Locomotor function is one of the keys to discharge home for patients who survived stroke. In severely impaired patients, locomotor function is more likely to recover than hand function [1]. Japan has suitable medical environment in studying long-term functional outcome of stroke since inpatient multidisciplinary rehabilitation has been covered by the national medical insurance system even for patients with stroke more than 6 months after the onset. Analysis of 1,056 patients with stroke based on the interval between stroke onset and admission to the rehabilitation hospital revealed that walking ability improved in 70.9% of nonambulatory patients who started inpatient multidisciplinary rehabilitation within 90 days after stroke. Improvement was also noted in 54.8% of patients who were admitted 91 to 180 days after the insult, and in 43.9% of patients more than 180 days. Improvement of activities of daily livings (ADLs) showed similar results. However assessment for ADLs does not necessarily reflect function of the affected upper extremity because patients learn to use the non-paretic arm to perform ADLs such as eating, writing, hygiene, and dressing. Functional outcome of the affected upper extremity with complete paralysis was not favorable. Although 29.7% of these patients improved, only 0.2% of them gained full functional use of the affected upper extremity. On the other hand, 37.5% of patients gained full functional use of the affected upper extremity, if they could grasp, hold, and release objects in the affected hand on admission. 43.8% of patients within 90 days, 31.3% of patients 91 to 180 days, and 21.7% of patients more than 180 days poststroke who retained reasonable function in the affected hand on admission gained full functional use of the affected upper extremity after inpatient rehabilitation [1].

These clinical observations for considerable differences of recovery curves between the upper extremity and gait raise a question whether neural mechanisms underlying functional recovery might be different between these two functional domains. To date functional neuroimaging studies using positron emission tomography (PET) and functional magnetic resonance imaging (fMRI) and neurophysiological studies using transcranial magnetic stimulation have provided abundant evidence that functional recovery after stroke depends on reorganization of the central nervous system (See [2] for review). Most of these studies investigated cerebral activations associated with movements of the paretic hand and changes of activation patterns related to functional recovery of the paretic hand. It should be noted that neural mechanisms underlying recovery also depend on time after the onset of stroke. In the acute phase of stroke, contribution of functional reorganization to recovery is likely to be masked by resolution of damaged lesion. In that period, dramatic recovery is mostly attributed to recanalization of the occluded artery or resolution of hematoma and edema that might result in subsequent re-functioning of reversibly damaged areas such as ischemic penumbra. This leads to the concept of “Time is brain” as emphasized in the brain attack campaign in the United States. Functional recovery usually slows down in the postacute phase. Residual cortico-spinal pathways might be needed to restore discrete movements of the paretic hand. For instance, absence of motor evoked potentials in hand muscles induced by transcranial magnetic stimulation in the acute phase predicts poor outcome of hand function since this reflect completely damage of the fast descending pathway for the primary motor cortex [3-5]. Patients with nearly complete hand paralysis due to total damages in the M1 and its descending pathways are unlikely to regain functional use of paretic hand. On the other hand, patients with some residual movements of paretic fingers have potential to improve even more than 1 year after the onset as mentioned above [1]. Further evidence is provided by results of studies regarding constraint-induced movement therapy for patients with chronic stroke where use of the unaffected hand is restricted using a sling or mitten for forced use of paretic hand [6-7]. This important observation is in accordance with experimental studies in primates showing that use-dependant plasticity is in the residual areas within the damaged primary motor cortex [8]. These suggest that improvement of impaired hand function due to damage in the primary motor cortex may depend on residual intact regions within the damaged primary motor cortex. Motor related areas other than the primary motor cortex such as the supplementary motor area and premotor cortex also play a crucial role in functional recovery. One of the common findings in functional neuroimaging studies using PET or fMRI is recruitment of these areas during motor tasks of well-recovered paretic hands [9-13]. Furthermore transcranial magnetic stimulation over the dorsal premotor cortex either in the ipsilesional or contralesional hemisphere induced a significant delay in simple reaction time in patients with stroke [14-15]. This indicates that recruitment of these areas might not be maladaptive.

On the other hand, there have been few studies regarding neural mechanisms underlying locomotor recovery after stroke. This is mainly due to technical limitation of conventional functional neuroimaging technique such as PET and fMRI that basically require subjects to stay still during measurements. A recently developed optical imaging technique using near-infrared spectroscopy (NIRS) had enabled measurement of cerebral function during dynamic movements including walking and running. In this chapter, neural mechanisms controlling human locomotion, human studies for normal and pathological gait using conventional neuroimaging techniques, principle of optical imaging technique, optical imaging studies for human locomotion, and optical imaging studies for hemiparetic gait in patients with stroke and clinical relevance of optical imaging studies in investigating neural mechanisms for locomotor recovery will be discussed.

# Neural Mechanisms Controlling Human Locomotion

Functional organization of the central nervous system controlling hand movements has been well documented. As discussed above, accumulated knowledge has been contributed to understanding neural mechanisms underlying functional recovery of hand after stroke. However less has been known about the cerebral mechanisms governing human locomotion. Experimental studies have indicated that bipedal movements during walking are controlled by cerebral cortex including motor neurons in the medial portion of the primary motor cortex [16-18]. Importantly locomotion is controlled by hierarchical structures including the cerebral cortex, basal ganglia, cerebellum, brainstem, and spinal cord [19-21]. Any lesion in these structures causes gait disturbance. Most striking difference between neural mechanisms controlling movements of hands and those controlling gait might be a role of interneurons in the spinal cord that generate rhythmic motor patterns. Experimental findings using quadripedal mammals such as cat have identified a neural network in the spinal cord, called central pattern generators (CPGs). To initiate locomotion, control locomotor speed, and adjust stepping, descending pathways from the brainstem locomotor regions via the reticulospinal pathway to the spinal cord are involved. Damage in the motor cortex impairs adaptive locomotion depending on visuomotor coordination such as stepping over an obstacle. The cerebellum might play an important role in adjusting deviations of actual movements from intended movements [22]. In human, unlike spinal cat, patients with complete spinal cord injury are unable to make spontaneous steppings. However it is evident that human infant, even an anencephalic infant, can make stepping movements immediately after birth with an appropriate support [23, 24]. This suggests the existence of the pattern generating neural circuits at least below the level of the brainstem. In general, spinal networks that contribute to human locomotion are more likely to depend on supraspinal centers than those in quadripedal animals [22]. Cortical mechanisms for human gait have been also studied by using transcranial magnetic stimulation. The tibialis anterior muscles are likely to be controlled by the corticospinal tract to an extent similar to hand muscles [25]. Although amplitudes of the motor evoked potentials evoked in the soleus muscle during walking were reduced compared with those during voluntary contraction, those from the tibialis anterior were comparable between these two conditions. These suggest that the flexor is more actively controlled by the corticospinal tract than the extensor during walking [26]. Using transcranial magnetic stimulation below motor threshold, Petersen and colleagues demonstrated that motoneuronal activities during walking were suppressed by activation of intracortical inhibitory neurons. These suggest that the primary motor cortex is directly controlling leg muscles during human walking [27] and that imaging of cortical activities during various locomotor tasks might contribute to further understanding of neural mechanisms of human locomotion.

## Neuroimaging Studies for Human Locomotion

Cerebral mechanisms for human locomotion have been studied using single photon emission tomography (SPECT), PET, and fMRI. Because of the technical limitations for motion artifacts, motor task paradigms mainly used for PET and fMRI are foot movements or imagery for locomotion. Fukuyama et al. took advantage of SPECT that reflect regional cerebra blood flow (rCBF) associated with movements when radioactive ligands are injected. Human walking was associated with significant activities in the primary sensorimotor cortex, supplementary motor area, visual cortex, cerebellar vermis, and the striatum [28]. Several PET studies have reported involvement of similar neuronal networks during locomotor related tasks. Bicycle movements activated the primary sensorimotor cortex, supplementary motor area, and anterior cerebellum. Imagination of the same task activated the supplementary motor area [29].

A number of fMRI studies using tasks of foot movements revealed comparable findings. Unilateral movements of foot extension and flexion were associated with activation in the medial sensorimotor cortex, which was greater with active than passive condition. The contrast of the preparation to move vs. active movement conditions revealed activation in the frontopolar region (BA10) and precuneus [30]. Task designs for foot movements appear to affect experimental findings. For instance, graded dorsiflexion produced graded BOLD signals in the primary sensorimotor and supplementary motor areas [31]. A PET study also found a significant correlation between electromyography (EMG) activities of the tibialis anterior muscle and rCBF in the cerebellum and the medial primary motor cortex during motor task of dorsal flexion of the foot. For plantar flexion a significant correlation was found between soleus EMG and rCBF in the left medial sensory cortex and motor cortex, left thalamus, and right cerebellum. Portion of peak activation in the primary motor cortex was 17 mm apart between dorsi- and plantar flexion. Dynamic contractions induced more extensive activation than tonic contractions [32]. These suggest that monitoring of the task performance is essential in using foot movement as a task to assess neural mechanisms for stroke recovery.

Neural mechanisms underlying motor learning of foot movement sequences have been studied [33, 34] using PET. In the early stage of learning, the dorsal premotor cortex, cerebellum, and left parietal lobe were involved. After practice, instead, the medial orbitofrontal cortex, striatum, left rostral anterior cingulate, and inferior parietal lobe were activated. Importantly mental practice of the sequence learning with motor imagery shared the similar structure to the learning with motor execution [34]. After intensive training using mental practice with motor imagery over several days, increase of rCBF in the orbitofrontal cortex correlated with improvement of the task performance [33]. Malouin et al. used various imagery tasks for locomotion including standing, initiation of gait, walking, and walking with obstacles. The common areas of activation in these tasks were the dorsal premotor cortex, precuneus, left dorsolateral prefrontal cortex, left inferior parietal lobule, and right posterior cingulate cortex. Increasing complexities of imagery were associated with recruitment of additional brain regions such as the precuneus, left supplementary motor area, the right parietal inferior cortex and left parahippocampal gyrus [35]. An fMRI study for imagined stance and locomotion compared to imagery for lying revealed similar activation patterns [36]. Imagery for standing induced activation in the thalamus, basal ganglia, and cerebellar vermis. Walking imagery involved the parahippocampal gyrus, fusiform gyrus, occipital visual areas, and cerebellum while running imagery caused larger cerebellar activation in the vermis and adjacent hemispheres. Cortical activation during imagined walking and running varied probably due to different individual strategies for imagery. It was suggested that automatic nature of running might be based on the spinal generators driven by the cerebellar locomotor region. During slow walking, spatial navigation, mediated by the parahippocampal cortex might be relatively important. These suggest that motor imagery for locomotion could also be useful in investigating neural mechanisms for human locomotion. However because of the technical limitation for canceling motion artifacts, there have been no data for actual walking in neuroimaging studies using PET or fMRI.

### Neuroimaging Studies for Pathological Human Gait

Using a task of ankle dorsiflexion, a pilot fMRI study in patients with ambulatory stroke suggested that the activation patterns might be modified by practice and consequent gain [37]. Since motor performance of the foot movement tasks can affect activation patterns as discussed above, the results might not be conclusive. Hanakawa et al. investigated rCBF patterns associated with pathological gait in patients with Parkinson's disease using SPECT [38, 39]. Patients showed decreased activation in the left medial frontal area, right precuneus and left cerebellar hemisphere with increased activities in the left temporal cortex, right insula, left cingulate cortex and cerebellar vermis. The reduced brain activities in the medial frontal motor areas appear to be associated with hypokinetic gait in Parkinson's disease [39]. Subsequently they analyzed changes in rCBF that can explain improved gait performance with visual cues provided by lines parallel to the direction of walking on the treadmill, so called, paradoxical gait. Patients with Parkinson's disease showed enhanced activation in the right dorsal premotor cortex with the visual cues, indicating that the area plays an important role in the improvement of gait performance such as decreased cadence induced by the visual stimuli [38]. Although there have been few studies regarding brain activation associated with pathological human gait, available studies imply that locomotor recovery might also depends on functional reorganization of the central nervous system.

## Optical Imaging Technique and its Principle

The noninvasive and flexible features of the optical imaging technique using NIRS enables stable real-time monitoring of cortical activation during dynamic motion including walking and running. The technique is based on the property of the near-infrared light. The light ranging from 650 nm to 900 nm penetrates the skull and bone and is mainly absorbed by chromophores including oxygenated hemoglobin (oxyHb), deoxygenated hemoglobin (deoxyHb), and cytochrome-c oxidase (cytox). NIRS can detect changes in cortical hemodynamics associated with neuronal activities by measuring changes in concentration of oxyHb, deoxyHb, and total hemoglobin (totalHb). Most commonly available NIRS system uses a continuous wave light that measures attenuation of near-infrared light. Other data acquisition approaches include time-resolved spectroscopy that assesses the distribution of photon arrival times using a pulsed light of picoseconds and frequency domain system using light of which amplitude is modulated at the rate of ten to hundreds of megahertz [40, 41]. NIRS system using continuous wave relies on modified Beer-Lambert Law in detecting changes in hemoglobin oxygenation (Figure 1A). The Beer-Lambert Law postulates that optical density is proportional to the concentration of absorbing chromophores and pathlength. However photon pathlength is usally longer than the actual distance because of tissue scattering. Thus differential pathlength factor (DPF) is introduced for the correction [42, 43]. DPF varies depending on type and site of the tissue. The modified Beer-Lambert Law is

$$A = \varepsilon CdB + G$$

where A is the optical density, ε is the extinction coefficient, C is the concentration of the chromophore, d is the distance between the light source and the detector, B is the DPF, and G is the attenuation of light accounting for scattering. If we measure A with at least two wavelengths of near-infrared light,

$$A_{\lambda 1} - A_{\lambda 2} = Cd(\varepsilon_{\lambda 1}B_{\lambda 1} - \varepsilon_{\lambda 2}B_{\lambda 2}) + (G\varepsilon_{\lambda 1} - G\varepsilon_{\lambda 2})$$

where $\lambda_1$ and $\lambda_2$ are two particular wave lengths.

If we assume that B and G remain constant ($B_{\lambda 1} = B_{\lambda 2}$ and $G_{\lambda 1} = G_{\lambda 2}$, the changes of optical density ($\Delta A$) caused by changes of the chromophore concentrations are determined as follows.

$$\Delta A_{\lambda 1 - \lambda 2} = \varepsilon_{\lambda 1 - \lambda 2}\Delta CdB = \varepsilon^{oxyHb}{}_{\lambda 1 - \lambda 2}\Delta[oxyHb]dB + \varepsilon^{deoxyHb}{}_{\lambda 1 - \lambda 2}\Delta[deoxyHb]dB + \varepsilon^{cytox}{}_{\lambda 1 - \lambda 2}\Delta[cytox]dB$$

Cytochrome-c oxidase usually remains constant except extreme condition such as severe hypoxia [44]. Thus if ε and B are determined, changes of oxyHb and deoxyHb concentrations can be calculated using at least two wavelengths. The ε value of each chromophore can be calculated experimentally although DPF cannot be determined in commonly available NIRS systems using continuous wave. Instead DPF is only measured by using ultra-short (picosecond) pulse of light. Therefore the unit for changes of hemoglobin oxygenation measured by using continuous wave NIRS system is the product of concentration and pathlength e.g., milli-mole x centimeter. Instead assumption that DPF value is constant (approximately 6 for brain tissue) can be applied [45] to determine approximate values. Typical task related hemodynamic changes detected by NIRS include increase in oxyHb and totalHb levels and decrease in deoxyHb levels. Changes in oxyHb are larger than those in deoxyHb.

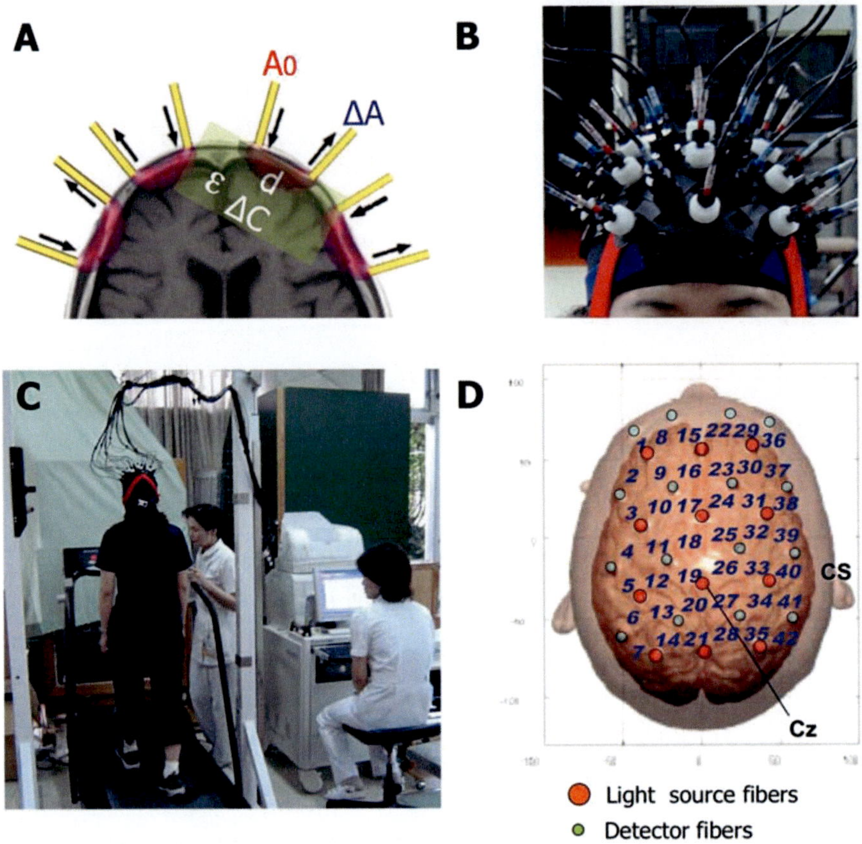


The technique relies on modified Beer-Lambert Law, which postulates that the changes in optical density are caused by changes in the chromophore concentration such as oxygenated and deoxygenated hemoglobin.

$\Delta A = -\log(A/A_0) = \varepsilon \Delta C d B$

A is the detected optical signal, $A_0$ is the optical input, ΔA is the change in optical density, ε is the extinction coefficient, ΔC is the change in concentration of the chromophore, d is the distance between the light source and the detector, B is the differential pathlength factor.

B. The light source fibers (red) and detector fibers (blue) was placed tightly on the skull using a custom-made head holder cap, with interoptode distance set to 3.0 cm. the optical fibers.

C. Optical imaging system (Shimadzu, OMM-2001, Japan). A subject is performing a walking task on the treadmill while fibers are suspended from a weight-balancer system to avoid motion-related artifacts.

D. In this setting using 12 light source fibers and 16 detector fibers result in simultaneous 42 channel recording. Location of each optode was superposed on the brain surface image with assigned channel numbers labeled as Channel 1 to Channel 42. The light-source fiber next to the posterior one in the center row was located in the Cz position according to the 10-20 international system. An anatomical 3-D T1-weighted MRI scan was performed with marking the optode location on the skull by vitamin D capsules. The anatomical MRI was normalized to a standard stereotaxic space, using a Montreal Neurological Institute (MNI) brain template, which corresponds to the space described by Talairach and Tournoux (1988). The normalization was performed using SPM99 (Wellcome Department of Cognitive Neurology, London, UK).

Figure 1. A. Theory of optical imaging using NIRS.

Both the blood oxygenation-dependent (BOLD) fMRI [46] and NIRS [47] detect hemodynamic changes assumed to link with neural activities [48]. Although BOLD fMRI measures only deoxyHb levels, NIRS can detect both oxyHb and deoxyHb values as mentioned above. Correlation between BOLD signals and deoxyHb or oxyHb levels measured from NIRS signals has been controversial in experiments simultaneously recording BOLD and NIRS signals [49-52].

Several reports demonstrating significant correlation between BOLD signals and deoxyHb levels in NIRS did not analyze oxyHb values. Strangman and colleague suggested that the superior contrast-to-noise ratio for oxyHb relative to deoxyHb measured from NIRS signals, rather than physiology related to BOLD signal interpretation since there were correlations between BOLD changes and all optical measures, with oxyHb providing the strongest correlation after several factors including partial volume errors, wavelength dependence of the partial volume effect, tissue model errors, and spatial incongruence between oxyHb and deoxyHb concentration changes were accounting for [51]. On the other hand, Schroeter and colleague applied general linear model to analyze NIRS data and found that the model is particularly feasible for deoxyHb [53]. In an experimental rat brain perfusion model, oxyHb is the most sensitive indicator of changes in CBF, while deoxyHb level varied depending on the degree of changes in venous blood oxygenation and volume [54]. One possible explanation for these discrepancies might be that NIRS is more likely to reflect hemodynamic changes in capillaries while BOLD fMRI reflects those in small veins [55].

## Advantage and Limitation of Optical Imaging Technique

There are several advantages of optical imaging using NIRS over other neuroimaging techniques such as PET and fMRI. Measurement setting for NIRS recording is highly flexible to enable measurement during dynamic movements such as walking, running, and reaching [56, 57]. It is also suitable to examine infants and even newborn babies at the bedside because of its portability [58-62]. Real-time monitoring of ongoing changes in oxyHb, deoxyHb, and totalHb with time resolution of few hundred seconds enables researcher to optimize experimental designs without delay. However there are also several limitations that should be born in mind. It is difficult to determine precise anatomical location of the measured cortical region under the skull between two optodes. Okamoto et al used the international 10-20 system to create a three-dimensional probabilistic anatomical location map of optodes [63] in the standard Montreal Neurological Institute and Talairach stereotactic coordinates [64]. Information regarding hemodynamic changes is principally limited to that from the cerebral cortices. There is no information from deep brain areas, cerebellum or the brainstem. Measured signals possibly include those from generalized or extracortical origins. NIRS signals of the intracranial origin increase as the interoptode distance of light source and detector increases while those of the extracranial origin decrease [65]. However larger interoptode distance results in decrease in light intensity. Thus interoptode distance of 3 to 4 cm is usually used [41]. In a block design experiment especially using motor tasks, signals outside of the brain such as those related to breathing, heart rate, and arterial pressure fluctuations might induce a systemic increase in oxygenation and blood volume [40, 66, 67]. In studying patients with ischemic stroke, impaired hemodynamic response might complicate the data obtained by optical imaging as well as those from fMRI [68]. Changes in cerebral blood supply in the affected hemisphere, especially in the areas surrounding the lesion might influence NIRS measurements. BOLD response has been shown to be modified in the time course of functional recovery [69]. To minimize such problem, a certain control task might help to interpret the signal changes [41]. Combination of neurophysiological method such as transcranial magnetic stimulation with NIRS might provide additional information to detect hemodynamic-electrical decoupling [69, 70].

## Optical Imaging Studies of Human Locomotion

To date optical imaging studies have replicated previous findings from fMRI and PET studies using motor [71-73], visual [74-76] and cognitive tasks [77-81] in healthy subjects. In patients with stroke, optical imaging has been used to assess functional reorganization associated with recovery of paretic hand [82] and aphasia [83]. These studies might provide the rationale of the use optical imaging in studying cerebral function in humans. However optical imaging might be most useful in mapping the human brain during locomotor tasks, such as gait [56] and even running [57], as well as in mapping the brain of neonates and children [58-62] for which use of fMRI and PET is not feasible.

In optical imaging studies for human locomotion [56,57], we used a 30 to 42-channel NIRS imaging system (OMM-2001, Shimadzu, Kyoto, Japan, Figure 1B, 1C) depending on the number of detector fibers and light source fibers, using continuous wave laser diodes with wavelengths of 780, 805, and 830 nm. The system detects the absorption spectrum of hemoglobin that depends on its oxygenation state and cortical changes in oxyHb, deoxyHb, and totalHb. Each optode with interoptode distance set to 3.0 centimeters was placed tightly on the skull using a custom-made holder cap and the optical fibers were suspended from a weight-balancer system to avoid motion-related artifacts during locomotor tasks on the treadmill (Figure 1B, 1C). An anatomical 3-D MRI scan while marking the optode position on the skull by vitamin D capsules, revealed that the optodes covered an area over fronto-parietal cortices including the primary sensorimotor cortex, supplementary motor area, and premotor cortex with 30-channel measurement. Measurements with 36 or 42-channel system also included the prefrontal cortices and pre-supplementary motor areas (Figure 1D, Figure 2A).

A block design that comprises 30 seconds of rest period alternating with 30 seconds of locomotion period for 3 to 5 repetitions was employed for locomotor tasks on the treadmill. Averaged changes in oxyHb, deoxyHb, and totalHb levels during walking on the treadmill at 1 km/hr from the channel that covers the medial portion of the left primary sensorimotor cortex are shown in Figure 2B and 2C. Levels of oxyHb in the channel started to increase 3 to 5 seconds after the task onset of walking at 1 km/hr, reached a plateau at 5 to 10 s, and returned to the baseline 3 to 5 seconds after the end of the task. There were few changes in deoxyHb levels. Consequently totalHb showed similar time course as oxyHb. Increase of

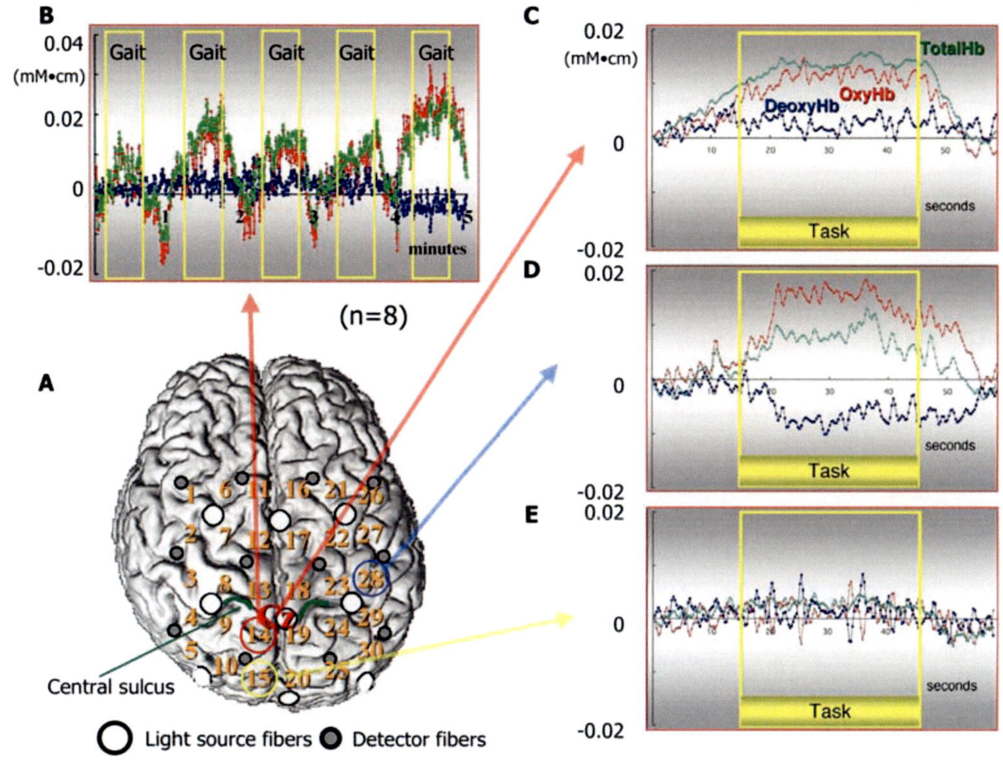


A. Location of optodes for 30 channel recording superposed onto a rendered surface MRI image of a subject and assigned channel numbers.

B. Whole time series of oxyHb (red), deoxyHb (blue), and totalHb (green) levels (mM□cm) during gait at 1 km/hr (n=8) obtained from the channel covering the left medial sensorimotor cortex. The time series is composed of 30 second task period alternating with 30 second rest period for 5 repetitions. Averaged data of 8 healthy subjects are shown. Task related increase of oxyHb is clearly shown although there are some variations across the task cycles. There are few changes in deoxyHb levels. Consequently the time course of totalHb is similar to that of oxyHb.

C. Changes of oxyHb (red), deoxyHb (blue), and totalHb (green) levels during one task cycle averaged from the 5 task cycles plotted in Figure 2B. After averaging the data, increase in oxyHb levels started approximately 2 seconds before the task and again there was a small increase approximately 5 seconds after starting the task. The apparent increase of oxyHb prior to task point might be caused by anticipation of the task with task repetitions since the increase disappears if time for rest period was pseudo-randomized. There were few changes in deoxyHb levels. TotalHb curve is similar to oxyHb curve.

D. Averaged time course (n= 8) of oxyHb (red), deoxyHb (blue), and totalHb (green) levels during arm swing without walking from the channel covering the right lateral sensorimotor regions. The increase in oxyHb started 3 to 5 seconds after the task was started. There was task related decrease in deoxyHb levels. The changes are smaller than those in oxyHb levels. E. In the channel covering the medial parietal regions, there were no significant task related changes as expected. (Miyai et al., 2001b, Copyright© 2001, Elsevier Science, Reprinted by Permission Elsevier Science).

Figure 2.

oxyHb and totalHb levels tended to begin earlier as subjects repeated the task cycles. This is probably due to anticipation of task initiation since such increase in the pre-task period disappears with a task design of pseudo-randomized resting perionda. In the same experimental setting, deoxyHb levels in the lateral channels covering hand-arm area of the primary sensorimotor cortex showed task related decrease along with increase in oxyHb levels in another task of swinging arms while subjects were standing still (Figure 2D). In the channel covering the medial parietal regions (Figure 2E), there were no significant task related changes in these parameters during either walking or arm swing without walking [56].

Cortical maps depicting increases in cortical oxyHb levels were obtained after adapting the linear interpolation to the simultaneously acquired 30 to 42 channel data from neighboring source-detector pairs. Each map was corrected to match the anatomical location of the source-detector pairs on the brain surface and was overlaid on anatomical MRI surface images (Figure 3). Comparison of oxyHb-based activation maps revealed that different types of locomotor task activated distinct cortical networks [56]. Walking on the treadmill at 1 km/hr induced bilateral cortical activation in the medial sensorimotor cortex and supplementary motor area. This finding is in accordance with previous SPECT studies [28, 39]. Alternating arm swing while a subject standing still on the treadmill activated the lateral portion of the primary sensorimotor cortex. Dorsi- and plantar flexions of the foot joint were associated with more localized activation in the medial sensorimotor cortex, comparable with fMRI or PET findings using similar tasks of foot movements [30-32]. Execution of gait performance and gait imagery in the first-person perspective induced similar activation patterns, although gait imagery appeared to induce more rostral and more circumscribed activation centered in the supplementary motor area compared with gait execution. Activation patterns based on task related decrease in deoxyHb levels are similar to those based on increase in oxyHb levels in the tasks of arm swing and foot movements, and but activated areas are smaller in deoxyHb maps than in oxyHb maps (Figure 3B). Few changes are detected in deoxyHb maps during gait execution and gait imagery. BOLD fMRI results using the same task of foot movements or gait imagery with the spine posture in the same subject, were similar to results of optical imaging based on changes of oxyHb levels (Figure 3C). Thus execution and imagery of gait appear to share the common structures in the medial frontal regions. These findings were also in accordance with PET and fMRI studies using locomotor imagery tasks [35,36] and PET findings of motor execution and imagery of foot movements in the learning process of the sequence [33, 34].

Locomotor tasks on the treadmill at different speeds commonly activated the medial frontal regions. However there appear to be no linear relationships between activities in the sensorimotor cortex and locomotor speeds or cadence. Using the same optical imaging system, Suzuki et al. investigated changes of regional activation in the frontal cortices as assessed by changes in oxyHb levels during walking at 3 and 5 km/hr and running at 9 km/hr on a treadmill [57]. During the acceleration period of locomotion on the treadmill immediately before reaching the steady speed, oxyHb levels increased in the frontal regions. The changes were greater at the higher locomotor speed in the prefrontal cortex and premotor cortex, but there were less speed-associated changes in the sensorimotor cortices. The medial prefrontal activation was the most prominent during the acceleration phase of the running task (Figure 4). However keeping walking or running at a steady speed for a longer period (more than 60 seconds) was associated with subsequent decrease of oxyHb and

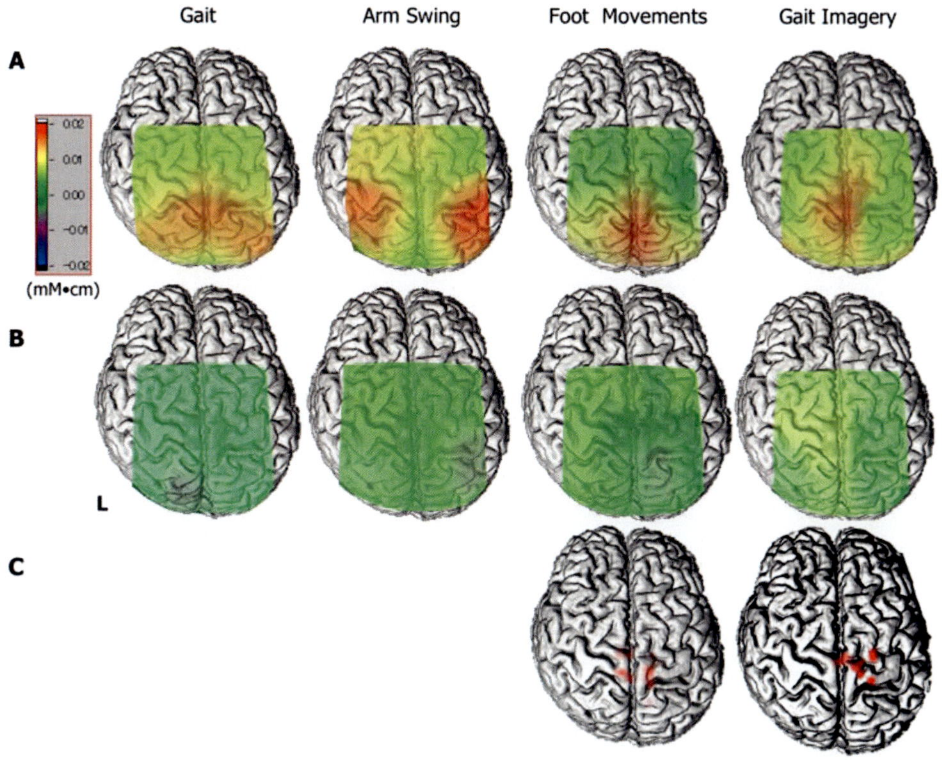


A: Cortical mappings on based on task related increase of oxyHb levels (30 channel recording). After adapting the linear interpolation to the 30 data for averaged changes of oxyHb from five cycles of each task simultaneously acquired from neighboring source-detector pairs, the images were corrected to match the anatomical location of the optodes on the brain surface and finally overlaid on anatomical MRI surface images. Different locomotor tasks are associated with distinct cortical activation patterns. During walking on the treadmill moving at 1 km/hr, the activation center is located in the medial sensorimotor cortex and the supplementary motor area. Activations are also seen in the lateral regions. Arm swinging without walking is associated with activities in the lateral sensorimotor cortex while there is no apparent activation in the medial regions. Alternating movements of dorsiflexion and plantar flexion of the feet also activate the medial sensorimotor cortex and the supplementary motor area but the activated areas appear to be more circumscribed compared with walking related activation. Gait imagery shares similar structures with walking and foot movements but appears to activate more rostral regions than foot movements do. The scale **indicates the color coordinates of concentration changes (mMol□cm).**

B. Cortical mappings based on task related decrease of deoxyHb levels. Activation patterns are similar to those based on oxyHb changes during arm swing and foot movements, and but distributed areas are smaller in deoxyHb maps than in oxyHb maps. Few changes are detected in deoxyHb maps during gait and gait imagery.

C: Activated areas during foot movements and gait imagery detected by BOLD-fMRI in the same subject. Task designs are the same as those used in optical imaging except the subjected performed the task with the spine position. The supplementary motor area and medial primary motor cortex were activated during both tasks. These activation patterns were similar to those of optical imaging.

L: Left. (Adapted from Miyai et al., 2001b, Copyright© 2001, Elsevier Science, Reprinted by Permission Elsevier Science).

Figure 3. Representative data for cortical activation during various locomotor tasks.

totalHb levels [57]. These suggest that maintaining walking or running condition might need less cortical control than adapting to speed changes in human locomotion and that the prefrontal and premotor cortices are involved in adapting to locomotor speed on the treadmill. These areas might predominantly participate in adaptive control of running rather than walking. In contrast, previous neuroimaging studies regarding hand movements showed a positive relationship between activities in the primary sensorimotor cortex and force or frequency of finger movements [84-86].

Such non-linear relationship in locomotion might be attributed to the hierarchical structures of locomotor control consisting of the spinal central pattern generators and supraspinal multiple motor centers such as the cerebellum, subthalamic locomotor region, mesencephalic locomotor region, ventral tegmental field, and dorsal tegmental fields as discussed above [19-21].

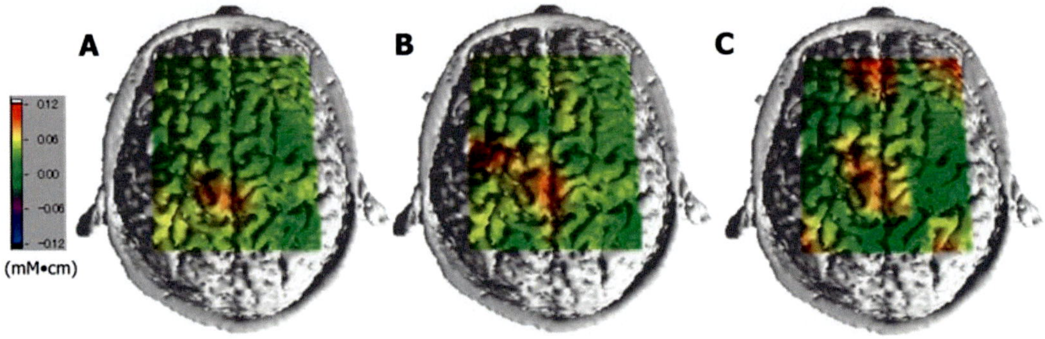


**Each mapping is based on increases in oxyHb levels (mM□cm) during the acceleration phase of** walking or running on the treadmill.

A. During walking at 3 km/h, the activation mostly centered in the medial sensorimotor cortex. The patterns are similar to those seen at 1 km/hr (See Figure 3).

B. During walking at 5 km/hr, the medial sensorimotor cortex appears to be activated to be similar to the similar extent as activated at 3 km/hr. The activation in the left dorsal premotor cortex becomes prominent at this speed.

C. During running at 9 km/h, the cortical vicinity including the prefrontal cortex and pre-supplementary motor area, as well as the premotor cortex and the medial sensorimotor cortex, show prominent activations. Although the left premotor activation appears to be prominent in this representative subject, the lateralities of activation in the premotor and prefrontal regions were inconsistent between subjects.

(Suzuki et al., 2004, Copyright© 2004, Elsevier Science, Reprinted by Permission Elsevier Science).

Figure 4. Cortical activation patterns during walking and running at different locomotor speeds.

Tendency toward greater demands for the subcortical structures during automated locomotor performance is also supported by the findings that cerebellar activations in the cerebellar vermis and adjacent hemispheres were more predominant during imagery for running than that for walking or standing. Automated locomotion might basically depend on the CPGs in the spinal cord driven by the cerebellar locomotor region [36]. Thus these findings might be in accordance with the idea that the main controller of locomotion might shift from the cortical to the subcortical levels. On the other hand, the frontal lobes and basal ganglia loops are involved in higher motor control when one is faced with complex environmental conditions. Experimental lesions of the motor cortex do not prevent animals from walking on a smooth floor although they lead to impairment on tasks requiring a high degree of visuomotor coordination, such as stepping over an obstacle [22]. Tendency toward more demands for cortical regions other than the primary sensorimotor cortex during relatively complex locomotor tasks is supported by PET findings indicating that imagery for obstacle avoidance during waking induces enhanced activities in the bilateral precuneus, the left supplementary motor area, the right parietal inferior cortex and the left parahippocampal gyrus compared with imagery for simple walking [35].

### Cortical Mapping of Pathological Gait in Hemiparetic Stroke

In patients with stroke, hemiparetic gait is characterized by decreased speed and cadence, asymmetry of swing and stance phase, abnormal synergic patterns of the affected upper and lower limbs during the whole gait cycles [87, 88]. Such abnormalities of gait are primarily due to the damage in the primary motor cortex in the unilateral cerebral hemisphere and/or its descending motor pathway including the corona radiata, internal capsule, cerebral peduncle, and ventral brainstem. Based on the findings for healthy subjects, we evaluated cortical activation patterns associated with hemiparetic gait in patients with stroke, using the same optical imaging system [89, 90]. Basic differences of cortical activation patterns between normal gait and hemiparetic gait were 1) asymmetry of activation in the medial sensorimotor cortex and 2) recruitment of other cortical areas, such as the premotor cortex and the prefrontal regions in patients with stroke (Figure 5 and 6). The observed activation patterns appeared to depend on the severity of hemiparesis as well as on the location and size of the cerebral lesion. In patients with ambulatory stroke due to capsular lesion, hemiparetic gait was associated with asymmetrical activation in the sensorimotor cortex, with less activation in the affected hemisphere than in the unaffected hemisphere (Figure 5 and 6). In patients with severe impairment due to combined damage in the cerebral cortex and subcortical regions including the whole internal capsule and the basal ganglia, recruitment of the premotor cortex, especially in the affected hemisphere, was also characteristic finding during assisted hemiplegic gait [89, 91].

## Role of the Sensorimotor Cortex in Locomotor Recovery after Stroke

In patients with stroke revealed that cortical activation patterns during hemiparetic gait as assessed by increase in oxyHb levels were similar to those in healthy subject in that activities centered in the medial sensorimotor cortex. However patients showed asymmetrical activation in the sensorimotor cortex that was less in the affected hemisphere compared with unaffected hemisphere ([89, 90] See Figure 5). These findings are expected since unilateral descending motor pathways subserving locomotor control were disrupted in patients with hemiparetic stroke. Serial optical imaging study revealed that activities in the medial sensorimotor cortex were more symmetrical when hemiparetic gait improved after 2 to 3 months of rehabilitative intervention (Figure 6).

For further analysis for clinical relevance of this finding, symmetry of regional activities was evaluated using laterality index defined as (ΔoxyHb in the affected hemisphere - ΔoxyHb in the unaffected hemisphere) / (ΔoxyHb in the affected hemisphere + ΔoxyHb in unaffected hemisphere) in the medial sensorimotor cortex. Positive laterality index indicates dominant activities in the affected hemisphere and vice versa. Laterality index of gait was defined as (time for swing phase of the sound leg - time for swing phase of the paretic leg) / (time for swing phase of the sound leg + time for swing phase of the paretic leg).

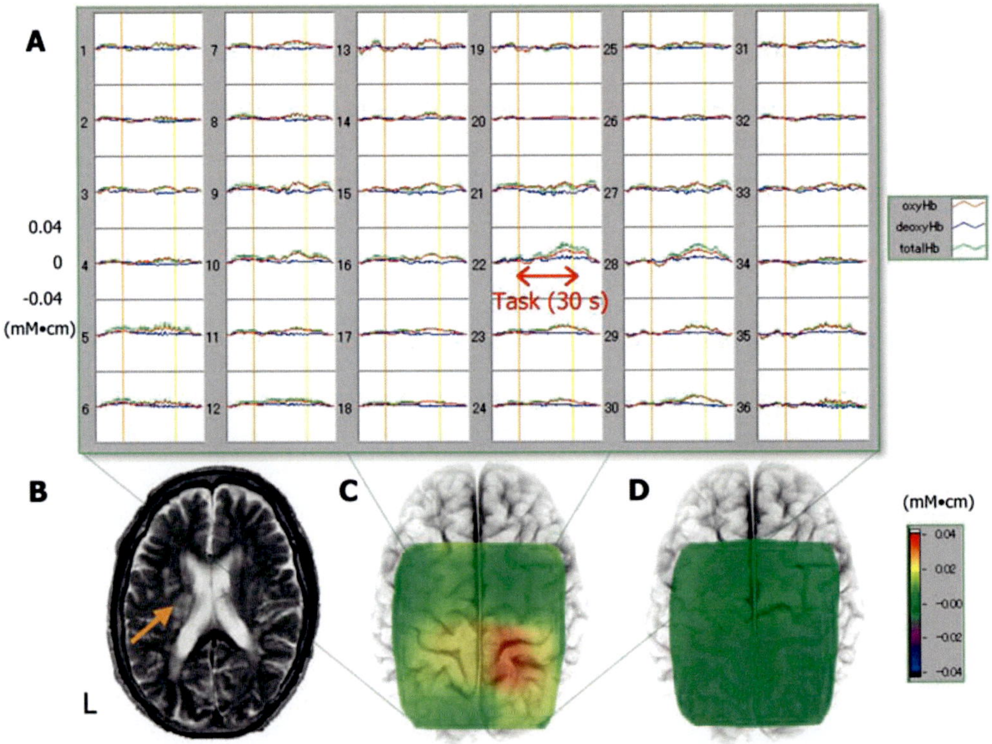


A. Averaged time courses of changes in oxyHb, deoxyHb, and totalHb during hemiplegic gait on the treadmill at 1 km/hr from 36 simultaneously recorded channels. Walking task consists of 30 seconds of walking period alternating with 30 seconds of rest period for 3 repetitions. There are task related increases in oxyHb and totalHb levels at approximately 5 s after starting the task and decreases at 5 s after the end of the task. Few changes can be detected in the levels of deoxyHb. Changes in oxyHb and deoxyHb are greater in the channels covering the right medial frontal regions than those covering the left regions in the affected hemisphere.

B. The corresponding cortical mapping of this case based on task related increase of oxyHb shows asymmetrical sensorimotor activation less in the affected hemisphere.

C. Cortical mapping based on task related changes of deoxyHb appear to be less sensitive in detecting activation.

Figure 5. An example of optical imaging during hemiparetic gait on the treadmill in a patient with left subcortical infarction (53 year-old male, right handed, 53 days poststroke).

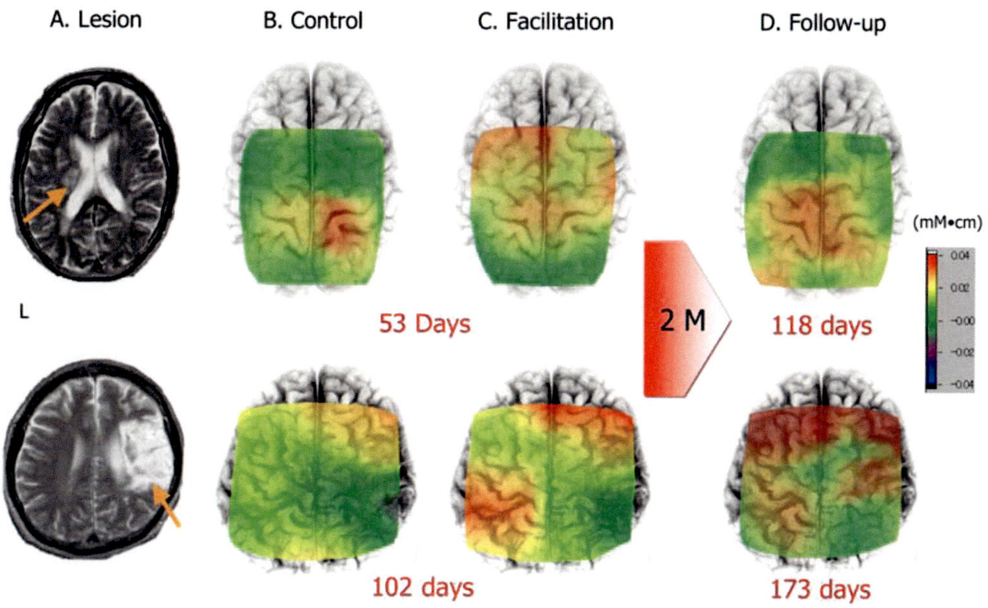


Upper row: Changes of cortical activation patterns in a 53 year-old, right handed male with mild right hemiparesis (See also Figure 5). A. T2 weighted MRI shows a small ischemic lesion in the left corona radiata (arrow). B. During minimally assisted gait by mechanically assisting stepping of the paretic leg on the treadmill at 1 km/hr on 53 days poststroke, the sensorimotor activation is asymmetrical with less activation in the affected hemisphere than in the unaffected hemisphere. C. A different intervention immediately alters cortical activation patterns. During assisted gait using facilitation technique that facilitates swing and stance of the paretic leg by providing sensorimotor stimulation to the pelvis (See also Figure 7), the sensorimotor activation appears to be symmetrical with enhanced activation in the premotor and prefrontal areas. D. Follow-up imaging after 2 months of intensive inpatient rehabilitation when patient reached independent level (118 days poststroke) revealed symmetrical activation in the medial sensorimotor cortex during unassisted walking on the treadmill at 1 km/hr. Activation patterns are similar to those observed during walking with facilitation technique before inpatient rehabilitation although prefrontal activation appear to be smaller than before. These suggest that symmetrical sensorimotor activation is associated with locomotor recovery and that induced activation patterns by facilitation technique might be beneficial for recovery.

Lower row: Changes of cortical activation patterns in a 58 year old, right handed male with severe left hemiparesis. A. T2 weighted MRI shows diffuse infarction in the territory of the right middle cerebral artery (arrow). B. On 102 days poststroke, the patient needed 20 % of partial body weight support to perform the locomotor tasks (0.2 km/hr). During gait assisted by a therapist who mechanically assisted the swing of the paretic leg (B), mild activations are observed in the premotor and prefrontal regions in the affected hemisphere and the fronto-parietal regions in the unaffected hemisphere. C. Enhanced activation in the premotor and prefrontal cortex in the affected hemisphere and the primary sensorimotor cortex in the unaffected hemisphere are immediately observed during assisted walking using facilitation technique (See also Figure 7). Note that there is no activation in the damaged cortical regions. D. Follow-up imaging during unassisted walking at 0.2 km/hr with 10 % of partial body weight support after 2 months of intensive inpatient rehabilitation when patient could walk with a cane supervised by others (173 days poststroke) revealed similar activation patterns as seen during assisted walking by using facilitation technique earlier. There are enhanced activations in the premotor cortex in the affected hemisphere, sensorimotor cortex in the unaffected hemisphere, and bilateral prefrontal regions. These suggest that the premotor cortex in the affected hemisphere might play a important role in locomotor recovery especially in severe cases. Similar to the upper case, activation patterns induced by facilitation technique earlier are similar to those seen after locomotor recovery. (Adapted from Miyai et al., 2003b, Copyright© 2003, Lippincott Williams and Wilkins, Reprinted by Permission).

Figure 6. Changes of cortical activation patterns associated with locomotor recovery and rehabilitative interventions.

Consequently there was a significant correlation between the changes of the two laterality indices, indicating that improvement of asymmetrical activities in the primary sensorimotor cortex is one of the neural mechanisms underlying locomotor recovery after stroke [90]. Significant relationship between changes in a physiological parameter of gait and changes in cortical oxyHb levels might support clinical relevance of measuring oxyHb as a marker for cortical activation associated with gait.

Relatively increased involvement of the affected hemisphere had bee also found in the course of functional recovery of the paretic hand. Several longitudinal neuroimaging studies using PET or fMRI showed that laterality index of activations in the primary sensorimotor cortex and premotor cortex during movements of the paretic hand turned to be positive. This indicates that functional recovery of paretic hand is associated with relatively increased activities of the motor related areas in the affected hemisphere [92-95] although amount of activation appear to decrease finally in these areas [96]. Reorganization is also evident within the primary motor cortex. Intracortical microstimulations revealed an increase of the hand representation within the partially damaged primary motor cortex in adult squirrel monkeys after they underwent rehabilitative training following an experimental cortical lesion [8]. Transcranial magnetic stimulation revealed an increased motor output areas to the affected hand muscles in patients with chronic stroke after constraint induced movement therapy [6]. An attempt to expand the hand area within the primary motor cortex by combining rehabilitative training and functional deafferentation of the proximal muscles of the affected upper extremity using regional anesthesia resulted in functional improvement of the distal muscles of the affected upper extremity in patients with chronic stroke [97]. Thus, residual capacity for reorganization in the primary motor cortex in the affected hemisphere appears to be one of the determinants for favorable outcome of hand function after stroke. However it remains to be determined whether locomotor recovery is accompanied by reorganization of foot areas within the primary motor cortex in the affected hemisphere.

In contrast, the primary motor cortex in the unaffected hemisphere might play a limited role in functional recovery of the paretic hand except cases that sustained brain damage in perinatal periods and rare adults cases with predominant uncrossed components of the descending motor pathways. In neonates, the ipsilateral and contralateral motor evoked potentials of the upper extremity muscles to transcranial magnetic stimulation have comparable latencies, amplitudes, and thresholds. The ipsilateral responses usually attenuate from 3 to 18 months although children with hemiplegic cerebral palsy due to brain damages in the perinatal period show sustained ipsilateral responses [98]. It should be noted, however, activations of the ipsilateral pathways still have clinical relevance to functional recovery following adult stroke since patients with stroke in the unilateral hemisphere showed exacerbated motor function of the recovered limbs when they developed a new stroke in the other hemisphere [99].

## Role of Other Motor Related Areas in Locomotor Recovery after Stroke

Optical imaging during hemiparetic gait also demonstrated recruitment of other cortical areas including the dorsal premotor cortex and prefrontal regions especially in patients with larger lesions and relatively severe hemiparesis ([89, See Figure 5 and 6). A subsequent follow-up study revealed that the premotor activation during hemiparetic gait was more prominent after locomotor function improved [90]. These observations are comparable with findings from previous studies regarding poststroke recovery [100, 101]. Among severely impaired patients due to diffuse infarction in the territory of the middle cerebral artery, those with lesion involving the premotor cortex had worse locomotor outcome that those without premotor damage [101]. In contrast, patients with capsular stroke and with MRI evidence for Wallerian degeneration of the pyramidal tract below the level of the lesion demonstrated comparable final locomotor outcome to those without evidence for Wallerian degeneration, although the former group of patients showed delayed improvement [102]. These suggest that the descending pathways from motor areas other than the primary motor cortex could compensate for the damage in the corticospinal pathways from the primary motor cortex. Indeed parallel motor pathways to the final effectors in the spinal cord from the primary motor cortex, premotor cortex, and supplementary motor area are known to exist [103, 104]. The premotor cortex and supplementary motor areas are also involved in control of the contralateral proximal musculature and bilateral axial musculature [105, 106]. Preserved function of the proximal part of the lower extremities and the trunk might provide basic ability for locomotion. Axial and proximal muscles are controlled by the corticospinal pathways bilaterally whereas distal muscles are principally controlled by the contralateral corticospinal pathways [107, 108]. This implies that the limbs might receive discordant efferent commands from both hemispheres and neural-crosstalk among the motor-related areas [109] might play an important role in controlling human gait. In addition, the right parieto-premotor activation was shown to be involved in execution of limb-independent antiphase movements of hands or feet [110]. The early phase of learning of an explicitly known sequence of foot movements was associated with increases in rCBF bilaterally in the dorsal premotor cortex and cerebellum as well as in the left inferior parietal lobule (34). Thus the premotor regions might be also involved in controlling complex movements of the lower extremities. Probably these areas are more likely to be recruited in patients with partial recovery since even simple stepping might be a relatively complex task for these patients. Finally the premotor and supplementary motor areas appear to be involved in the purposeful modification and initiation of locomotion through connections with the subcortical structures as discussed above [19-21]. Thus, both functional neuroimaging studies and lesion studies suggest that the premotor cortex as well as the primary motor cortex and their descending pathways might be involved in the mechanisms underlying locomotor recovery after stroke.

Altered activations in multiple motor-related areas are also commonly seen in the course of functional recovery of the paretic hand after stroke. Cortical activation patterns during movements of the completely recovered hand include recruitment of the peri-infarct area in the primary motor cortex of the affected hemisphere, the premotor cortex and supplementary motor area in the affected hemisphere, and combination of these areas in the undamaged hemisphere [9-13]. However roles of these motor-related areas in functional recovery of the paretic hand appear partly to depend on degree of impairment. In patients with infarction in the territory of the middle cerebral artery, improvement of finger movements was associated with bilateral activation of the premotor cortex [100]. When patients with capsular infarct and MRI evidence for Wallerian degeneration reached similar functional level as those without Wallerian degeneration, the former group showed persistent premotor activation in the affected hemisphere during grasping tasks of the paretic hand [111]. Transcranial magnetic stimulation has been also used to explore a role of the premotor cortex in the preparation and execution of hand movements in normal subjects and patients with stroke. Transcranial magnetic stimulation applied to the dorsal premotor cortex in the unaffected hemisphere, 100 ms after the cue to move, induced a significant delay in simple reaction time of finger movements in patients with right hemiparesis. Furthermore the slowing of reaction time correlated with the degree of motor impairment and the relative hemispheric lateralization of fMRI activation in the dorsal premotor cortex. These findings were not observed in controls [14], indicating that the recruitment of the premotor cortex in the unaffected hemisphere might be an adaptive response to the brain damage and functionally relevant change. A similar experiment was done to investigate a role of the dorsal premotor cortex in the affected hemisphere in functional recovery of the paretic hand. In chronic patients with subcortical stroke representing with good recovery, transcranial magnetic stimulation applied to the dorsal but not ventral premotor cortex in the affected hemisphere, 120 ms after the cue to move, elicited clear delays in simple reaction time in the paretic hand. Motor evoked potentials after stimulation of the dorsal premotor cortex in the affected hemisphere were larger and had shorter latency than those after stimulation of the primary motor cortex in the affected hemisphere. There results indicate that the dorsal premotor cortex of the affected hemisphere can reorganize to be involved in execution of hand movements usually assigned to the function of the primary motor cortex [15]. Findings from experimental models also support this idea. In adult primates with experimental lesion in the unilateral sensorimotor cortex, transient inhibition of the premotor cortex in the damaged hemisphere by using microinjections of the GABA-agonist muscimol suppressed the recovered manual dexterity of the affected while transient inactivation of the hand/arm areas in the primary motor cortex had no effect [112]. In adult squirrel monkeys, damage in the primary motor cortex induced reorganization of the ventral premotor cortex that was not injured. Greater sparing of the hand area in the primary motor cortex resulted in less expansion of the hand area in the ventral premotor cortex [113].

## Rehabilitative Interventions Alter Cortical Activation during Hemiparetic Gait

Multiple structures including the primary motor cortex, premotor cortex and supplementary motor area as well as the sensorimotor cortex appear to be involved in locomotor recovery as well as recovery of the paretic hand after stroke as discussed above. Improved symmetry of sensorimotor activation and enhanced activation of the premotor cortex might be associated with improved gait performance [89, 90]. Impairment of locomotion due to partial damage in these structures is more likely to be compensated than impairment of hand function for a longer period after the insult [1] probably because gait performance is bipedal in nature and is centrally controlled in a hierarchical manner. These observations raise a question whether rehabilitative interventions might alter the brain activation patterns in the way similar to those seen in the course of locomotor recovery. Optical imaging might be suitable to test this hypothesis since it enables real-time monitoring of cortical activities during locomotor training. If this is the case, optical imaging will provide an effective tool to establish "brain-based" strategies for neurorehabilitation. Thus, we investigated the immediate effect of a number of rehabilitative interventions to test if they modify cortical activation patterns as well as physiological parameters of gait. Consequently it was shown rehabilitative interventions including therapeutic handling such as a facilitation technique, and partial body weight support (BWS) during locomotor training might modify activation patterns. More importantly some of the modified patterns immediately induced by rehabilitative interventions appear to be similar to those seen when patients restored locomotor function after a few months of inpatient rehabilitation.

## Effect of Sensorimotor Stimulation Using Facilitation Technique on Cortical Activation in Patients with Stroke

We compared to immediate effects of a number of techniques to assist hemiparetic patients to walk on the treadmill on cortical activation patterns. Therapists can mechanically assist patients to make their steps by holding the paretic foot. Other options to help patients might be facilitation technique (Figure 7) and partial body weight support (BWS). In facilitation technique therapists provide patients sensorimotor stimulation by pressing the hip forward and backward to prevent hyperextension of the knee in the stance phase, assisting flexion of the knee for initiation of the swing phase with the body weight well over the intact leg, and preventing the pelvis from being hitched up as the hemiparetic leg moved forward [114, 115]. Compared with mechanical assistance, facilitation technique induced enhanced overall activation in motor-related cortical areas, particularly in the premotor cortex of the affected hemisphere and improved asymmetry of activation in the sensorimotor cortex along with improvement of gait asymmetry and increased cadence [88, 89]. Furthermore activation patterns re-examined after 2 or 3 months of inpatient rehabilitation when patients could walk with little assistance were similar to those seen during assisted gait using facilitation technique before inpatient rehabilitation (Figure 6). These suggest that sensorimotor stimulation provided by therapists might play a role in reorganizing brain function.

Patient 1 in Figure 6 is a right-handed 53 year-old male with mild right hemiparesis due to subcortical infarction in the left corona radiata. Optical imaging 53 days poststroke revealed that hemiparetic gait on the treadmill (1.0 km/hr) with minimal mechanical assistance of the paretic leg was associated with asymmetrical activation in the sensorimotor cortex with less activation in the affected hemisphere. However when the patient walked assisted by the therapist using facilitation technique, the sensorimotor cortex showed symmetrical activation, indicating that sensorimotor stimulation from the pelvis might affect cortical activation patterns as well as gait performance.

Additionally enhanced activations were seen in the premotor and prefrontal regions predominantly in the affected hemisphere. Follow-up imaging after approximately 2 months of inpatient rehabilitation was done on 118 days poststroke when the patient could walk indoor independently. During walking unassisted, there was symmetrical activation in the medial sensorimotor cortex. Another patient, a right-handed 58 year-old male, with large infarction in the territory of the right middle cerebral artery showed similar findings in terms of modified activation patterns induced by rehabilitative interventions (Figure 6).

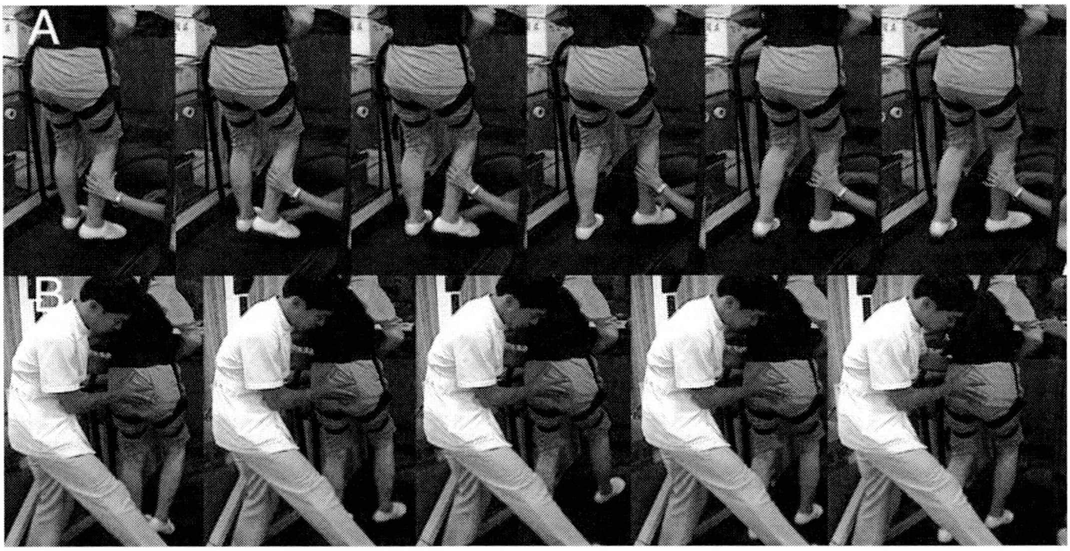


A. Mechanical assistance. A therapists mechanically assist a patients make their steps by holding their paretic legs.

B. Facilitation technique. A therapist provide patients sensorimotor stimulation by pressing the hip forward and backward to prevent hyperextension of the knee in the stance phase, assisting flexion of the knee for initiation of the swing phase with the body weight well over the intact leg, and preventing the pelvis from being hitched up as the hemiparetic leg moved forward (Bobath, 1978; Davis, 2000). Thus the patient can make her steps without direct assistance of the paretic foot. Note that the patient wears a parachute harness for partial body weight support but just for safety in the case.

Figure 7. Different types of rehabilitative interventions for locomotor training on the treadmill.

Because of severe motor impairment, he needed 20% of BWS using a parachute harness as well as assistance by a therapist to walk on the treadmill moving at 0.2 km/hr. On 102 days poststroke, walking with BWS and moderate mechanical assistance in making steps of the paretic leg, induced only a small sensorimotor activation. Instead activation was evident in the premotor and prefrontal regions in the affected hemisphere that are intact. While walking assisted by using facilitation technique as well as BWS, there were enhanced activations in the sensorimotor cortex in the unaffected hemisphere, and the premotor and prefrontal cortex in the affected hemisphere. The patient could walk with a cane and supervised by others after approximately 2 months of inpatient rehabilitation. Follow-up imaging on 173 days poststroke during walking with BWS and minimal mechanical assistance revealed enhanced activations in the sensorimotor cortex in the affected hemisphere and the premotor and prefrontal cortex in both hemispheres. These patterns were similar to those seen while patient walked assisted by using facilitation technique earlier (102 days after the onset). Based on these observations it is suggested that an optimized intervention might induce favorable activation patterns in the earlier stages before patients show considerable improvement in gait performance.

Sensorimotor stimulation that modifies afferent inputs from the hip joints has been shown to improve gait performance of hemiparetic or paraparetic patients. In patients with hemiparetic stroke, a clinical neurophysiological study demonstrated that facilitation technique immediately induced a more balanced walking pattern with a prolonged single stance period of the affected leg, an unobstructed hip movement, enhanced weight acceptance and a faster gait [115]. Crucial roles of proprioceptive afferent inputs from the hip joints similar to those provided by therapists in facilitation technique as well as those from load receptors in the generation of locomotor activities have been shown in patients with complete spinal cord injury, trained with partial BWS on the treadmill [116]. Dietz and colleagues analyzed EMG patterns of leg muscles during treadmill walking mechanically induced by driven gait orthosis with 70 % of BWS. In patients with complete spinal cord injury, locomotor movements from the hips provided by the orthosis were sufficient to elicit leg EMG patterns similar to those of healthy subjects. Locomotor movements restricted to the ankles, however, did not induce such EMG activities. There also found that inputs from load receptor was the other essential factor. Moreover, bilateral leg muscle activations were induced by unilateral locomotion in normal subjects but not in patients with spinal cord injury. This suggests that supraspinal structures including the cerebellum and cerebral cortex are essential for interlimb coordination in human locomotion. Similarly interlimb coordination of wrist and foot movements has been shown to be associated with enhance cortical activation, especially activation in the supplementary motor area [117]. Modification of cortical activation patterns associated with locomotor recovery from longitudinal study of optical imaging might also support this notion [90].

## Effect of Body Weight Support on Cortical Activation in Patients with Stroke and Parkinson's disease

Enhancement of the CPGs in the spinal cord might be also crucial for locomotor recovery [118]. Locomotor training on the treadmill with partial BWS by means of an overhead harness with a pelvic belt and thigh provides nonambulatory patients or even patients who are unable to stand with opportunities for gait training. Although details of rehabilitative interventions tend to be in the "black-box" [119], the strategy is easy to describe in terms of degree of body weight support, treadmill speed, training time, frequency of training etc., and can be replicated in any rehabilitation facility. Several studies have suggested that treadmill training with partial BWS might be effective in improving locomotor outcome of patients with spinal cord injury [120-122], stroke [123-125], cerebral palsy [126], and Parkinson's disease [127, 128] although there is controversy. A randomized controlled trial comparing the effect of treadmill training with and without BWS in stroke also showed greater efficacy of the former training than the latter [125]. In patients with Parkinson's disease, patients could tolerate a higher speed when walking on the treadmill with partial BWS as compared to walking without BWS [127]. These suggest that the favorable locomotor outcome after treadmill training with partial BWS might be attributed to BWS itself rather than to forced walking on the treadmill. Enhancement of the CPGs has been postulated as a mechanism for the efficacy of treadmill training with partial BWS [129]. However it remains unknown whether BWS alters activities of the supraspinal structures including the cerebral cortex.

In patients with subcortical stroke, optical imaging showed that BWS reduced activation in the sensorimotor cortex (Figure 8). BWS induced changes of the sensorimotor activation significantly correlated with those of cadence [90, 91].

This indicates that BWS might decrease demands for activities of sensorimotor cortex in controlling locomotion at the same cadence. Improvement of asymmetry in sensorimotor activation as assessed by laterality index also correlated with improved asymmetry of time for swing phase during hemiparetic gait. In control subjects, BWS tended to increase overall activation but did not modify gait parameters and there was no correlation between gait parameters and sensorimotor activation [91,130-131]. Thus these findings are in accordance with the hypothesis that improvement of hemiparetic gait during treadmill training with partial BWS might be associated with the shift of main controller of locomotion from the cortical to subcortical levels including the CPGs in the spinal cord as patients walked with less effort and more automatically. Along this line, speed dependent treadmill training, a sprint training at maximum speed as tolerated, has been also shown to improve gait disorders due to hemiparetic stroke [132], ataxia [133], acute vestibulopathy [134], and Parkinsonism [135]. Similarly it might be probable that the automatic spinal locomotor program might dominate in controlling locomotion during locomotion at higher speed [134].

In patients with early Parkinson's disease (Hoehn-Yahr stage 2.5 or 3), findings from optical imaging indicate that BWS is also likely to modify cortical activation patterns [130]. Basic cortical activation patterns as assessed by task-related increase of oxyHb levels during gait at 1 km/hr on the treadmill without BWS were also altered in Parkinson's disease. In agreement with previous SPECT study [39], optical imaging demonstrated a reduced regional activation ratio of the supplementary motor area/sensorimotor cortex in patients with Parkinson's disease compared with controls. BWS immediately induced increase in the regional activation ratio as well as decrease in cadence in patients but not in controls. Changes of the ratio induced by BWS negatively correlated with changes of cadence in Parkinson's disease [130]. These suggest that improved short step gait in patients with Parkinson's disease might be associated with modified cortical control of gait. Relatively enhanced activation in the supplementary motor area might be associated with improved motor control based on internal cues [136, 137] while improved gait performance by visual cues in Parkinson's disease induced increased activation in the premotor cortex [38]. The enhanced activation in the supplementary motor area might also reflect better interlimb coordination during gait with BWS since improved coordination of wrist and foot movements in different directions is associated with extra activation of the supplementary motor areas, as compared to movements in the same direction [117].

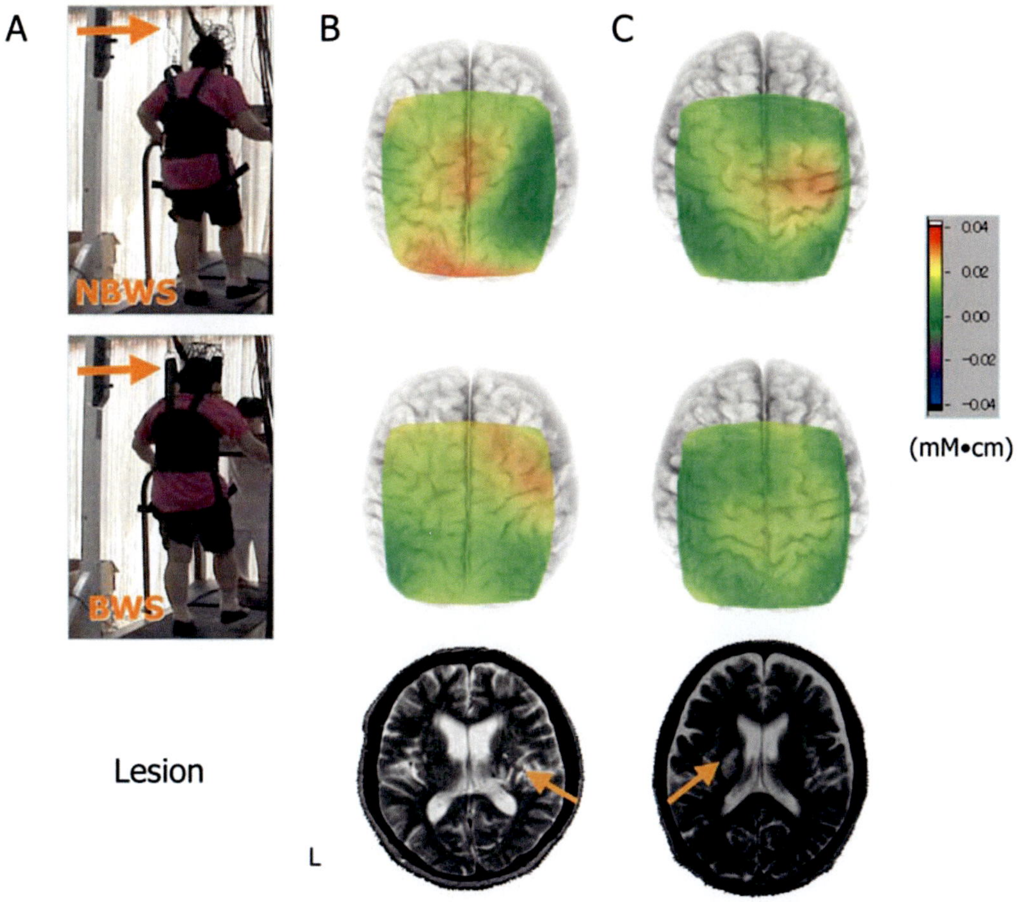


A. Examples of treadmill training with and without BWS (NBWS). Note the suspenders are tight in BWS condition (arrows).

B. A 58 year old male with a hemorrhagic lesion (108 days poststroke) in the right internal capsule and thalamus (arrow). In NBWS condition, activations as assessed by increased levels of oxyHb are seen in the sensorimotor cortex and premotor cortex less in the affected hemisphere than in the unaffected hemisphere as well as the supplementary motor area. In BWS condition, the sensorimotor and supplementary motor activations appear to be decreased, but there are enhanced activations in the premotor cortex in the affected hemisphere and prefrontal regions.

C. A 60 year old male with an ischemic lesion (60 days poststroke) in the left corona radiata (arrow). In NBWS condition, there are asymmetrical activations in the sensorimotor and premotor cortex that are less in the affected hemisphere. In BWS condition, these activations appear to be more symmetrical with reduced overall activations.

Figure 8. Effect of partial body weight support (BWS) on cortical activation patterns in patients with stroke.

## Monitoring Rehabilitation by Using Optical Imaging: A Future Perspective of Neurorehabilitation

Based on these observations, it is likely that rehabilitative interventions alter brain activation patterns associated with locomotor controls. Alterations occur immediately and possibly some degree of carry-over effect might lead to long-term reorganization. However further studies are needed to determine activation patterns associated with favorable outcome since there are considerable individual variations. Individual variations might also depend on side, site and size of lesion, severity of motor impairment, time after the onset, and degree of sensory and visual deficit. Optical imaging using continuous wave has high temporal resolution of one hundred seconds that enables real-time monitoring rehabilitation. Monitoring brain activation during rehabilitative interventions using optical imaging might allow us to evaluate rationale for using a certain rehabilitation strategy from the aspect of cerebral reorganization. For instance, therapists and patients can learn how symmetrical activations are during locomotor training and knowledge of result might be helpful in modifying rehabilitative strategies optimized for each patient.

## Conclusion

Optical imaging technique provides a new tool for assessing brain mechanisms underlying locomotor recovery after stroke. A comparison of the findings from neuroimaging studies regarding hand recovery after stroke and those the current optical imaging studies indicates that more symmetrical activation in the sensorimotor cortex and recruitment of other motor related areas including the premotor cortices might be closely related to restoration of gait after hemiparetic stroke. Furthermore it is probable that rehabilitative interventions might alter cerebral activation patterns associated with locomotion. Optical imaging technique might also contribute to establishing brain-based as well as evidence-based strategies for neurorehabilitation.

## References

[1] Yagura H, Miyai I, Seike Y, et al. Benefit of inpatient multidisciplinary rehabilitation up to 1 year after stroke. *Arch. Phys. Med. Rehabil.* 2003;84:1687-1691.

[2] Ward N, Frackowiak RSJ. The cerebral basis of functional recovery. In: Frackowiak RSJ, Friston KJ, Frith CD, Dolan RJ, Price CJ, Zeki S, Ashburner J, Penny W, eds. *Human brain function*, 2nd edition, San Diego, CA: Academic Press 2004; 105-123.

[3] Delvaux V, Alagona G, Gerard P, et al. Post-stroke reorganization of hand motor area: a 1-year prospective follow-up with focal transcranial magnetic stimulation. *Clin. Neurophysiol.* 2003;114:1217-1225.

[4] Escudero JV, Sancho J, Bautista D, et al. Prognostic value of motor evoked potential obtained by transcranial magnetic brain stimulation in motor function recovery in patients with acute ischemic stroke. *Stroke* 1998;29:1854-1859.

[5] Pennisi G, Alagona G, Rapisarda G, et al. Transcranial magnetic stimulation after pure motor stroke. *Clin. Neurophysiol.* 2002;113:1536-1543.

[6] Liepert J, Bauder H, Wolfgang HR, et al. Treatment-induced cortical reorganization after stroke in humans. *Stroke.* 2000;31:1210-1216.

[7] Taub E, Miller NE, Novack TA, et al. Technique to improve chronic motor deficit after stroke. *Arch. Phys. Med. Rehabil.* 1993;74:347-354.

[8] Nudo RJ, Wise BM, SiFuentes F, et al. Neural substrates for the effects of rehabilitative training on motor recovery after ischemic infarct. *Science.* 1996;272:1791-1794.

[9] Chollet F, DiPiero V, Wise RJ, et al. The functional anatomy of motor recovery after stroke in humans: a study with positron emission tomography. *Ann. Neurol.* 1991;29:63-71.

[10] Weiller C, Chollet F, Friston KJ, et al. Functional reorganization of the brain in recovery from striatocapsular infarction in man. *Ann. Neurol.* 1992;31:463-472.

[11] Weiller C, Ramsay SC, Wise RJ, et al. Individual patterns of functional reorganization in the human cerebral cortex after capsular infarction. *Ann. Neurol.* 1993;33:181-189.

[12] Cramer SC, Nelles G, Benson RR, et al. A functional mri study of subjects recovered from hemiparetic stroke. *Stroke.* 1997;28:2518-2527.

[13] Cao Y, D'Olhaberriague L, Vikingstad EM, et al. Pilot study of functional MRI to assess cerebral activation of motor function after poststroke hemiparesis. *Stroke.* 1998;29:112-122.

[14] Johansen-Berg H, Rushworth MF, Bogdanovic MD, et al. The role of ipsilateral premotor cortex in hand movement after stroke. *Proc. Natl. Acad. Sci. USA.* 2002;99:14518-14523.

[15] Fridman EA, Hanakawa T, Chung M, Hummel F, Leiguarda RC, Cohen LG. Reorganization of the human ipsilesional premotor cortex after stroke. *Brain.* 2004;127:747-758.

[16] Ferrier, D. 1876. *The Functions of the Brain.* Smith, Elder, London.

[17] Leyton ASF, Sherrington ES. Observation on the excitable cortex of the chimpanzee, orangutan, and gorilla. *Q. J. Exp. Physiol.* 1917;11: 135-222.

[18] Penfield W. *The Cerebral Cortex of Man: A Clinical Study of Localization of Function.* Macmillan, New York. 1950.

[19] Armstrong DM. The supraspinal control of mammalian locomotion. *J. Physiol.* 1988;405:1-37.

[20] Drew T. Motor cortical cell discharge during voluntary gait modification. *Brain Res.* 1988;457:181-187.

[21] Nutt JG, Marsden CD, Thompson PD. Human walking and higher-level gait disorders, particularly in the elderly. *Neurology* 1993;43:268-279.

[22] Pearson K, Gordon J. Locomotion. In: Kandel ER, Schwartz JH, Jessell TM (eds) *Principles of neural science*, 737-755, McGraw-Hill, New York, 2000.

[23] Thelen E. Developmental origins of motor coordination: Leg movements in human infants. *Dev. Psychobiol.* 1985;18:1-22.

[24] Forssberg H. Ontogeny of human locomotor control. I. Infant stepping, supported locomotion and transition to independent locomotion. *Exp. Brain Res.* 1985;57:480-493.

[25] Petersen NT, Pyndt HS, Nielsen JB. Investigating human motor control by transcranial magnetic stimulation. *Exp. Brain Res.* 2003;152:1-16.

[26] Capaday C, Lavoie BA, Barbeau H, et al. Studies on the corticospinal control of human walking. I. Responses to focal transcranial magnetic stimulation of the motor cortex. J. *Neurophysiol.* 1999;81:129-139.

[27] Petersen NT, Butler JE, Marchand-Pauvert V, et al. Suppression of emg activity by transcranial magnetic stimulation in human subjects during walking. *J. Physiol.* 2001;537:651-656.

[28] Fukuyama H, Ouchi Y, Matsuzaki S, et al. Brain functional activity during gait in normal subjects: A spect study. *Neurosci Lett.* 1997;228:183-186.

[29] Christensen LO, Johannsen P, Sinkjaer T, et al. Cerebral activation during bicycle movements in man. *Exp. Brain Res.* 2000;135:66-72.

[30] Sahyoun C, Floyer-Lea A, Johansen-Berg H, et al. Towards an understanding of gait control: Brain activation during the anticipation, preparation and execution of foot movements. *Neuroimage.* 2004;21:568-575.

[31] MacIntosh BJ, Mraz R, Baker N, et al. Optimizing the experimental design for ankle dorsiflexion fmri. *Neuroimage.* 2004;22:1619-1627.

[32] Johannsen P, Christensen LO, Sinkjaer T, Nielsen JB. Cerebral functional anatomy of voluntary contractions of ankle muscles in man. *J. Physiol.* 2001;535:397-406.

[33] Jackson PL, Lafleur MF, Malouin F, et al. Functional cerebral reorganization following motor sequence learning through mental practice with motor imagery. *Neuroimage.* 2003;20:1171-1180.

[34] Lafleur MF, Jackson PL, Malouin F, et al. Motor learning produces parallel dynamic functional changes during the execution and imagination of sequential foot movements. *Neuroimage.* 2002;16:142-157.

[35] Malouin F, Richards CL, Jackson PL, et al. Brain activations during motor imagery of locomotor-related tasks: A pet study. *Hum. Brain Mapp.* 2003;19:47-62.

[36] Jahn K, Deutschlander A, Stephan T, et al. Brain activation patterns during imagined stance and locomotion in functional magnetic resonance imaging. *Neuroimage.* 2004;22:1722-1731.

[37] Dobkin BH, Firestine A, West M, et al. Ankle dorsiflexion as an fmri paradigm to assay motor control for walking during rehabilitation. *Neuroimage.* 2004;23:370-381.

[38] Hanakawa T, Fukuyama H, Katsumi Y, et al. Enhanced lateral premotor activity during paradoxical gait in parkinson's disease. *Ann. Neurol.* 1999;45:329-336.

[39] Hanakawa T, Katsumi Y, Fukuyama H, et al. Mechanisms underlying gait disturbance in parkinson's disease: A single photon emission computed tomography study. *Brain.* 1999;122 (Pt 7):1271-1282.

[40] Boas DA, Franceschini MA, Dunn AK, et al Noninvasive imaging of cerebral activation with diffuse optical tomography, In Frostig ed, *In vivo optical imaging of brain function,* CRC press, Boca Raton, p193-221, 2002.

[41] Villringer A, Obrig H. Near-infrared spectroscopy and imaging, In Toga, Mazziotta eds, *Brain mapping. The methods,* 2nd ed, Academic Press, San Diego, p141-158, 2002.

[42] Duncan A, Meek JH, Clemence M, et al. Optical pathlength measurements on adult head, calf and forearm and the head of the newborn infant using phase resolved optical spectroscopy. *Phys. Med. Biol.* 1995;40:295-304.

[43] Duncan A, Meek JH, Clemence M, et al. Measurement of cranial optical path length as a function of age using phase resolved near infrared spectroscopy. *Pediatr. Res.* 1996;39:889-894.

[44] Hoshi Y, Hazeki O, Kakihana Y, et al. Redox behavior of cytochrome oxidase in the rat brain measured by near-infrared spectroscopy. *J. Appl. Physiol.* 1997;83:1842-1848.

[45] van der Zee P, Cope M, Arridge SR, et al. Experimentally measured optical pathlengths for the adult head, calf and forearm and the head of the newborn infant as a function of interoptode spacing. *Adv. Exp. Med. Biol.* 1992;316, 143– 153.

[46] Ogawa S, Tank DW, Menon R, et al. Intrinsic signal changes accompanying sensory stimulation: Functional brain mapping with magnetic resonance imaging. *Proc. Natl. Acad. Sci. USA*. 1992;89:5951-5955.

[47] Frostig RD, Lieke EE, Ts'o DY, et al. Cortical functional architecture and local coupling between neuronal activity and the microcirculation revealed by in vivo high-resolution optical imaging of intrinsic signals. *Proc. Natl. Acad. Sci. USA*. 1990;87:6082-6086.

[48] Roy CS, Sherrington CS. On the regulation of the blood-supply of the brain. *J. Physiol.* London. 11, 1890; 85–108.

[49] Kleinschmidt A, Obrig H, Requardt M, et al. Simultaneous recording of cerebral blood oxygenation changes during human brain activation by magnetic resonance imaging and near-infrared spectroscopy. *J. Cereb. Blood Flow Metab.* 1996;16:817-826.

[50] Mehagnoul-Schipper DJ, van der Kallen BF, Colier WN, et al. Simultaneous measurements of cerebral oxygenation changes during brain activation by near-infrared spectroscopy and functional magnetic resonance imaging in healthy young and elderly subjects. *Hum. Brain Mapp.* 2002;16:14-23.

[51] Strangman G, Culver JP, Thompson JH, et al. A quantitative comparison of simultaneous bold fmri and nirs recordings during functional brain activation. *Neuroimage.* 2002;17:719-731.

[52] Toronov V, Walker S, Gupta R, et al. The roles of changes in deoxyhemoglobin concentration and regional cerebral blood volume in the fmri bold signal. *Neuroimage.* 2003;19:1521-1531.

[53] Schroeter ML, Bucheler MM, Muller K, et al. Towards a standard analysis for functional near-infrared imaging. *Neuroimage.* 2004;21:283-290.

[54] Hoshi Y, Kobayashi N, Tamura M. Interpretation of near-infrared spectroscopy signals: A study with a newly developed perfused rat brain model. *J. Appl. Physiol.* 2001;90:1657-1662.

[55] Yamamoto T, Kato T. Paradoxical correlation between signal in functional magnetic resonance imaging and deoxygenated haemoglobin content in capillaries: A new theoretical explanation. *Phys. Med. Biol.* 2002;47:1121-1141.

[56] Miyai I, Tanabe HC, Sase I, et al. Cortical mapping of gait in humans: A near-infrared spectroscopic topography study. *Neuroimage*. 2001b;14:1186-1192.

[57] Suzuki M, Miyai I, Ono T, et al. Prefrontal and premotor cortices are involved in adapting walking and running speed on the treadmill: An optical imaging study. *Neuroimage*. 2004;23:1020-1026.

[58] Bartocci M, Winberg J, Ruggiero C, et al. Activation of olfactory cortex in newborn infants after odor stimulation: A functional near-infrared spectroscopy study. *Pediatr. Res*. 2000;48:18-23

[59] Isobe K, Kusaka T, Nagano K, et al. Functional imaging of the brain in sedated newborn infants using near infrared topography during passive knee movement. *Neurosci. Lett.* 2001;299:221-224.

[60] Hintz SR, Benaron DA, Siegel AM, et al. Bedside functional imaging of the premature infant brain during passive motor activation. *J. Perinat. Med.* 2001;29:335-343.

[61] Taga G, Konishi Y, Maki A, et al. Spontaneous oscillation of oxy- and deoxy-hemoglobin changes with a phase difference throughout the occipital cortex of newborn infants observed using non-invasive optical topography. *Neurosci. Lett.* 2000;282:101-104.

[62] Taga G, Asakawa K, Maki A, et al. Brain imaging in awake infants by near-infrared optical topography. *Proc. Natl. Acad. Sci. USA*. 2003;100:10722-10727.

[63] Okamoto M, Dan H, Sakamoto K, et al. Three-dimensional probabilistic anatomical cranio-cerebral correlation via the international 10-20 system oriented for transcranial functional brain mapping. *Neuroimage*. 2004;21:99-111.

[64] Talairach J, Tournoux P. *Co-planar Stereotaxic Atlas of the Human Brain. Thieme*, Stuttgart. 1988.

[65] Germon TJ, Evans PD, Barnett NJ, et al. Cerebral near infrared spectroscopy: Emitter-detector separation must be increased. *Br. J. Anaesth.* 1999;82:831-837.

[66] Jasdzewski G, Strangman G, Wagner J, et al. Differences in the hemodynamic response to event-related motor and visual paradigms as measured by near-infrared spectroscopy. *Neuroimage.* 2003;20:479-488.

[67] Wobst P, Wenzel R, Kohl M, et al. Linear aspects of changes in deoxygenated hemoglobin concentration and cytochrome oxidase oxidation during brain activation. *Neuroimage.* 2001;13:520-530.

[68] Hamzei F, Knab R, Weiller C, et al. The influence of extra- and intracranial artery disease on the bold signal in fMRI. *Neuroimage.* 2003;20:1393-1399.

[69] Binkofski F, Seitz RJ. Modulation of the bold-response in early recovery from sensorimotor stroke. *Neurology*. 2004;63:1223-1229.

[70] Noguchi Y, Watanabe E, Sakai KL. An event-related optical topography study of cortical activation induced by single-pulse transcranial magnetic stimulation. *Neuroimage*. 2003;19:156-162.

[71] Hirth C, Obrig H, Villringer K, et al. Non-invasive functional mapping of the human motor cortex using near-infrared spectroscopy. *Neuroreport.* 1996;7:1977-1981.

[72] Obrig H, Hirth C, Junge-Hulsing JG, et al. Length of resting period between stimulation cycles modulates hemodynamic response to a motor stimulus. *Adv. Exp. Med. Biol.* 1997;411:471-480.

[73] Colier WN, Quaresima V, Oeseburg B, et al. Human motor-cortex oxygenation changes induced by cyclic coupled movements of hand and foot. *Exp. Brain Res.* 1999;129:457-461.

[74] Kato T, Kamei A, Takashima S, et al. Human visual cortical function during photic stimulation monitoring by means of near-infrared spectroscopy. *J. Cereb. Blood Flow Metab.* 1993;13:516-520.

[75] Meek JH, Elwell CE, Khan MJ, et al. Regional changes in cerebral haemodynamics as a result of a visual stimulus measured by near infrared spectroscopy. *Proc. R. Soc. Lond B. Biol. Sci.* 1995;261:351-356.

[76] Takahashi K, Ogata S, Atsumi Y, et al. Activation of the visual cortex imaged by 24-channel near-infrared spectroscopy. *J. Biomed. Opt.* 2000;5:93-96.

[77] Villringer A, Planck J, Hock C, et al. Near infrared spectroscopy (nirs): A new tool to study hemodynamic changes during activation of brain function in human adults. *Neurosci. Lett.* 1993;154:101-104.

[78] Hock C, Muller-Spahn F, Schuh-Hofer S, et al. Age dependency of changes in cerebral hemoglobin oxygenation during brain activation: A near-infrared spectroscopy study. *J. Cereb. Blood Flow Metab.* 1995;15:1103-1108.

[79] Watanabe E, Maki A, Kawaguchi F, et al. Non-invasive assessment of language dominance with near-infrared spectroscopic mapping. *Neurosci. Lett.* 1998;256:49-52.

[80] Sato H, Takeuchi T, Sakai KL. Temporal cortex activation during speech recognition: An optical topography study. *Cognition.* 1999;73:B55-66.

[81] Hoshi Y, Oda I, Wada Y, et al. Visuospatial imagery is a fruitful strategy for the digit span backward task: A study with near-infrared optical tomography. *Brain Res. Cogn. Brain Res.* 2000;9:339-342.

[82] Kato H, Izumiyama M, Koizumi H, et al. Near-infrared spectroscopic topography as a tool to monitor motor reorganization after hemiparetic stroke: A comparison with functional MRI. *Stroke.* 2002;33:2032-2036.

[83] Sakatani K, Xie Y, Lichty W, et al. Language-activated cerebral blood oxygenation and hemodynamic changes of the left prefrontal cortex in poststroke aphasic patients: A near-infrared spectroscopy study. *Stroke.* 1998;29:1299-1304.

[84] Dettmers C, Fink GR, Lemon RN, et al. Relation between cerebral activity and force in the motor areas of the human brain. *J. Neurophysiol.* 1995;74:802-815.

[85] Kawashima R, Inoue K, Sugiura M, et al. A positron emission tomography study of self-paced finger movements at different frequencies. *Neuroscience.* 1999;92:107-112.

[86] Waldvogel D, van Gelderen P, Ishii K, et al. The effect of movement amplitude on activation in functional magnetic resonance imaging studies. *J. Cereb. Blood Flow Metab.* 1999;19:1209-1212.

[87] Roth EJ, Merbitz C, Mroczek K, et al. Hemiplegic gait. Relationships between walking speed and other temporal parameters. *Am. J. Phys. Med. Rehabil.* 1997;76:128-133.

[88] Davis PM. *Steps to follow*, 2nd ed. New York: Springer, 2000.

[89] Miyai I, Yagura H, Oda I, et al. Premotor cortex is involved in restoration of gait in stroke. *Ann. Neurol.* 2002;52:188-194.

[90] Miyai I, Yagura H, Hatakenaka M, et al. Longitudinal optical imaging study for locomotor recovery after stroke. *Stroke.* 2003;34:2866-2870.

[91] Miyai I. Cortical networks associated with locomotion in man and patients with hemiparetic stroke. In Swinnen SP, Duysens J eds. *Neurobehavioral determinants of interlimb coordination,* Kluwer Academic Publishers, MA, 2004, p.109-128.

[92] Calautti C, Leroy F, Guincestre JY, et al. Dynamics of motor network overactivation after striatocapsular stroke: A longitudinal pet study using a fixed-performance paradigm. *Stroke.* 2001;32:2534-2542.

[93] Carey JR, Kimberley TJ, Lewis SM, et al. Analysis of fmri and finger tracking training in subjects with chronic stroke. *Brain.* 2002;125:773-788.

[94] Feydy A, Carlier R, Roby-Brami A, et al. Longitudinal study of motor recovery after stroke: Recruitment and focusing of brain activation. *Stroke.* 2002;33:1610-1617.

[95] Marshall RS, Perera GM, Lazar RM, et al. Evolution of cortical activation during recovery from corticospinal tract infarction. *Stroke.* 2000;31:656-661.

[96] Ward NS, Brown MM, Thompson AJ, et al. Neural correlates of motor recovery after stroke: A longitudinal fMRI study. *Brain.* 2003;126:2476-2496.

[97] Muellbacher W, Richards C, Ziemann U, et al. Improving hand function in chronic stroke. *Arch. Neurol.* 2002;59:1278-1282.

[98] Eyre JA, Taylor JP, Villagra F, et al. Evidence of activity-dependent withdrawal of corticospinal projections during human development. *Neurology.* 2001;57:1543-1554

[99] Fisher CM. Concerning the mechanism of recovery in stroke hemiplegia. *Can. J. Neurol. Sci.* 1992;19:57-63.

[100] Seitz RJ, Hoflich P, Binkofski F, et al. Role of the premotor cortex in recovery from middle cerebral artery infarction. *Arch. Neurol.* 1998;55:1081-1088.

[101] Miyai I, Suzuki T, Kang J, Kubota K, Volpe BT. Middle cerebral artery stroke that includes the premotor cortex reduces mobility outcome. *Stroke.* 1999;30:1380-1383.

[102] Miyai I, Suzuki T, Kii K, Kang J, Kubota K. Wallerian degeneration of the pyramidal tract does not affect stroke rehabilitation outcome. *Neurology.* 1998;51:1613-1616.

[103] Fink GR, Frackowiak RS, Pietrzyk U, Passingham RE. Multiple nonprimary motor areas in the human cortex. *J. Neurophysiol.* 1997;77:2164-2174.

[104] Fries W, Danek A, Scheidtmann K, Hamburger C. Motor recovery following capsular stroke. Role of descending pathways from multiple motor areas. *Brain.* 1993;116 :369-382.

[105] Freund HJ, Hummelsheim H. Lesions of premotor cortex in man. *Brain.* 1985;108 :697-733.

[106] Halsband U, Ito N, Tanji J, et al. The role of premotor cortex and the supplementary motor area in the temporal control of movement in man. *Brain.* 1993;116:243-266.

[107] Kuypers HG. A new look at the organization of the motor system. *Prog. Brain Res.* 1982;57:381-403.

[108] Davidoff RA. The pyramidal tract. *Neurology.* 1990;40:332-339.

[109] Swinnen SP. Intermanual coordination: From behavioural principles to neural-network interactions. *Nat. Rev. Neurosci.* 2002;3:348-359.

[110] de Jong BM, Leenders KL, Paans AM. Right parieto-premotor activation related to limb-independent antiphase movement. *Cereb. Cortex.* 2002;12:1213-1217.

[111] Miyai I, Suzuki T, Mikami A, et al. Patients with capsular infarct and Wallerian degeneration demonstrate persistent regional premotor cortex activation on functional MRI. *J. Stroke Cereb. Dis*. 2001;10:210-216.

[112] Liu Y, Rouiller EM. Mechanisms of recovery of dexterity following unilateral lesion of the sensorimotor cortex in adult monkeys. *Exp. Brain Res.* 1999;128:149-159.

[113] Frost SB, Barbay S, Friel KM, et al. Reorganization of remote cortical regions after ischemic brain injury: A potential substrate for stroke recovery. *J. Neurophysiol.* 2003;89:3205-3214.

[114] Bobath B. *Adult hemiplegia. Evaluation and treatment*, 2nd ed. William Heinemann Medical Books Ltd, London, England; 1978.

[115] Hesse S, Jahnke MT, Schaffrin A, et al. Immediate effects of therapeutic facilitation on the gait of hemiparetic patients as compared with walking with and without a cane. *Electroencephalogr. Clin. Neurophysiol.* 1998;109:515-522.

[116] Dietz V, Muller R, Colombo G. Locomotor activity in spinal man: Significance of afferent input from joint and load receptors. *Brain.* 2002;125:2626-2634.

[117] Debaere F, Swinnen SP, Beatse E, et al. Brain areas involved in interlimb coordination: A distributed network. *Neuroimage*. 2001;14:947-958.

[118] Wickelgren I. Teaching the spinal cord to walk. *Science.* 1998;279:319-321.

[119] Duncan P, Studenski S, Richards L, et al. Randomized clinical trial of therapeutic exercise in subacute stroke. *Stroke.* 2003;34:2173-2180.

[120] Visintin M, Barbeau H. The effects of body weight support on the locomotor pattern of spastic paretic patients. *Can. J. Neurol. Sci.* 1989;16:315-325.

[121] Wernig A, Muller S. Laufband locomotion with body weight support improved walking in persons with severe spinal cord injuries. *Paraplegia*. 1992;30:229-238.

[122] Wernig A, Nanassy A, Muller S. Maintenance of locomotor abilities following laufband (treadmill) therapy in para- and tetraplegic persons: Follow-up studies. *Spinal Cord*. 1998;36:744-749.

[123] Hesse S, Bertelt C, Schaffrin A, et al. Restoration of gait in nonambulatory hemiparetic patients by treadmill training with partial body-weight support. *Arch. Phys. Med. Rehabil*. 1994;75:1087-1093.

[124] Hesse S, Bertelt C, Jahnke MT, et al. Treadmill training with partial body weight support compared with physiotherapy in nonambulatory hemiparetic patients. *Stroke.* 1995;26:976-981.

[125] Visintin M, Barbeau H, Korner-Bitensky N, et al. A new approach to retrain gait in stroke patients through body weight support and treadmill stimulation. *Stroke.* 1998;29:1122-1128.

[126] Schindl MR, Forstner C, Kern H, et al. Treadmill training with partial body weight support in nonambulatory patients with cerebral palsy. *Arch. Phys. Med. Rehabil.* 2000;81:301-306.

[127] Miyai I, Fujimoto Y, Ueda Y, et al. Treadmill training with body weight support: Its effect on parkinson's disease. *Arch. Phys. Med. Rehabil.* 2000;81:849-852.

[128] Miyai I, Fujimoto Y, Yamamoto H, et al. Long-term effect of body weight-supported treadmill training in parkinson's disease: A randomized controlled trial. *Arch. Phys. Med. Rehabil.* 2002;83:1370-1373.

[129] Duysens J, Pearson KG. From cat to man: basic aspects of locomotion relevant to motor rehabilitation. *NeuroRehabilitation* 1998;10: 107-118.

[130] Miyai I, Yagura H, Hatakenaka M, et al. *Effect of body weight support on cortical activation during gait in patients with hemiparetic stroke and healthy subjects.* Program No. 824.2. 2003 Abstract Viewer/Itinerary Planner. Washington, DC: Society for Neuroscience.

[131] Miyai I. Locomotor training with partial body weight support in patients with Parkinson's disease and stroke: Its efficacy and neural mechanisms. *Geriatrics and Gerontology International* 2004;4:S205–S206.

[132] Pohl M, Mehrholz J, Ritschel C, et al. Speed-dependent treadmill training in ambulatory hemiparetic stroke patients: A randomized controlled trial. *Stroke.* 2002;33:553-558.

[133] Fatar M, Baezner H, Griebe M, Stroick M, Hennerici M. Cerebellar stroke with speed-dependent gait ataxia. *Stroke.* 2003;34:e178.

[134] Brandt T, Strupp M, Benson J. You are better off running than walking with acute vestibulopathy. *Lancet.* 1999;354:746.

[135] Pohl M, Rockstroh G, Ruckriem S, Mrass G, Mehrholz J. Immediate effects of speed-dependent treadmill training on gait parameters in early parkinson's disease. *Arch. Phys. Med. Rehabil.* 2003;84:1760-1766.

[136] Mushiake H, Inase M, Tanji J. Neuronal activity in the primate premotor, supplementary, and precentral motor cortex during visually guided and internally determined sequential movements. *J. Neurophysiol.* 1991;66:705-718.

[137] Halsband U, Matsuzaka Y, Tanji J. Neuronal activity in the primate supplementary, pre-supplementary and premotor cortex during externally and internally instructed sequential movements. *Neurosci. Res.* 1994;20:149-155.

In: State-of-the-Art Imaging in Stroke, Volume 2
Editor: Bernhard Schaller, pp. 75-86
ISBN 978-1-60021-499-8


*Chapter III*

# Neuroimaging of Depressive Disorders Associated with Cerebrovascular Disease

***Ricardo E. Jorge, Andres A. Capizzano and Robert G. Robinson***
Department of Psychiatry
Roy J. and Lucille A. Carver College of Medicine
University of Iowa

## A. Introduction

Depressive disorders associated with cerebrovascular disease can be classified into two major groups, those that occur during the subacute and chronic stages of a clinically apparent stroke and are known as post-stroke depression (PSD), and those that are associated with the presence of ischemic lesions in the deep white matter and basal ganglia that had not been clinically attested (i.e., *silent* stroke). Silent ischemic events are one of the major determinants of late life depression, an association that has been previously formulated in the concept of *"vascular depression"*. In the present chapter we will analyze neuroimaging correlates of these two groups of depressive disorders.

## B. Post-Stroke Depression

Depression is among the most common psychiatric disorders that occur after stroke. The frequency of post-stroke depression (PSD) depends upon several factors including the criteria and instruments used to assess depression, whether it is assessed in clinical or community samples or whether patients are studied during the sub-acute post-stroke period or later during its clinical course. Overall, pooling the data of the most relevant studies, the mean prevalence in hospitalized acute stroke patients was 22% for major depression and 17% for minor depression. In outpatient populations, the mean prevalence was 23% for major depression, and 35% for minor depression; while in community samples the mean prevalence for major depression was 13% and minor depression was 10% [1].

Neuroimaging studies in PSD have mostly focused in establishing a relationship between the location of brain lesion and the likelihood of developing depression. Mood disorders might be conceptualized as resulting from the disruption of distributed networks that regulate mood, motivation and emotion. In this context, it is reasonable to hypothesize that strategic lesions along these networks would be associated with functional alterations that lead to PSD. However, accounting for the fact that diverse lesions can produce the same type of functional abnormality and structurally identical lesions might result in completely different activation patterns, the association of specific brain lesions with complex behavioral disorders such as depression is difficult to establish. Although conventional CT and MRI scans fall short to provide the information required to address this complexity, most of the previous studies published on this topic used these neuroimaging methods. Newer radiological techniques including functional magnetic resonance imaging (fMRI) and metabolic studies such as magnetic resonance spectroscopy (MRS) hold the promise of increasing our insight into the physiology of emotion and mood, and how these physiological mechanisms are affected by the occurrence of cerebrovascular lesions.

## Interhemispheric and Intrahemispheric Lesion Location as Risk Factors for PSD

Approximately two decades ago, Robinson et al., examined the effect of unilateral ischemic lesions on depression in a series of patients who had no known risk factors for depression and were admitted to hospital after an acute stroke. Major or minor depression was found in 14 of 22 patients with left hemisphere lesions and two of 14 patients with right hemisphere lesions ($p < 0.01$) [2]. The patients were further grouped according to whether they had anterior and posterior lesions using the anatomical criteria that the anterior border of the lesion was located in the frontal lobe. In addition to the increased frequency of depression in patients with left hemisphere lesions, those patients with left anterior injuries were found to have a significantly greater frequency of major depression than patients with any other lesion location. These findings were replicated in another study of 45 patients with single ischemic lesions restricted to either cortical or subcortical structures in the right or left hemisphere [3]. Patients with subcortical lesions had infarcts limited to the basal ganglia, thalamus, or internal capsule while patients with cortical lesions had ischemic damage of the cortex or underlying white matter. Patients with lesions of the left hemisphere had significantly higher rates of depression than patients with right hemisphere lesions, regardless of the cortical or subcortical location of the lesion ($p < 0.01$). All five patients with left cortical anterior lesions involving the frontal lobe had depression as compared to only two out of 11 patients with left cortical posterior lesions ($p < 0.01$). Moreover, four of the 6 patients with left subcortical anterior lesions had depression as compared to one among 7 patients with left subcortical posterior lesions ($p < 0.01$) (Figure 1). In a subsequent study,

Starkstein et al. compared patients with lesions limited to the basal ganglia / internal capsule with those having right or left thalamic lesions. Caudate and/or putamen lesions produced major depression in 7 out of 8 patients with left hemisphere lesions but in only one of 7 patients with right hemisphere lesions. None of the patients with thalamic lesions had major depression ($p < 0.001$)[4].

The largest study examining clinical pathological correlations in patients with PSD was reported by Vataja et al. [5]. Twelve to 20 weeks following stroke, 275 patients were examined using the Structured Interview for Clinical Assessment in Neuropsychiatry (SCAN) and DSM-IV diagnostic criteria for depressive disorders. Of the 275 patients, 83 (30%) had prior strokes and 54 (20%) had a history of depression. A logistic regression analysis showed an association between PSD and ischemic lesions in the genu of the internal capsule on the left side (odds ratio 3.2, 95% confidence interval=1.0-10.1) as well as in the pallidum of either side (odds ratio 1.6, 95% confidence interval =1.1-2.3). These authors have recently published a secondary analysis of their data focusing on 70 patients with single ischemic lesions. Basal ganglia lesions were the major anatomical correlate of PSD. When a separate analysis of each hemisphere was done, lesions of the left caudate and pallidum were significantly associated with depression while lesions of these structures in the right hemisphere were not [6].

However, other studies have not find a consistent relationship between left sided lesions and a greater likelihood to develop depressive disorders. For example, a study of 88 Australian patients seen in a rehabilitation hospital 8.4 weeks (average) following stroke found that 43% of patients with left hemisphere lesions had major or minor depression and 38% of patients with right hemisphere lesions had depression [7]. Similarly, Eastwood [8] examined 87 patients admitted to rehabilitation hospital 12 weeks (average) after stroke. Of 28 patients with left hemisphere lesions, 50% had either major or minor depression while among 45 patients with right hemisphere stroke 62% had major or minor depression. Thus, both of these studies conducted in rehabilitation settings failed to show a lateralized effect of hemispheric brain injury on frequency of depression.

Carson et al. [9] reported a meta-analysis of studies that examined the association between PSD and lesion location. The authors concluded that there is no consistent support for the hypothesis that the risk of depression after stroke is affected by the location of the brain lesion. A more recent meta-analytical study, however, concluded that the association between left hemisphere lesion location and PSD was dependent upon whether patients were sampled as inpatients or from the community and whether they were examined during the acute as compared to chronic period following stroke. Inpatients during the acute stroke had significant associations between left hemisphere lesions and poststroke depression (OR 1.36 CI 11.05-1.76 inpatients; OR 2.14 CI 1.50-3.04 acute patients) [10].

Shimoda and Robinson examined the effect of time since stroke on the relationship between lesion location and depression among 142 patients with single stroke lesions followed up to 2 years [11]. The frequency of depression in patients with right and left hemisphere lesions during the initial evaluation and at the short- and long-term follow-up is shown in (Figure 2). During the initial evaluation, patients with left hemisphere stroke had a significantly higher prevalence of DSM-IV defined depressive disorders than patients with right hemisphere stroke ($p = 0.0006$). At short-term and long-term follow-up, however, there were no significant differences between right and left hemisphere lesion groups in terms of the frequency of major or minor depression. Moreover, a meta-analysis performed by Dr. Robinson's group showed that, when the effect of left anterior versus right anterior lesion location on the risk of major depression was compared, the odds ratio was 2.18 (95% confidence interval 1.44-3.3), supporting the hypothesis that depressive disorders are more frequent in patients with left sided lesions over the first two months following stroke [12].

## Correlation between the Severity of Depression and Anterior-Posterior Lesion Location

A clinical-pathological correlation between the severity of depression, as measured by depression rating scales, and the distance of the lesion from the frontal pole on CT or MRI scan images was first reported in 1981 [13]. This finding was subsequently replicated in other studies performed by the same group of investigators. In the right hemisphere, however, correlation was in the opposite direction with more posterior lesions being associated with more severe depressive symptoms.

Did this correlation also varied over time after the index stroke? Shimoda et al. , examined this issue among 60 patients with single ischemic lesions who were followed up over 2 years [11]. Correlations between the severity of depression and the proximity of the lesion to the frontal pole were significant during the initial evaluation and short -term follow-up. However, at long-term follow-up (i.e., 12 to 24 months), this significant correlation was lost. On the other hand, among patients with right hemisphere stroke, both lesion volume and proximity of the lesion to the occipital pole correlated with the severity of depression.

Similar findings have now been reported by other investigators in Canada, UK, Germany, and Australia. Some studies found that the correlation between the severity of depression and the proximity of the lesion to the frontal pole applied to combined right and left hemisphere lesion groups [14, 15] while others found this to be the case only among patients with left-sided lesions [8, 16].

A recent meta-analysis of studies which examined patients during the first 6 months following stroke reported that the correlation between the proximity of the lesion to the frontal pole and severity of depression was significantly stronger for the left hemisphere than the right hemisphere [12].

## Relationship between Depression and Ischemic Lesions in the Anterior Versus Posterior Cerebral Circulation

Starkstein et al., compared depression associated with infarcts of the posterior circulation (PC) (i.e., vertebral-basilar arteries supplying the brainstem, cerebellum, thalamus, occipital lobes and medial aspect of the temporal lobes) and infarcts of the middle cerebral artery circulation (MCA) [17].

Among 37 patients in the PC group, 27% were found to be depressed immediately after the acute lesion. Among 42 patients with MCA lesions, 48% developed depressive disorders immediately after the stroke. This higher frequency of depression among the MCA compared with the PC group just failed to reach statistical significance ($p = 0.054$).

At 6 months follow-up, 82% of the patients with MCA lesions who were depressed in hospital remained depressed (Figure 2). Among patients with PC lesions who were depressed at the in-hospital evaluation only 20% remained depressed at the 6 months follow-up ($p < 0.05$). At 1 or 2 years follow-up, the percentage of patients with continued depression was 68% for the MCA group and zero for the PC group ($p < 0.05$). Although the significantly shorter course of depression in the PC as compared to the MCA group might be hypothesized to result from the PC group having smaller lesion volumes than the MCA group, there was no significant correlation between lesion volume and the severity of depression for the combined group of MCA and PC lesion patients either in hospital or at 1 or 2 years follow-up (Figure 3).

## Post Stroke Depression Associated with Right Hemisphere Lesions

A substantial proportion of patients with right hemisphere lesions develop depression following stroke. Starkstein et al., examined the clinical correlates of depression associated with right hemisphere lesions to compare them with the clinical correlates of left hemisphere lesion location [18]. The study included a consecutive series of 93 patients who had stroke lesions of the right hemisphere. Of these 93 patients, 28 patients developed a depressive disorder during the first few weeks following stroke. Patients with depression (both major and minor) showed a significantly higher frequency of lesions involving either the right parietal cortex ($p = 0.02$) or the right lateral frontal cortex $p < 0.01$). In addition, patients with major depression had a significantly higher frequency of psychiatric disorder among their first- or second-degree relatives compared with other diagnostic groups. This finding, however, was not replicated by other studies [7].

Finset et al. [19] found that among 42 patients with single right hemisphere lesions, ischemic damage involving white matter underlying the parietal cortex was associated with a higher frequency of depression (five of 13 patients) than lesions in any other location in the right hemisphere (7 of 29 patients) ($p < 0.02$). House et al. [14] reported on a group of 21 patients with CT-verified right hemisphere lesions examined one month following their first stroke. Of the three patients with major depression following a right hemisphere lesion, all of them had a right posterior lesion (i.e., three major depressions of 8 patients with right posterior injury) compared with none of the patients with right anterior ($n = 7$) or right intermediate ($n = 6$) lesion locations ($p < 0.03$). Sinyor et al. [15] examined 16 patients with single CT-verified right hemisphere lesions studied an average of 56 days post-stroke. There was a significant quadratic relationship between depression scores and the distance between the anterior border of the lesion and the frontal pole in patients with right hemisphere lesions (i.e., patients with the most anterior and most posterior lesions of the right hemisphere had the highest depression scores, $p < 0.05$). Another study by Stern and Bachman [20] examined 19 patients with CT-verified single right hemisphere lesions an average of 16 months poststroke. Lesions were classified as dorsal or ventral, frontal or nonfrontal. Dysphoric mood was significantly more severe in patients with right ventral non-frontal as compared with right ventral frontal lesions. This suggests that right temporal lesions are associated with depressed mood. Finally, Astrom et al. [21] and Eastwood et al. [8] found no association between lesion location in the right hemisphere and the existence of PSD.

# C. Take-Home-Message

Current evidence suggests that, during the first two months following stroke, the frequency of major depression following left frontal or left basal ganglia stroke is more than two times as great as that associated with right anterior lesions or left parietal-occipital lesions. Similarly, over the first 6 months following stroke, the available evidence is consistent with the presence of a significant correlation between the proximity of the lesion to the left frontal pole and severity of depressive symptoms. Studies of specific areas of brain injury have found that depressive disorder is more common following basal ganglia as compared with thalamic stroke and with middle cerebral artery compared with posterior circulation strokes.

## Vascular Depression

The presence of cerebrovascular disease constitutes an important risk factor for the occurrence of geriatric depression and may account for part of its clinical heterogeneity [22]. A causal relationship between cerebrovascular disease and late life depression is supported by diverse epidemiological studies. For instance, results from the Rotterdam study suggest that atherosclerosis and depression are associated in the elderly [23].

In addition, the high frequency of depression in patients with hypertension, diabetes or coronary artery disease, and the high frequency of depression following stroke are consistent with this view. Moreover, a family history of mood disorders is less frequently observed among patients with vascular depression suggesting that genetic vulnerability plays a lesser role in the pathogenesis of this disorder [24].

Recent studies have focused on the clinical implications of white and gray matter hyperintensities detected by Magnetic Resonance Imaging (MRI) (Figures 4, 5, 6). Elderly depressed patients show higher volume of white matter T2 signal hyperintensities (WMHs) than non-depressed age matched controls [25]. Deep WMHs are recognized markers of ischemic damage to the white matter [26] and, in elderly depressed patients, such ischemic lesions tend to be located in the dorsolateral prefrontal cortex [27] These findings have been replicated in other studies of geriatric depression that controlled for age, sex, and the presence of cerebrovascular risk factors [28, 29]. For instance, in a large community-based population study of 3600 subjects (i.e., Cardiovascular Health Study), vascular lesions involving the basal ganglia were significantly associated with the presence of depressive symptoms [30]. However, multiple regression analysis of the data revealed that, when measures of physical disability and cognitive impairment were added to the models, MRI-changes were no longer significantly related to depression measures, suggesting that the functional consequences of cerebrovascular disease may be the causal pathway by which basal ganglia and non-basal-ganglia lesions are associated with depressive symptoms [30]. The Cardiovascular Health Study investigators also examined whether baseline structural brain disease was associated with persistence or worsening of depressive symptoms as well as new onset of depression among patients who were not depressed at the initial evaluation. Large cortical white-matter lesions, severe sub-cortical white-matter disease, and lacunar basal ganglia infarcts were associated with depressive symptoms over the course of the study. In addition, worsening of depression was associated with sub-cortical white-matter lesions [31].

Taylor et al. conducted a longitudinal, morphometric MRI study among vascular depression patients to examine if progression of WMH over 2 years influences depression outcomes. WMH volume was measured using a semi-automated segmentation process. The authors reported that depressed patients who showed sustained remission of their symptoms had significantly less increases in WMH volume (11.5%) than did the group of patients with persistent depression (31.6%) ($P$ = .01). This finding suggest that the pathological changes associated with progressive vascular disease are etiologically related with mood disturbance and, probably, with cognitive decline [32].

When compared with findings from non-depressed control subjects, conventional magnetic resonance imaging (MRI) scans of elderly depressed patients display brain volume decreases in critical brain regions, such as the prefrontal lobe, the hippocampus, and the head of the caudate nucleus [33].

Recent imaging studies in vascular depression intend to assess subtler degrees of white matter damage by means of newer techniques such as diffusion tensor imaging (DTI) and magnetic resonance spectroscopy (MRS). Water diffusion in white matter is anisotropic, i.e. it depends on the direction of molecular movement. This anisotropy depends upon the integrity of axonal membranes and myelin sheaths and can be reliably estimated by DTI [34]. Thus, this technique provides a quantitative method to assess the structural integrity of white matter fiber bundles [35]. It has been shown that WMHs display increased apparent diffusion coefficients (ADCs) and reduced fractional anisotropy (FA) both in depressed geriatric patients and elderly controls [36]. Furthermore, in late life depression, DTI shows reduction in FA of frontal white matter between 10 and 15 mm above the anterior-posterior commissural line -containing fibers of the cortical-striatal pathways- in patients who do not respond to antidepressant medication [37]. Proton magnetic resonance spectroscopic imaging ($^1$H MRSI) is a non-invasive technique that depicts the anatomic distribution of metabolites including N-acetyl-aspartate (NAA), creatine and phosphocreatine (Cr), choline containing compounds (Cho), and myoinositol (mI). NAA is concentrated solely in neurons in the mature nervous system, so it has been used as a surrogate of neuronal density and neuronal metabolism [38]. There have been few spectroscopic studies of depressive disorders associated with cerebrovascular disease. For instance, Charles et al. [39] reported increases in Cho/Cr ratios in a large voxel in the subcortical region (including the caudate, internal capsule, and parts of the temporal lobe) in patients with late-life major depression compared to controls. Interestingly, these changes normalized with treatment. Murata et al. [40] reported lower NAA/Cr ratios in the dorsolateral prefrontal white matter of elderly depressed patients that were associated with the presence of WMSHs in the deep white matter. Another recent study reported that elderly depressed patients had increased ratios of Cho and mI with respect to Cr (Cho/Cr and mI/Cr) in white matter regions, with NAA levels comparable to those seen in age-matched controls [41]. Finally, a pilot study of two-dimensional MRS in late life major depression detected gender differences in the metabolic distribution of prefrontal white matter, along with a trend toward raised mI, phosphor-ethanolamine and glutamate in depressed patients [42].

## References


[1] Robinson RG., *The Clinical Neuropsychiatry of Stroke*. 1998, Cambridge: Cambridge University Press. pp 491.

[2] Robinson, RG, et al., Mood disorders in stroke patients: importance of location of lesion. *Brain*, 1984. 107:81-93.

[3] Starkstein S., Robinson RG, Price TR. Comparison of cortical and subcortical lesions in the production of post-stroke mood disorders. *Brain,* 1987, 110:1045-1059.

[4] Starkstein SE, et al., Differential mood changes following basal ganglia versus thalamic lesions. *Arch. Neurol.*, 1988, 45:725-730.

[5] Vataja R., et al., Magnetic resonance imaging correlates of depression after ischemic stroke. *Arch. Gen. Psychiatry*, 2001, 58:925-931.

[6] Vataja R, et al., Poststroke depression and lesion location revisited. *J. Neuropsychiatry Clin. Neurosci.* 2004, 16:156-162.

[7] Morris PLP, Robinson RG, Raphael B. Prevalence and course of depressive disorders in hospitalized stroke patients. *Intl. J. Psychiatr. Med.*, 1990. 20:349-364.

[8] Eastwood MR, et al., Mood disorder following cerebrovascular accident. *Br. J. Psychiatry*, 1989, 154:195-200.

[9] Carson AJ, et al., Depression after stroke and lesion location: a systematic review. *Lancet,* 2000. 356: 122-126.

[10] Bhogal, SK, et al., Lesion location and poststroke depression. Systematic review of the methodological limitations in the literature. *Stroke*, 2004, 35:794-802.

[11] Shimoda K, Robinson RG, The relationship between post-stroke depression and lesion location in long-term follow-up. *Biol. Psychiatry,* 1999, 45:187-192.

[12] Narushima K, Kosier JT, Robinson RG. A reappraisal of post-stroke depression, intra and inter-hemispheric lesion location using meta-analysis. *J. Neuropsychiatry Clin. Neurosci.*, 2003, 15: 422-430.

[13] Robinson RG, Szetela B. Mood change following left hemispheric brain injury. *Ann. Neurol.*, 1981, 9:447-453.

[14] House A, et al., Mood disorders after stroke and their relation to lesion location. A CT scan study. *Brain*, 1990, 113:1113-1130.

[15] Sinyor D, et al., Post-stroke depression and lesion location: an attempted replication. *Brain*, 1986. 109:539-546.

[16] Morris PLP, Robinson RG, Raphael B. Lesion location and depression in hospitalized stroke patients: evidence supporting a specific relationship in the left hemisphere. *Neuropsychiatry Neuropsychol Behav. Neurol.*, 1992, 3:75-82.

[17] Starkstein SE, et al, Depressive disorder following posterior circulation compared with middle cerebral artery infarcts. *Brain,* 1988, 111:375-387.

[18] Starkstein SE, et al., Mood changes after right hemisphere lesion. *Br. J. Psychiatry,* 1989, 155:79-85.

[19] Finset A., et al., Depressed mood and intra-hemispheric location of lesion in right hemisphere stroke patients. *Scand. J. Rehabil. Med.*, 1989, 21: 1-6.

[20] Stern RA, Bachman DL. Depressive symptoms following stroke. *Am. J. Psychiatry*, 1991, 148: 351-356.

[21] Astrom M, Adolfsson R, Asplund K. Major depression in stroke patients: a 3-year longitudinal study. *Stroke*, 1993. 24:976-982.

[22] Alexopoulos GS, et al., Vascular depression hypothesis. *Arch. Gen. Psychiatry*, 1997. 54:915-922.

[23] Tiemeier H, et al., Relationship between atherosclerosis and late-life depression: the Rotterdam Study. *Arch. Gen. Psychiatry*, 2004. 61:369-76.

[24] Alexopoulos GS, et al. Clinically defined vascular depression. *Am. J. Psychiatry,* 1997, 154: 562-565.

[25] Coffey CE. Subcortical hyperintensity on magenetic resonance imaging: A comparison of normal and depressed elderly subjects. *Am. J. Psychiatry*, 1990, 147:187-189.

[26] Fazekas F. et al., Pathologic correlates of incidental MRI white matter signal hyperintensities. *Neurology*, 1993, 43:1683-9.

[27] Thomas AJ, et al. Ischemic basis for deep white matter hyperintensities in major depression: a neuropathological study. *Arch. Gen. Psychiatry*, 2002. 59: 785-92.

[28] Greenwald BS, et al. Neuroanatomic localization of magnetic resonance imaging signal hyperintensities in geriatric depression. *Stroke*, 1998, 29: 613-617.

[29] Pohjasvaara, T. et al. Clinical features of MRI-defined subcortical vascular disease. *Alzheimer Dis. Assoc Disord,* 2003. 17:236-242.

[30] Steffens DC, et al. Cerebrovascular disease and depression symptoms in the cardiovascular health study. *Stroke*, 1999. 30:2159-2166.

[31] Steffens DC, Krishnan KR, Crump C. Cerebrovascular disease and evolution of depressive symptoms in the cardiovascular health study. *Stroke*, 2002. 33:1636-1644.

[32] Taylor WD, et al. White matter hyperintensity progression and late-life depression outcomes. *Arch. Gen. Psychiatry,* 2003. 60:1090-6.

[33] Ballmaier M., et al. Anterior cingulate, gyrus rectus, and orbitofrontal abnormalities in elderly depressed patients: an MRI-based parcellation of the prefrontal cortex. *Am. J. Psychiatry,* 2004. 161: 99-108.

[34] Beaulieu C. The basis of anisotropic water diffusion in the nervous system - a technical review. *NMR Biomed.*, 2002. 15:435-55.

[35] Basser P.J., Jones DK. Diffusion-tensor MRI: theory, experimental design and data analysis - a technical review. *NMR Biomed.*, 2002. 15:456-67.

[36] Taylor WD, et al. Evidence of white matter tract disruption in MRI hyperintensities. *Biol. Psychiatry,* 2001. 50:179-83.

[37] Alexopoulos GS. et al. Frontal white matter microstructure and treatment response of late-life depression: a preliminary study. *Am. J. Psychiatry,* 2002. 159:1929-32.

[38] Birken DL, Oldendorf WH. N-acetyl-L-aspartic acid: a literature review of a compound prominent in 1H-NMR spectroscopic studies of brain. *Neurosci. Biobehav. Rev.*, 1989, 13:23-31.

[39] Charles HC, et al. Brain choline in depression: in vivo detection of potential pharmacodynamic effects of antidepressant therapy using hydrogen localized spectroscopy. *Prog. Neuropsychopharmacol Biol. Psychiatry*, 1994. 18:1121-7.

[40] Murata T, et al. MRI white matter hyperintensities, (1)H-MR spectroscopy and cognitive function in geriatric depression: a comparison of early- and late-onset cases. *Int. J. Geriatr. Psychiatry,* 2001. 16:1129-35.

[41] Kumar A, et al. Frontal white matter biochemical abnormalities in late-life major depression detected with proton magnetic resonance spectroscopy. *Am. J. Psychiatry*, 2002. 159:630-6.

[42] Binesh N. et al. Neurochemistry of late-life major depression: a pilot two-dimensional MR spectroscopic study. *J. Magn. Reson. Imaging*, 2004. 20:1039-45.

[43] Robinson RG., *The Clinical Neuropsychiatry of Stroke*. 1998, Cambridge: Cambridge University Press. pp 491.

[44] Robinson, RG, et al., Mood disorders in stroke patients: importance of location of lesion. *Brain*, 1984. 107:81-93.

[45] Starkstein S., Robinson RG, Price TR. Comparison of cortical and subcortical lesions in the production of post-stroke mood disorders. *Brain,* 1987, 110:1045-1059.

[46] Starkstein SE, et al., Differential mood changes following basal ganglia versus thalamic lesions. *Arch. Neurol.*, 1988, 45:725-730.

[47] Vataja R., et al., Magnetic resonance imaging correlates of depression after ischemic stroke. *Arch. Gen. Psychiatry*, 2001, 58:925-931.

[48] Vataja R, et al., Poststroke depression and lesion location revisited. *J. Neuropsychiatry Clin. Neurosci*. 2004, 16:156-162.

[49] Morris PLP, Robinson RG, Raphael B. Prevalence and course of depressive disorders in hospitalized stroke patients. *Intl. J. Psychiatr. Med.*, 1990. 20:349-364.

[50] Eastwood MR, et al., Mood disorder following cerebrovascular accident. *Br. J. Psychiatry*, 1989, 154:195-200.

[51] Carson AJ, et al., Depression after stroke and lesion location: a systematic review. *Lancet,* 2000. 356: 122-126.

[52] Bhogal, SK, et al., Lesion location and poststroke depression. Systematic review of the methodological limitations in the literature. *Stroke*, 2004, 35:794-802.

[53] Shimoda K, Robinson RG, The relationship between post-stroke depression and lesion location in long-term follow-up. *Biol. Psychiatry,* 1999, 45:187-192.

[54] Narushima K, Kosier JT, Robinson RG. A reappraisal of post-stroke depression, intra and inter-hemispheric lesion location using meta-analysis. *J. Neuropsychiatry Clin. Neurosci.*, 2003, 15: 422-430.

[55] Robinson RG, Szetela B. Mood change following left hemispheric brain injury. *Ann. Neurol.*, 1981, 9:447-453.

[56] House A, et al., Mood disorders after stroke and their relation to lesion location. A CT scan study. *Brain*, 1990, 113:1113-1130.

[57] Sinyor D, et al., Post-stroke depression and lesion location: an attempted replication. *Brain*, 1986. 109:539-546.

[58] Morris PLP, Robinson RG, Raphael B. Lesion location and depression in hospitalized stroke patients: evidence supporting a specific relationship in the left hemisphere. *Neuropsychiatry Neuropsychol Behav. Neurol.*, 1992, 3:75-82.

[59] Starkstein SE, et al, Depressive disorder following posterior circulation compared with middle cerebral artery infarcts. *Brain,* 1988, 111:375-387.

[60] Starkstein SE, et al., Mood changes after right hemisphere lesion. *Br. J. Psychiatry,* 1989, 155:79-85.

[61] Finset A., et al., Depressed mood and intra-hemispheric location of lesion in right hemisphere stroke patients. *Scand. J. Rehabil. Med.*, 1989, 21: 1-6.

[62] Stern RA, Bachman DL. Depressive symptoms following stroke. *Am. J. Psychiatry*, 1991, 148: 351-356.

[63] Astrom M, Adolfsson R, Asplund K. Major depression in stroke patients: a 3-year longitudinal study. *Stroke*, 1993. 24:976-982.

[64] Alexopoulos GS, et al., Vascular depression hypothesis. *Arch. Gen. Psychiatry*, 1997. 54:915-922.

[65] Tiemeier H, et al., Relationship between atherosclerosis and late-life depression: the Rotterdam Study. *Arch. Gen. Psychiatry*, 2004. 61:369-76.

[66] Alexopoulos GS, et al. Clinically defined vascular depression. *Am. J. Psychiatry,* 1997, 154: 562-565.

[67] Coffey CE. Subcortical hyperintensity on magenetic resonance imaging: A comparison of normal and depressed elderly subjects. *Am. J. Psychiatry*, 1990, 147:187-189.

[68] Fazekas F. et al., Pathologic correlates of incidental MRI white matter signal hyperintensities. *Neurology*, 1993, 43:1683-9.

[69] Thomas AJ, et al. Ischemic basis for deep white matter hyperintensities in major depression: a neuropathological study. *Arch. Gen. Psychiatry*, 2002. 59: 785-92.

[70] Greenwald BS, et al. Neuroanatomic localization of magnetic resonance imaging signal hyperintensities in geriatric depression. *Stroke*, 1998, 29: 613-617.

[71] Pohjasvaara, T. et al. Clinical features of MRI-defined subcortical vascular disease. *Alzheimer Dis. Assoc Disord,* 2003. 17:236-242.

[72] Steffens DC, et al. Cerebrovascular disease and depression symptoms in the cardiovascular health study. *Stroke*, 1999. 30:2159-2166.

[73] Steffens DC, Krishnan KR, Crump C. Cerebrovascular disease and evolution of depressive symptoms in the cardiovascular health study. *Stroke*, 2002. 33:1636-1644.

[74] Taylor WD, et al. White matter hyperintensity progression and late-life depression outcomes. *Arch. Gen. Psychiatry,* 2003. 60:1090-6.

[75] Ballmaier M., et al. Anterior cingulate, gyrus rectus, and orbitofrontal abnormalities in elderly depressed patients: an MRI-based parcellation of the prefrontal cortex. *Am. J. Psychiatry,* 2004. 161: 99-108.

[76] Beaulieu C. The basis of anisotropic water diffusion in the nervous system - a technical review. *NMR Biomed.*, 2002. 15:435-55.

[77] Basser P.J., Jones DK. Diffusion-tensor MRI: theory, experimental design and data analysis - a technical review. *NMR Biomed.*, 2002. 15:456-67.

[78] Taylor WD, et al. Evidence of white matter tract disruption in MRI hyperintensities. *Biol. Psychiatry,* 2001. 50:179-83.

[79] Alexopoulos GS. et al. Frontal white matter microstructure and treatment response of late-life depression: a preliminary study. *Am. J. Psychiatry,* 2002. 159:1929-32.

[80] Birken DL, Oldendorf WH. N-acetyl-L-aspartic acid: a literature review of a compound prominent in 1H-NMR spectroscopic studies of brain. *Neurosci. Biobehav. Rev.,* 1989, 13:23-31.

[81] Charles HC, et al. Brain choline in depression: in vivo detection of potential pharmacodynamic effects of antidepressant therapy using hydrogen localized spectroscopy. *Prog. Neuropsychopharmacol Biol. Psychiatry*, 1994. 18:1121-7.

[82] Murata T, et al. MRI white matter hyperintensities, (1)H-MR spectroscopy and cognitive function in geriatric depression: a comparison of early- and late-onset cases. *Int. J. Geriatr. Psychiatry,* 2001. 16:1129-35.

[83] Kumar A, et al. Frontal white matter biochemical abnormalities in late-life major depression detected with proton magnetic resonance spectroscopy. *Am. J. Psychiatry,* 2002. 159:630-6.

[84] Binesh N. et al. Neurochemistry of late-life major depression: a pilot two-dimensional MR spectroscopic study. *J. Magn. Reson. Imaging*, 2004. 20:1039-45.

In: State-of-the-Art Imaging in Stroke, Volume 2
Editor: Bernhard Schaller, pp. 87-142
ISBN 978-1-60021-499-8


*Chapter IV*

# Poststroke Dementia and Imaging

*V. Mok[1], W. W. M. Lam[2], Y. L. Chan[2] and Ka Sing Wong[1]*
[1]Department of Medicine and Therapeutics
[2]Department of Radiology and Organ Imaging,
Chinese University of Hong Kong, Shatin, Hong Kong, China

## A. Introduction

Stroke increases the risk of dementia by approximate 2-9 times [1-5]. World wide, vascular dementia (VaD) is the second commonest cause of dementia [6-7]. Presence of poststroke dementia (PSD) reduces survival among stroke survivors and increases risk of long term stroke recurrence [8-10]. Varying severity levels of cognitive impairment affects functional outcome independent of physical impairment [11-14]. With an ageing population, burden of PSD is expected to rise. Although PSD is prevalent, relevant to mortality and morbidity, and is potentially more preventable than Alzheimer's disease (AD), it has received less attention relative to poststroke physical impairment or to AD. It is not until the last decade that more attention has been paid to PSD.

Historically, in the late 19$^{th}$ century, VaD was considered to be the commonest cause of dementia. It was thought that dementia was due to a relentless strangulation of the brain's blood supply, resulting in degeneration of the brain and dementia [15]. In the middle of the 20$^{th}$ century, pathological studies have begun to reveal that senile plaques and neurofibrillary tangles, rather than vascular lesions, were key findings among most of the elderly demented patients with atrophic brains. In the early 70s, VaD was thought to be uncommon and the mechanism of VaD was attributed to multiple small or large cerebral infarcts (multi-infarct dementia) [15]. In recent decades, advances of neuroimaging have enhanced greatly our understanding on VaD, its complexity far exceeds that of the concept of multi-infarct dementia [16,17]. We aim to review the current understanding of PSD and its imaging. Poststroke dementia will first be defined. Following that, foundational issues of PSD including its classification, pathology, prevalence, and cognitive pattern will be reviewed. This sets the background for discussing the imaging aspects relevant to PSD.

## B. Defining Poststroke Dementia

Dementia comes from the Latin word, *de mens*, which means "without mind". In general, it refers to deterioration of cognitive abilities that are severe enough to interfere daily activities. Various sets of diagnostic criteria for dementia have been proposed over the decades. The most commonly used criteria worldwide are the various editions of the Diagnostic and Statistical Manual of Mental Disorders (DSM) and the International Classification of Diseases (ICD). Albeit emphasis of each set of criteria varies slightly, they share similar framework that requires 3 elements: (1) memory impairment; (2) impairment of one or more cognitive domain, e.g. executive dysfunction, aphasia, apraxia, or agnosia; and (3) the cognitive impairment is severe enough to interfere social functions, such as work or social activities.

In this review, PSD is defined as the presence of dementia noted after stroke, irrespective of presence of preexisting dementia, prior stroke history, mechanisms for dementia, or the latency between stroke and onset of dementia. Stroke is commonly defined according to the World Health Organization as rapidly developing clinical signs of focal (or global) disturbance of cerebral function, with symptoms lasting 24 hours or longer or leading to death, with no apparent cause other than vascular origin. Since majority of the recent studies have evaluated the presence of dementia at 3 months poststroke, those studies that have evaluated dementia longer than 3 months poststroke will be described as delayed PSD in this review [3,18,19]. Most studies on PSD have used various editions of DSM or ICD to define dementia poststroke.

Poststroke dementia is a broader phenomenon than VaD. The current usage of VaD refers to patients whose dementia is wholly or at least partially attributed to cerebrovascular disease (CVD). Various sets of diagnostic criteria for VaD have been proposed over the decades (table 1), including the Hachinski Ischemic Score (HIS) [20], DSM IV [21], ICD-10 [22], State of California Alzheimer's Disease Diagnostic and Treatment Centers (ADDTC) [23], and the National Institute for Neurological Disorders and Stroke with the Association Internationale pour la Recherche et l'Enseignement en Neurosciences (NINDS-AIREN) [16]. The presence of dementia and evidence for CVD (e.g. history of stroke, focal neurological signs, neuroimaging evidences of CVD) are 2 key elements of these criteria. Most criteria also emphasize evidences for the relationship between CVD and dementia, e.g. dementia onset within 3 months of stroke, abrupt or stepwise cognitive deterioration, fluctuating course, or neuroimaging features that are relevant to dementia. Supporting features for and suspicious features against the diagnosis for VaD are also included in some of the criteria [16, 23]. As will be discussed later, specific imaging criteria have also been incorporated into some of these criteria [16]. Note that not all patients with VaD have history of overt stroke. Overall, these criteria identify different frequencies and clusters of patients [16] with varying sensitivity and specificity [16]. The NINDS-AIREN criteria are probably the most stringent and specific (80%), yet least sensitive (58%) [24, 25], while the DSM IV criteria are the most liberal [24]. Terms such as "probable", "possible", "mixed", or "definite" VaD have been used in various criteria to describe the certainty of which the dementia is attributed to CVD [16,23]. In general, definite VaD requires pathological verification. Recently, diagnostic criteria have also been proposed for a subtype of VaD (subcortical VaD) for use in clinical trials (table 1e).

**Table 1. Diagnostic criteria for vascular dementia**

| 1a. Hachinski Ischemi Score | |
|---|---|
| Features | Score |
| Abrupt onset | 2 |
| Stepwise deterioration | 1 |
| Fluctuating course | 2 |
| Nocturnal confusion | 1 |
| Relative preservation of personality | 1 |
| Depression | 1 |
| Somatic complaints | 1 |
| Emotional incontinence | 1 |
| History of hypertension | 1 |
| History of strokes | 2 |
| Evidence of associated atherosclerosis | 1 |
| Focal neurological symptoms | 2 |
| Focal neurological signs | 2 |

Score > 7 = VaD, score <4 = AD

| 1b. The NINDS-AIREN criteria |
|---|
| *Probable VaD* (include all of the following) |
| 1. Dementia = cognitive decline manifested by impairment in memory + 2 or more other cognitive domains that are severe enough to interfere daily activities independent to physical deficits related to stroke |
| 2. Cerebrovascular disease (CVD) =<br>a. Presence of focal signs on neurological examination, such as hemiparesis, lower facial weakness, Babinski sign, sensory deficit, hemianopsia, dysarthria, etc. consistent with stroke (with or without history of stroke); AND<br>b. Evidence of relevant CVD by brain imaging (CT or MRI) including multiple large-vessel strokes or a single strategically placed infarct (angular gyrus, thalamus, basal forebrain, PCA or ACA territories), as well as multiple basal ganglia and white matter lacunes or extensive periventricular white matter lesions or combinations thereof. |
| 3. A relationship between the above two disorders, manifested or inferred by the presence of one or more the following:<br>a. onset of dementia within 3 months following a recognized stroke;<br>b. abrupt deterioration in cognitive functions; or fluctuating, stepwise progression of cognitive deficits |
| *Possible VaD* |
| 1. Dementia (as above) +<br>2a. Focal neurological signs in the absence of imaging confirmation, OR<br>2b. absence of clear temporal relationship between dementia and stroke, OR<br>2c. subtle onset and variable course (plateau or improvement) of cognitive deficits and evidence of relevant CVD |

**Table 1. Diagnostic criteria for vascular dementia (Continued)**

| **1c The ADDTC criteria for ischemic vascular dementia** |
|---|
| *Probable ischemic VaD* (include all of the following) |
| 1. Dementia = decline of intellectual function sufficient to interfere broadly patient's usual daily activities, which is not isolated to a single narrow category of intellectual performance |
| 2. Evidence of two or more ischemic strokes by history, neurological signs, and/or neuroimaging studies (CT or T1-weighted MRI); or<br>Occurrence of a single stroke with a clearly documented temporal relationship to the onset of dementia |
| 3. Evidence of at least one infarct outside the cerebellum by CT or T1-weighted MRI |
| *Possible ischemic VaD* |
| 1. Dementia (as above) |
| 2a. A history or evidence of a single stroke (but not multiple strokes) without a clearly documented temporal relationship to the onset of dementia; or<br>2b. Binswanger's syndrome (without multiple strokes) that includes all of the followsing:<br>(i) early-onset urinary incontinence not explained by urologic disease, or gait disturbance (e.g. parkinsonian, magnetic, apraxic, or "senile" gait) not explained by peripheral cause,<br>(ii) vascular risk factors, and<br>(iii) extensive white matter changes on neuroimaging |

| **1d. The DSM IV criteria (include all of the following)** |
|---|
| 1. Dementia=decline in memory impairment + one or more domain of cognitive impairment that cause significant impairment in social or occupational functioning |
| 2. Focal neurological signs and symptoms (e.g. exaggeration of deep tendon reflexes, extensor plantar response, pseudobulbar palsy, gait abnormalities, weakness of an extremity) or laboratory evidence indicative of cerebrovascular disease (e.g. multiple infarctions involving cortex and underlying white matter) that are judged to be etiologically related to the disturbance |

| **1e. Criteria for subcortical vascular dementia (include all of the following)** |
|---|
| *Cognitive syndrome including both:*<br>a. Dysexecutive syndrome: impairment in goal formulation, initiation, planning, organizing, sequencing, executing, set-shifting and maintenance, abstracting<br>b. Memory deficit (may be mild): impaired recall, relative intact recognition, less severe forgetting, benefit from cues<br>c. Which indicate deterioration from a previous higher level of functioning and are interfering with complex (executive) occupational and social activities not due to physical effects of cerebrovascular disease alone |
| *Cerebrovascular disease including both:*<br>a. Evidence of relevant cerebrovascular disease by brain imaging (see table 4b)<br>b. Presence or a history of neurological signs as evidence for cerebrovascular disease such as hemiparesis, lower facial weakness, Babinski sign, sensory deficit, dysarthria, gait disorder, extrapyramidal signs consistent with subcortical brain lesion(s) |

Given that it is the most prevalent and homogeneous subtype of VaD, recent authorities have suggested that future clinical trials should focus on this entity, rather than mixing various subtypes of VaD together [26]. These criteria are modified from NINDS-AIREN criteria, which put greater emphasis on executive dysfunction and lesser emphasis on the presence of stroke history because executive dysfunction in subcortical VaD may be prominent and overt stroke episode may not occur in subcortical VaD [27]. Note that in these criteria cognitive deterioration that is severe enough to interfere "complex" or "executive" occupational and social activities is already sufficient to fulfill the severity requirement for dementia. Specific imaging criteria are also included in this set of criteria. The specificity and sensitivity of this set of criteria await further evaluation from pathology study.

Different to VaD, PSD refers to presence of dementia noted after stroke that may or may not be attributed to stroke or CVD. Dementia post stroke may be due to other dementing illnesses, e.g. AD. Vascular dementia may be considered as a subtype of PSD. In this review, PSD will be emphasized, yet studies on VaD that have included stroke patients will also be covered.

Note that stroke affecting specific brain regions can induce cognitive impairment that is restricted only to a particular cognitive domain, such as aphasia, apraxia or agnosia [28, 29], or is subtle [30]. The cognitive profile of these cases may not fulfill the standard diagnostic criteria for dementia either because the spectrum of affected cognitive domains is not broad enough or the impact of cognitive symptoms to social function is not severe enough. Although failure to recognize cases with poststroke cognitive impairment that falls short of dementia may underestimate the full impact of CVD or may hinder application of potential preventive treatment [31], for the purpose of this review, this category will not be emphasized.

## C. Classification of Poststroke Dementia

To date, a consensus on the clinical classification of PSD that is derived from its mechanisms and is also relevant to its management is not available mainly because its exact mechanisms are yet uncertain. It is currently believed that PSD may involve complex interactions between vascular etiologies, brain lesions, brain atrophy, co-existing dementing diseases and the host factors [17]. The classification framework will certainly evolve as we gain better understanding on the mechanisms of PSD. At present, we propose to classify PSD according to the vascular etiology and the etiology for dementia.

### Vascular Etiology

The vascular etiology of PSD includes both "stroke-related" and "concurrent" vascular etiology. Stroke-related vascular etiology covers present or previous stroke(s). Concurrent vascular etiology covers vascular etiology that may explain non-stroke related vascular lesion, e.g. arteriosclerosis that contributes to white matter changes (WMC) or vascular etiology that explains "silent" infarct. Similar to stroke etiology, the vascular etiology of PSD can be classified into large artery disease, small vessel disease (SVD), cardioembolism, miscellaneous causes, hemorrhage, and PSD of undetermined vascular etiology.

**Table 2. Classification of poststroke dementia**

| 1. Vascular etiology (stroke-related or concurrent vascular etiology) | |
|---|---|
| *Subtypes* | *Brain lesions associated with the vascular etiology* |
| a. Large artery disease | cortical / large subcortical territorial infarct<br>borderzone infarct (anterior, posterior, superior, internal), lacunar infarct |
| b. Small Vessel Disease | |
| *lipohyalinosis* | lacunar infarct (smaller) |
| *atherosclerosis* | lacunar infarct (larger) |
| *arteriosclerosis* | WMC |
| c. Cardioembolism | cortical / large subcortical territorial infarct (frequently multiple),<br>borderzone infarct (anterior, posterior, superior, internal), lacunar infarct |
| d. Hemorrhage, e.g. | |
| *SVD related* | deep (along territory of deep penetrating artery) |
| *cerebral amyloid angiopathy* | superficial or lobar |
| e. Miscellaneous, e.g. | |
| *CADASIL* | lacunar infarct, WMC |
| *hemodynamic* | borderzone infarct |
| *cerebral amyloid angiopathy (non-hemorrhagic)* | lacunar infarct, WMC |
| f. Undetermined etiology | Variable |
| 2. Etiology of dementia | |
| a. Poststroke VaD | The dementia is secondary to the stroke and/or concurrent vascular etiologies; current diagnostic criteria for probable VaD can be applied; e.g. of poststroke VaD are subcortical VaD or strategic infarct dementia |
| b. Poststroke mixed dementia | The concurrent presence of AD that explains mostly or partially the dementia syndrome poststroke |
| c. Poststroke other dementia | The concurrent present of other non-vascular and non-AD related dementia syndrome, e.g. frontal temporal dementia, dementia with Lewy bodies |

### *1. Large Artery Disease*

Large artery disease refers to atherosclerosis affecting extra or intracranial large artery. In Caucasians, it commonly affects extracranial carotid artery, while in Asians, Blacks, and Hispanics, it commonly affects intracranial large artery, in particular, middle cerebral artery (MCA) [32]. Types of brain lesions associated with extracranial carotid atherosclerotic disease are heterogeneous, and may include cortical territorial infarct, large subcortical infarct, borderzone infarct (internal, anterior, posterior, superior borderzone) and even lacunar infarct. Although brain lesions associated with MCA atherosclerotic disease are similar to that with carotid artery stenosis, our recent study demonstrated that the former was associated more commonly with subcortical lacunar infarcts, which were often scattered as chain-like fashion along the internal, anterior or posterior borderzone [33]. If the infarct hits at "strategic" areas or is of adequate size or frequency, it may induce PSD. Strategic area refers to cerebral cognitive eloquent area, which if it is affected, will cause cognitive impairment. Examples of "strategic" areas are thalamus, angular gyrus, genu of the left internal capsule, left anterior corona radiata, anterior corpus callosum, inferior medial temporal lobe, hippocampus, frontal lobe, and caudate nucleus [34-37]. Less commonly, large artery disease may involve multiple arteries sequentially, inducing multiple brain lesions, and result in multi-infarct dementia.

### *2. Cardioembolism*

Emboli from the heart are frequently large, causing impaction at intracranial large artery, resulting in extensive cortical territorial infarct. Scattered emboli may occlude multiple or bilateral arteries simultaneously, inducing multiple large infarcts. Or that recurrent embolic stroke occurs at different times, causing cumulative large brain lesions. The end results of multiple large infarcts may again be multi-infarct dementia. Note that as in large artery disease, types of brain lesions associated with cardioembolism are also heterogeneous, including lacunar infarcts, large subcortical infarct or borderzone infarcts. If infarct hits at strategic areas or is extensive or multiple, dementia may result (figure 1).

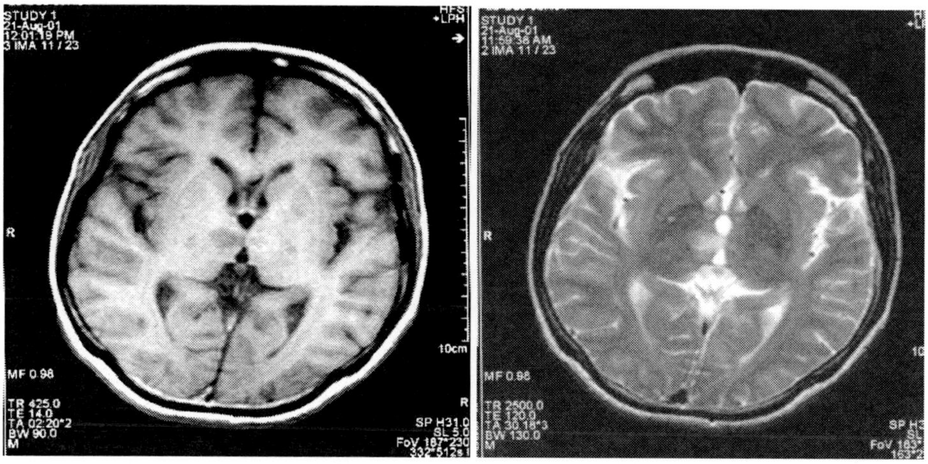


1a. T1-weighted MRI 1b. T2-weighted MRI

Figure 1. Strategic infarct dementia secondary to cardioembolic stroke

A 45-year-old female presented with acute confusion, gaze palsy, and fluctuating consciousness without motor problems. MRI shows bilateral paramedian thalamic infarcts (hypointense on T1- [figure 1a] and hyperintense on T2-weighted [figure 1b] imaging, the left sided lesion is smaller and appears more subtle than the right one; smaller infarcts are also noted lateral to the paramedian thalamic infarcts). Investigation revealed underlying apical hypertrophic cardiomyoapthy and paroxysmal atrial fibrillation. At 3 months poststroke, she remained apathetic along with memory complaints and poor attention span. Her MMSE was 25/30 then. The cognitive impairment affected her daily functioning as a housewife. This case represents a cardioembolic stroke (vascular etiology) causing multiple infarcts at strategic areas (bilateral thalamic infarcts), resulting in a dementia syndrome that has a strong component of executive dysfunction. Both the history and MRI fulfill the NINDS-AIREN criteria for probable VaD.

### *3. Small Vessel Disease*

Small vessel disease is used here to include only the commonest types of small artery pathologies that are most prevalent among the elderly with vascular risk factors. These include lipohyalinosis (or complex SVD), arteriosclerosis (or simple SVD) and the small vessel variant of atherosclerosis (microatheroma). Other vascular etiologies, e.g. amyloid angiopathy, which also affect small vessels, will not be classified as SVD here. Small vessel disease affects both deep and superficial long penetrating arteries that supply the subcortical and brainstem regions. The brain lesion associated with lipohyalinosis or atherosclerosis is lacunar infarct that is located in the subcortical or brainstem region. Brain lesion associated with arteriosclerosis is WMC, which are located in the deep white matter or periventricular region. White matter change is commonly referred as "leukoaraiosis", where "*leuko*" is "white" and "*araiosis*" means rarefaction. Since present imaging modalities and techniques are not able to visualize small artery lesions, SVD in vivo is diagnosed by presence of radiological lacunar infarcts and/or WMC in the absence of large artery disease, cardioembolism and other miscellaneous causes. Note also that it is only lacunar infarct that is related to overt stroke episode, while arteriosclerosis and WMC are not directly responsible for the stroke event. Although arteriosclerotic related WMC are most prevalent in lacunar stroke, it also exists in other stroke subtypes.

Binswanger's disease [38] and lacunar state (état lacunaire or lacunar dementia) [39] are probably the commonest examples of SVD that are associated with dementia (figure 2). Brain lesions characteristic of Binswanger's disease are diffuse WMC, yet sparing the U fibers; while that of lacunar state, are multiple lacunar infarcts. Although it has been considered as two distinct entities historically, authorities have recently believed that they are varying manifestations of the same disease [40]. Subcortical VaD has been used to describe these 2 entities collectively. Apart from the above more severe forms of SVD, focal SVD inducing an isolated lacunar infarct that is located in a strategic area, such as genu of the internal capsule, caudate or thalamus, can also induce PSD in the absence of diffuse SVD [35-37].

### *4. Hemorrhage*

In this review, hemorrhagic stroke refers only to intracerebral hemorrhage (ICH). Although subdural, epidural and subarachnoid hemorrhages are all related to dementia, these non-ICH related hemorrhages will not be discussed in this review. Perhaps the commonest form of ICH in the elderly is associated with SVD and hypertension. The brain lesion is usually located in the "deep" cerebral or cerebellar region. If hemorrhage occurs at strategic area, such as thalamus, cognitive impairment or dementia may result [41, 42]. Size of the haematoma or presence of ventricular extension may affect severity of cognitive impairment [41]. Yet, concurrent vascular etiology (e.g. SVD) and brain lesions (e.g. WMC and lacunar infarcts) can also contribute to the dementia syndrome. Cerebral amyloid angiopathy (CAA) affects small artery and has particular relevance to PSD. It is commonly associated with recurrent "superficial" lobar hemorrhages and dementia [43]. The lobar hemorrhage in CAA classically occurs in the absence of hypertension among elderly patient. It is also found commonly in patients with AD. Rarely, CAA is associated with hereditary cerebral hemorrhages. However, the mechanism for CAA related ICH in inducing dementia is complex. Apart from the direct effect of recurrent cerebral hemorrhages, CAA may induce dementia due to concurrent AD and/or its associated concurrent brain lesions, namely WMC and lacunes [44, 45]. Other forms of ICH may include iatrogenic (e.g. warfarin related) and less commonly, arteriovenous malformations, intracranial venous thrombosis or microangiomas. In general, its relevance to PSD is related to the site, size and extent (ventricular extension) of the haematoma.

### *5. Miscellaneous Vascular Etiology*

Miscellaneous subtypes of vascular etiology mainly comprise of rare forms of stroke disorders or CVD. Typical brain lesions may be associated with these diseases. Vascular etiologies of these miscellaneous subtypes of PSD can be further classified into hereditary, e.g. cerebral autosomal dominant arteriopathy with subcortical infarcts and leukoencephalopathy (CADASIL) [46], non-hemorrhagic form of CAA, autoimmune vasculitis (e.g. systemic lupus erythematosus), hemodynamic (e.g. hypoxic-ischemic encephalopathy, severe heart failure, orthostatic hypotension, post-coronary artery bypass graft) or hypercoagulable state, e.g. antiphospholipd syndrome.

### *6. Undetermined Vascular Etiology*

Poststroke dementia of undetermined vascular etiology refers to case where extensive imaging and laboratory evaluations reveal no vascular etiology that can account for the stroke. Patients are commonly young, free of vascular risk factors, having stroke related cortical or large subcortical infarct(s). In many cases, the mechanism is presumed to be embolic in nature as angiography fail to reveal intra or extracranial large artery disease. Yet, cardiac investigation is also unrevealing. Stroke with unknown vascular etiology was found to be associated with PSD [47, 48].

## Etiology of Dementia

In a patient with PSD, after determining the vascular etiology and brain lesion, the second step is to determine how much does the vascular related brain lesion contribute to the dementia syndrome poststroke, or in other word, is to determine the etiology of dementia. Dementia after stroke may not be related to stroke or other vascular related etiology and brain lesion, but may be related to other dementing illnesses, e.g. AD. A simple way is to classify etiology of dementia into "poststroke VaD", "poststroke mixed dementia" and "poststroke other dementia".

### *1. Poststroke Vascular Dementia*

Poststroke VaD refers to dementia that is predominantly attributed to the stroke or other concurrent vascular etiologies and related brain lesions. However in practice, establishing this causal link between dementia and stroke or CVD is complex and consensus on the methods in doing so has not been reached. In principle, the occurrence of new onset cognitive deterioration poststroke [5, 48, 49] and/or presence of relevant radiological vascular related brain lesions suggest a strong vascular contribution. Relevant brain lesions include infarcts located at strategic sites, multiple territorial infarcts, or multiple lacunar infarcts associated with severe WMC. Many studies have used current diagnostic criteria of VaD as mentioned previously to classify poststroke VaD [11, 50] and imaging criteria defining relevant brain lesions have also been proposed. These criteria will be discussed in detail later. In poststroke VaD, the dementia syndrome can be the direct result of one stroke, the cumulative effects of multiple strokes (multi-infarct dementia), and/or the effects of other concurrent non-stroke related vascular etiology and related brain lesions, e.g. WMC or silent infarcts.

### *2. Poststroke Mixed Dementia*

Poststroke mixed dementia refers to the concurrent presence of AD in a stroke patient with dementia. In daily practice, it is clinically determined by a diagnosis of AD prestroke or a history of progressive prestroke cognitive impairment in the absence of relevant radiological cerebral vascular lesions, e.g. extensive WMC or multiple silent lacunes, which probably already exist prestroke. In mixed dementia, the index stroke episodes may or may not worsen the cognitive impairment poststroke. Information regarding the prestroke cognitive status is usually obtained through closed informants of patients. Instrument such as the Informant Questionnaire on Cognitive Decline has been commonly used to evaluate objectively the presence of prestroke cognitive impairment or dementia [19, 51, 52]. Mixed dementia also covers case where progressive cognitive decline develops poststroke in the absence of further stroke and / or new relevant vascular related brain lesions. In such case, concurrent AD is implicated. Recent studies have shown that vascular brain lesions (e.g. lacunar infarct) may also interact synergistically with Alzheimer's pathology in aggravating the cognitive severity of patients with Alzheimer's pathology [53, 54].

### *3. Poststroke Other Dementia*

The last subtype of PSD is poststroke other dementia. It refers to the presence of other non-vascular and non-AD related dementing illness (e.g. dementia with Lewy bodies or chronic alcoholism) that either exists already prestroke or develops poststroke, and may or may not contribute to the dementia poststroke. In general, other dementia among patients with PSD is rare [48].

In summary, we propose a 2-step classification for PSD, i.e. first, to determine the stroke-related and/or concurrent vascular etiology, second, to determine how much the vascular component, or other dementing illnesses contribute to the dementia syndrome (i.e. etiology of dementia). In clinical practice, determining the etiology of dementia is probably the most difficult. However, attempt to classify PSD according to etiologies based on all available clinical data is still worthwhile as potential effective treatment and prevention rest on accurate knowledge on these aspects of PSD. To date, recent clinical studies have suggested that response to cognitive treatments vary according to vascular etiology and/or etiology for dementia. For example, effects of memantine or nimodipine may be better for subcortical VaD relative to that for large arterial related cortical VaD [55, 56], while acetylcholinesterase inhibitor may be more effective in mixed dementia over probable VaD [57].

# D. Pathology of Poststroke Dementia

The role of pathology in diagnosing and classifying PSD in conjunction with clinical information is less concrete than that in AD, where definite pathological markers (neuritic plaques and neurofibrillary tangles) exist [58]. At present, there is no consensus for the pathological diagnosis of PSD [59] and controversies regarding brain substrates that are representative of poststroke VaD remain. Yet, pathology still plays the definitive role in providing information on the presence, nature and extent of vascular lesions, brain lesions, brain atrophy and other concurrent pathologies, e.g. AD, which is relevant in the overall evaluation of PSD. It has been used as the gold standard to evaluate the validity of various clinical diagnostic criteria for VaD.[25, 60] Further pathological studies will certainly contribute in unraveling the mechanisms of PSD. Furthermore, with the advances of imaging techniques, more types of pathological lesions can now be visualized by imaging, which are previously not detectable by standard imaging modality. Hence, understanding the pathological lesions for PSD provide an important interface for interpretation of imaging findings or development of new imaging techniques.

In general, the size (large artery or penetrating small artery), site, types (e.g. atherosclerosis, arteriosclerosis, lipohyalinosis, amyloid angiopathy), and extent of the arterial pathologies are important in the evaluation of PSD. Relevant brain lesions include cortical or large subcortical territorial infarct, borderzone infarct, lacunar infarct, microinfarct, perivascular space, hemorrhage, cortical laminar necrosis, granular atrophy, microbleed, WMC, hippocampal sclerosis, brain atrophy, and other non-vascular related pathologies, e.g. Alzheimer or cortical Lewy bodies pathology [59, 61, 62]. The location, size, extent, and interaction of these lesions may affect its relevance to the dementia syndrome poststroke. The pathology related to PSD has been reviewed recently in detail.[63] A brief overview on key pathological substrates will be presented below.

## Lacunar Infarct

Pathologically, lacunar infarct refers to small cavity of size between 3-15mm, which is associated by either in-situ SVD (i.e. atherosclerosis or lipohyalinosis) or embolism from proximal sites causing occlusion of small vessels. Atherosclerosis affects small artery of size 200-800μm and induces larger lacunar infarct (>5mm) due to occlusion [64]. Lipohyalinosis affects arteries of size 40-200μm and may cause smaller lacunar infarct (3-7mm) possibly by occlusion and endothelial leakage associated with breakdown of blood brain barrier (BBB).[64, 65].

## Perivascular Space (Virchow-Robin Space)

Similar to lacunar infarct, perivascular space is also a cavity, which is commonly smaller than that related to lacunar infarct. It surrounds a penetrating artery and various hypotheses explain its occurrence, including brain atrophy, mechanical stress from the pulsatile arterioles, or interstitial fluid drainage disorder [64]. Imaging differentiation between lacunar infarct and perivascular space will be discussed later.

## White Matter Changes

White matter refers to myelinated axons and glial cells that are located in the deep and periventricular region. Long superficial and deep penetrating arteries originated from the superficial pial plexus and major intracerebral large arteries respectively supply the cerebral white matter. Given that the arteries are long and anastomoses are minimal or absent between deep and superficial penetrators, white matter region is vulnerable to hypoperfusion.

White matter changes describe both ischemic and non-ischemic related white matter pathology. Ischemic WMC consist of pallor of myelin, loss of oligodendrocytes, myelins and axons, cavitation with or without lipid-laden macrophages, and astrogliosis but without definite necrosis [63]. Arteriosclerosis is invariably found in these areas. Note that the strip of white matter that is located just beneath the cortex (U-fiber) is usually spared due probably to adequate perfusion by unaffected shorter vessels located adjacent to the cortex. The cause of the ischemia can be multi-factorial, which may include narrowed arteries related to arteriosclerosis, reduced cerebral blood flow (e.g. cardiac failure, severe carotid artery stenosis), hyperviscosity (e.g. hyperglycemia, polycythemia, hyperlipidemia) and/or impaired cerebral autoregulation [40] The WMC may also be due to endothelial leakage from artery secondary to BBB dysfunction as a result of SVD [65]. Furthermore, study has demonstrated that WMC may be indirectly due to impaired venous drainage associated with collagenous thickening affecting parenchymal veins or venules [66]. In general, ischemic WMC are visualized radiologically as confluent deep WMC or irregular / extending periventricular WMC [67].

Non-ischemic WMC refers mainly to the periventricular spongioform zone that is associated with paucity of myelin, disrupted subependymal lining, and gliosis [67]. The cause for it is probably due to altered periventricular fluid dynamics, which may simply be age-related with no pathological significance. On MRI, these pathological changes are seen as thin rim of caps or smooth halo [67]. Note that small punctate deep WMC shown on MRI might not be visible on autopsy specimens and hence pathological nature of these WMC are uncertain [67].

## Microinfarct

Microinfarct ranges from a few microns to 0.5mm and is characterized by loss of myleinated fibers in white matter or total loss of neurons in gray matter. Recent pathology studies have highlighted its relevance to PSD [59, 61]. At present, it cannot be visualized on current imaging modality.

## Granular Cortical Atrophy

It consists of multifocal cortical microinfarcts accompanied by focal gliosis, which are commonly found in the cortical borderzone between MCA and anterior cerebral artery. Cerebral hypoperfusion is implicated as the mechanism. Although cortical atrophy may be seen on imaging, identifying microinfarcts by current imaging is not yet possible. Hence granular cortical atrophy associated with microinfarcts remains a pathological diagnosis.

## Cortical Laminar Necrosis

Cortical laminar necrosis describes a particular pattern of severe ischemic injury that is characterized by an extensive band of necrosis along cortical layers most vulnerable to ischemia. It is commonly related to hypoxic ischemic encephalopathy associated with global cerebral hypoperfusion or hypoxia.

## Hippocampal Sclerosis

Hippocampal sclerosis in the elderly is characterized by severe neuronal loss and gliosis in the CA-1 and subiculum region of the hippocampus, with relative sparing of other hippocampal fields. It is currently believed to be due to ischemia secondary to systemic hypoperfusion or intrinsic CVD.

## Microbleed

Microbleed is characterized by hemosiderin around abnormal small vessel, with infarction of the surrounding tissue. Although it was once thought to be silent, a recent study using T2*-weighted gradient-echo (GE) magnetic resonance imaging (MRI) demonstrated its cognitive relevance among stroke patients independent of other ischemic lesions [68].

In principle, poststroke VaD is defined by the presence of relevant cerebral vascular lesions associated with no or minimal plaques or tangles,25, 60 while mixed dementia is defined as concurrent presence of both vascular related brain lesions and significant Alzheimer's pathology [63]. However, as mentioned before, consensus on detailed criteria regarding vascular related brain lesions related to VaD has not been reached.

# E. Frequency, Incidence, and Clinical Determinants of Poststroke Dementia

## Hospital-Based Studies at 3 Months Poststroke

The frequency of PSD in general (i.e. including those with prestroke dementia and prior stroke) at 3 months poststroke based on more recent hospital-based studies ranges from 20% – 32%.[5, 48-50, 69-71]. The frequency of new onset dementia poststroke at 3 months ranges from 9% – 16%, [50, 72] which is around half of that of PSD in general. If only patients with first ever stroke were included, the frequency ranges from 13%-29%, [49, 71, 73] which is slightly less than that of PSD in general. The frequency of PSD after hemorrhagic stroke is probably similar to that of ischemic stroke [69]. The frequency of PSD among different stroke subtypes varies only slightly, [48] although one study revealed that SVD increased PSD by 2.7 times relative to other stroke subtypes [70]. One must also aware that the frequency of PSD also varies with the set of diagnostic criteria that are used to define dementia. In a study among the same cohort of patients, frequency of PSD varied from 6% by ICD-10 to 25.5% by DSM-III [74].

Various clinical and imaging determinants interact to produce PSD. Imaging determinants will be discussed in a later section and the former will be discussed now. Various hospital-based studies have yielded somehow similar clinical determinants of PSD based on multivariate regression analyses. Basic demographic determinants include old age, [2, 5, 48, 50, 69, 70, 72, 73, 75] low education, [2, 5, 49, 50, 70] and non-white population [2, 48, 70] Vascular risk factors predicting PSD include diabetes [48, 70, 73] atrial fibrillation, [5, 69, 75] and prior stroke [5, 48, 49, 70, 72] Stroke-related clinical features that determine PSD include aphasia [5, 49, 73, 75], major hemispheric stroke syndrome, [48, 49, 70] and stroke severity according to clinical scale [50, 69, 72]. Relevant stroke features include left sided cerebral infarct [5, 48, 70, 72] and MCA infarct [50, 73]. Prestroke cognitive and functional impairment also predict PSD [50, 69, 75].

## Delayed Poststroke Dementia

Cumulative incidence rate of new onset delayed PSD according to hospital-based studies ranges from about 16% at 1 to 2 year [47, 75] to around 20%-30% at 3 to 4 year [18, 19]. The relative risk of incident dementia associated with stroke as demonstrated by an early study was 3.83 [4]. A recent study found that VaD accounted for two-thirds of delayed PSD at 3 years follow up [19]. In another recent study, the PSD etiology was found to shift from predominantly AD with CVD type (mixed dementia) in the first 2 years and to VaD type later on [18].

Hospital-based incident studies have identified the following clinical determinants for delayed PSD: old age, [3, 4, 18, 19] low education, [3] diabetes mellitus, [19] previous stroke, [47] cerebral hypoxia associated with intercurrent medical illnesses, e.g. cardiopulmonary arrest, cardiac arrhythmias or epilepsy, [4] stroke severity at admission, [19] baseline intellectual function, [3] and prestroke cognitive impairment [19] Most of these factors are similar to that found in hospital-based studies of PSD at 3 months.

### Community-Based Studies

Few community-based studies have investigated the incidence of delayed PSD. An earlier study found that the cumulative incidence rate of new onset delayed PSD increased from 7% at 1 year to 48% at 25 year poststroke [76]The incidence of dementia in the first year was 9 times greater than expected and age, male sex, and second stroke were found to predict PSD based on multivariate model [76]. In another community study, incident rate of stroke related dementia was 21.3% at 2 years of follow up and elevated levels of low-density lipoprotein were associated with risk of stroke-related dementia [77]. In the more recent community-based Framingham study, stroke was found to double the risk of dementia relative to controls who were free of stroke and dementia [1] Interestingly, factors associated with lower risk of AD, namely young age, high education, and presence of 2 apolipoprotein E ε3 alleles, were found to predict delayed PSD. These findings highlight the long-term cognitive consequence of stroke, as stroke appears to nullify the lower prestroke risk of dementia among those with low risk for dementia.

## F. Cognitive Pattern of Poststroke Dementia

Different to AD, which has a unique cognitive pattern and progression; cognitive profile of PSD varies with its subtypes and sites of the brain lesions.

### Cognitive Pattern with Cortical Brain Lesions

Cognitive pattern of poststroke VaD associated with cortical brain lesions depends on the site of the lesion, and at times, the pattern may be "patchy". For example, cognitive impairment secondary to cardioembolism that induces multiple cortical infarcts involving mesial temporal lobe, dominant frontal-parietal lobe, and medial frontal lobe may present with amnesia, aphasia, ideomotor apraxia, and executive dysfunction. If non-dominant frontal-parietal cortex is affected, dressing apraxia, constructional apraxia, or agnosia may result. A classical Gerstmann's syndrome (agraphia, acalculia, right-left disorientation, finger agnosia) may result if the dominant parietal lobe (angular gyrus) is involved.

### Cognitive Pattern with Subcortical Brain Lesions

Subcortical infarcts affecting strategic areas, such as paramedian and polar region of the thalamus, caudate, inferior genu of the internal capsule, and anterior corona radiata commonly produce amnesia and executive dysfunction. The mechanism whereby lesions at subcortical structures produce amnesia and executive dysfunction is probably due to disruption of the frontal–subcortical or medial temporal limbic circuits [78].

Cognitive pattern of poststroke subcortical VaD typically has predominant executive dysfunction. The stroke-related physical deficits commonly include various lacunar syndromes, namely pure motor stroke, pure sensory stroke, ataxic hemiparesis, or hemiballism/chorea/athetosis. Other associated features of subcortical VaD may include urinary symptoms, mood disturbance (e.g. depression), parkinsonism, and gait abnormality [26].

## Executive Dysfunction in Poststroke Vascular Dementia

Recent study by Sachdev et al found that executive dysfunction was the predominant feature of poststroke VaD in general and was thought to be related the high prevalence of WMC in patients with poststroke VaD [11]. This study suggested that while large cortical infarcts do contribute to the dementia pattern, they are best regarded as being superimposed on a background of executive dysfunction in those with poststroke VaD [11].

Executive dysfunction refers to a set of loosely related cognitive functions that serve the purpose of coordinating higher order cognitive capabilities and emotion and regulating behavioral responses to environmental demands. It was originally described in patients with frontal lobe injuries, and later in those with subcortical lesions, probably related to disruption of various frontal-subcortical circuits [79]. Features of executive dysfunction may include impaired decision making, poor judgment, distractibility, emotion instability, failure to inhibit inappropriate response, failure of set-shifting, perseveration, poor initiation, poor abstraction, abulia, restricted emotion, deficient empathy, lack of planning, or executive memory loss. Executive memory loss describes memory loss that is due to defective retrieval mechanism, which is different to amnesia in AD, which is due to impaired encoding mechanism related to hippocampal lesion. Patients with executive memory loss will have better recognition memory when cues are given to help memory retrieval, whereas recognition memory remains poor in AD patients [80].

## Cognitive Progression in Poststroke Dementia

As mentioned before, poststroke VaD can be the result of a single stroke event or the cumulative effects of recurrent strokes and/or other vascular related brain lesions. The cognitive progression can be acute deterioration poststroke followed by recovery, [81] stepwise deterioration after recurrent strokes, [82] slow progressive deterioration, [83] fluctuating, or any combinations of the above. In general, the cognitive decline in patients with poststroke VaD is slower than those with AD but is faster than those without dementia poststroke [83].

# G. Imaging in Poststroke Dementia

Imaging has revolutionized our understanding and management of PSD. At the most elementary level, imaging helps to ascertain the presence of cerebrovascular lesions and to rule out surgically treatable dementias, e.g. subdural hemorrhage, tumor, or hydrocephalus. With the recent advances and availability of various imaging techniques, knowledge on the mechanisms of how vascular etiologies, brain lesions and other brain pathologies interact in producing PSD has been enhanced. A better knowledge on its mechanisms has shaped our present conceptual framework in classifying and diagnosing PSD, and in turn, imaging features have been incorporated into various diagnostic criteria for VaD [16, 26, 84].

Apart from the evaluation of the mechanisms and diagnosis of PSD, imaging has also been proved useful in clinical studies for PSD. In a recent multi-center drug study for probable VaD as defined by NINDS-AIREN criteria, besides fulfilling the criteria for having evidence of dementia, CVD, and the relationship between the two, fulfillment of specific imaging criteria based on MRI as confirmed by a blinded central reader was also essential for inclusion [85]. Given that accuracy of clinical judgment may vary with centers, imaging criteria probably provide the most objective mean to ensure the accuracy in diagnosis.

As will be discussed later, certain imaging features can be used as a prognostic indicator for cognitive progression [86] and have helped in providing insights for therapeutic interventions [87]. It has also been recently hypothesized that progression of WMC as shown by MRI, may help not only to reflect disease progression, but also to act as a surrogate marker in clinical trials on cerebral SVD [88].

# H. Basic Imaging Modalities and Methods in Poststroke Dementia

The type of imaging modalities and methods that are used in PSD depends first, on its ability in detecting and quantifying cerebral abnormalities that are relevant to PSD; and second, on the availability and expertise of the individual center. To date, the following imaging characteristics are found to be relevant to PSD: (1) type and distribution of the arterial lesions; (2) type, size, site, and number of vascular related brain lesions (e.g. hemorrhage, stroke-related infarct, borderzone infarct, silent infarct or WMC); (3) severity and distribution of cerebral atrophy (e.g. cortical, subcortical or regional atrophy); (4) severity and pattern of cerebral blood flow, glucose metabolism, and oxygen metabolism; and (5) cerebral vasoreactivity. In this section, imaging modalities and methods that have been used most commonly in practices or researches of PSD will be described.

**Table 3. Imaging variables (Computed Tomography and conventional Magnetic Resonance Imaging) relevant to study of poststroke dementia**

| *A. Stroke related brain lesions* | Remarks |
|---|---|
| Types | ischemic or hemorrhage |
| Sites | strategic sites |
| Relevance | symptomatic, silent, or old |
| Patterns | cortical, large subcortical, lacunar infarct or borderzone infarct |
| Laterality | dominant hemisphere |
| Multiplicity | single or multiple |
| Size | linear, planimetric, or volumetric |
| Extent | ventricular or subarachnoid extension for ICH |
| *B. Whit matter changes* | |
| Sites | periventricular and/or deep |
| Extent | visual grading of extent of WMC (thin cap or rim, halo, irregular, extending, punctate, patchy, or confluent), volumetric quantification* |
| *C. Brain atrophy* | |
| Cortical atrophy | sulci/fissures enlargement (visual, linear, planimetric, volumetric*), cortical gray matter global and regional (volumetric)* |
| Subcortical atrophy | ventricular enlargement (visual, linear, planimetric, volumetric) |
| General cerebral atrophy | ventricular brain ratio, ventricular cranial ratio (linear, planimetric, volumetric), total brain atrophy (volumetric) |
| Regional atrophy | hemispheric, frontal, parietal, temporal, hippocampal, corpus callosum (visual, planimetric* or volumetric*) |
| *D. Others* | |
| Perivascular space | FLAIR (hypointense) and T2-weighted MRI (hyperintense)* |
| Hippocampal sclerosis | coronal FLAIR and T2-weighted MRI (hyperintense)* |

* Applicable mainly for MRI.

These include computed tomography (CT), MRI (T1-, T2-, and proton density [PD] weighted, and fluid attenuation inversion recovery [FLAIR]), SPECT, PET, and xenon CT. Since the present clinical diagnostic and classification framework of PSD or VaD are based on findings from structural CT and the above MRI techniques, its methods in the evaluation of PSD will be described first (table 3). The last 3 modalities have been used mainly in research setting and a brief overview on the functions and findings of these standard functional imaging modalities will be given next. The physics and technical details of these imaging modalities are beyond the scope of this review. Following this section, imaging determinants and imaging criteria that are based on the above imaging modalities for PSD will be described respectively. Recent imaging applications on PSD (e.g. diffusion weighted imaging [DWI], diffusion tensor imaging [DTI], magnetization transfer imaging [MTI], T2*-weighted GE sequence, MR perfusion, and MR spectroscopy [MRS]) will be presented last. Although we recognize the importance of angiography techniques (digital subtraction angiography and CT and MR angiography) in the evaluation of vascular etiology for PSD, these techniques will not be covered in this review.

## Computed Tomography

Routine CT is able to provide essential data relevant to PSD. Despite rapid advances in MRI techniques, CT will remain an important imaging modality in the study of PSD especially among developing countries given its low cost, wide availability, and simplicity in both technique and interpretation. Computed tomography can accurately detect surgical treatable dementias, such as subdural hemorrhage or hydrocephalus. Limitations of CT relevant to PSD include poor visualization of small infarcts and infratentorial lesions. Furthermore, assessment of temporal region, although is possible, [89] is usually difficult due to bone-hardening artifact and coronal images of CT, which has better visualization for medial temporal or hippocampal region, are difficult to obtain [90]. Note that with the rapid advances in CT techniques, some of these limitations may be overcome. For e.g., with the recent application of multidetector CT, smaller infarct may be visualized given its better spatial resolution.

In general, standard methods in the evaluation of stroke are also applicable for the evaluation of PSD. Contrast enhanced CT imaging has no specific role in the evaluation of PSD except in occasional case where cerebral malignancy or infection needs to be ruled out in stroke patient with dementia. Issues relating to the detection of acute cerebral infarctions by CT will not be discussed in this review.

### *1. Brain Lesions*

Established cerebral infarcts appear as hypodense lesions on CT. Site (e.g. strategic sites), laterality (dominant versus non-dominant side) and pattern (e.g. lacunar, territorial cortical or large subcortical, borderzone) of the infarcts can be determined and involved vascular territories or mechanisms can then be implied. Differentiation between symptomatic, silent, or old infarct is mainly determined by correlation with clinical features. Lacunar infarct on CT is defined as a small, sharply demarcated round or oval hypodense area located along territory of small penetrating artery. Radiological limits for the size of lacunar infarct are commonly set between 3-20mm, which are larger than the pathological limits of 3-15mm. This is because surrounding edema of the infarct is also visualized by the neuoimaging. Although SVD is the commonest cause for lacunar infarct, subcortical lacunar infarct may also be associated with intra/extracranial large artery diseases and cardioembolism. Note that MCA atherosclerotic disease may not uncommonly induce subcortical lacunar infarcts due to blockage of the origin of a penetrating artery or microembolic phenomeon [32]. Hence, evaluation of intracranial large artery status by transcranial doppler ultrasound or CT / MR angiography is needed to assess the vascular etiology of lacunar infarct among ethnic groups (e.g. Asians, Blacks and Hispanics) where intracranial large artery disease is prevalent. This practice applies also to the use of MRI in the evaluation of lacunar infarcts. In evaluating ICH among those with PSD, apart from its site (e.g. strategic site, superficial or deep), laterality, and size, presence of ventricular/subarachnoid extension needs also to be assessed.

Linear measurement on the size of the ischemic or hemorrhagic lesion can be done manually and is usually represented by the greatest diameter of the lesion. Most of the CT workstation is able to quantify the surface area of the lesions at its greatest diameter. Volume of hematoma or infarcts can also be estimated via various formulas [41, 91] or by computerized automated methods [92]. The volume is the best measure in reflecting the size of the vascular lesion. Furthermore, various ratios of the infracted volumes over brain volume or brain volume minus ventricular volumes have been used in the study of PSD [93]. These ratios may be more relevant to cognitive impairment than the actual size of the lesions.

### *2. White Matter Changes*

On CT, WMC are defined as patchy or diffuse symmetric areas of intermediate density, i.e. density between that of normal white matter and that of CSF, with ill-defined margins, located in the periventricular and/or the deep (centrum semiovale) white matter region (figure 2a). Different visual methods in rating its severity have been devised and have been used in cross-sectional studies [93-96]. Standard template has commonly been used as reference to grade severity. Qualitatively, the severity of WMC may vary from punctuate or fuzzy hypodensity at around the frontal or occipital horns to diffuse periventricular hypodensity with ill-defined margins extending into the deep white matter. The sensitivity of detecting WMC by CT is less than that by MRI in particular when WMC are small or are located at the parieto-occipital and infratentorial regions [94]. Inter-rater agreement of visual rating scale based on CT is generally less than that based on MRI [94, 96] Using CT based visual rating method to monitor WMC progression longitudinally for research purpose is generally not advisable as inter/intra-rater agreement will deem to be low. In principle, visual rating is highly rater dependable and is best used by a single rater for assessment of the same patient. Quantitative method in assessment of WMC by CT has not been applied as the margin between normal and abnormal white matter is poorly delineated by CT. Albeit the above disadvantages, CT findings of WMC may correlate more with clinical severity than that of conventional MRI due to higher specificity in detecting severe WMC by CT, whereas small area of hyperintense white matter signals detected by MRI may have no clinical relevance [97].

Geroldi et al had recently devised a CT-based method to rate the cerebral load of SVD [98]. Apart from severity of WMC, measures of lacunes were also incorporated into the scale. They attempted to construct the rating method with reference to clinical severity. In this rating method, they scored three types of SVD separately: (1) diffuse leukoaraiosis; (2) patchy hypodensity that exists within the leukoaraiosis and fuzzy hypodensity that exists outside the context of leukoaraiosis; and (3) lacunes. Weighting was then assigned to the score of each type of SVD based on its correlation with a scale that measures severity of extrapyramidal signs. A continuous score and an ordinal class with higher values indicating greater severity of SVD were derived accordingly by a formula and statistical methods respectively. The scoring system was found to have good inter/intra-rater reliability and correlation with vascular risk factors and physical impairment. Furthermore, patients diagnosed to have severe SVD based on conventional method were found more often to have higher class while those with AD were found more often to have lower class.

Figure 2. Subcortical vascular dementia

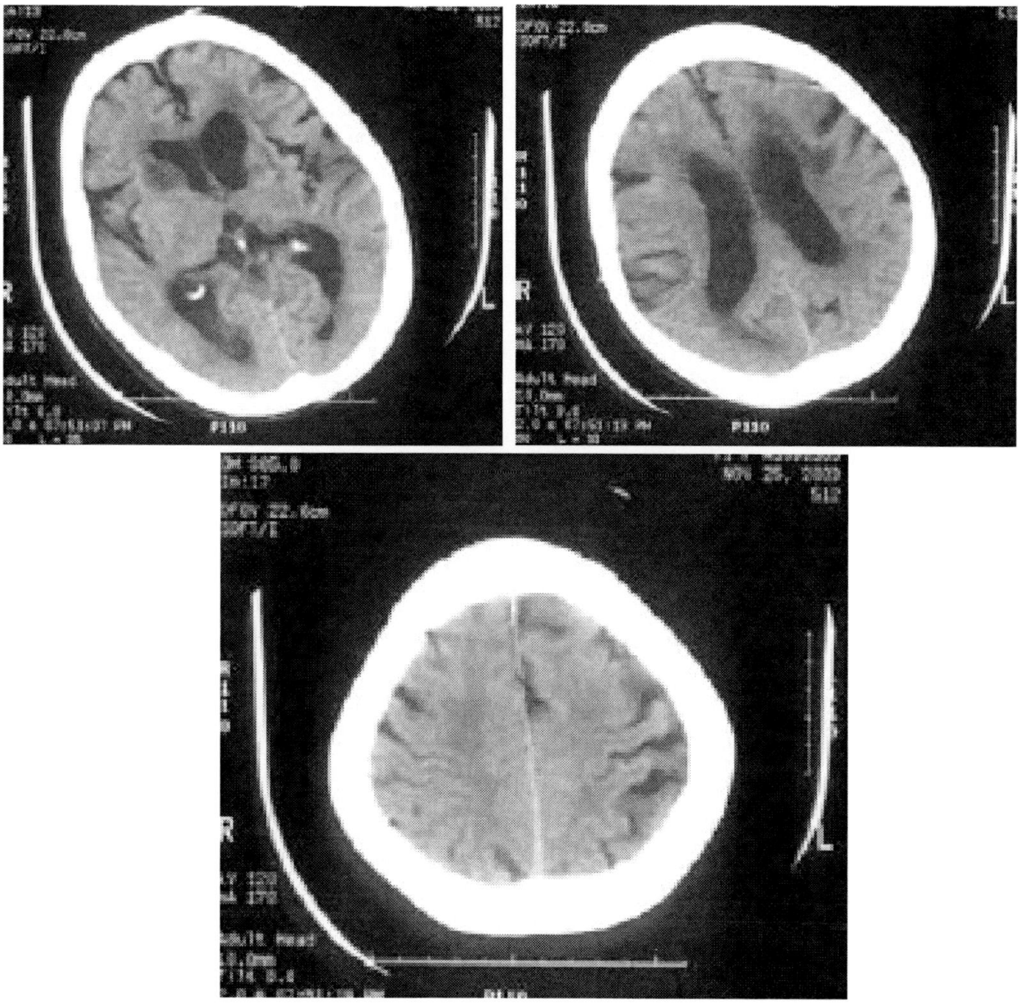

Figure 2a. Computed Tomography

Patient is a 73-year-old female with hypertension who presented with fall and acute confusion. Examination revealed small step gait with postural instability. Her MMSE was only 5/30. Initial CT (figure 2a) reveals multiple lacunar infarcts (more lacunar infarcts are present on other slices that are not shown here) and periventricular WMC extending into the centrum semiovale, with left side slightly more sever than the right side.

Note that radiological WMC are not only related to vascular etiology, and can be related to non-ischemic etiologies, e.g. multiple sclerosis, cerebral malignancy, or post radiation. Hence, acquiring patients' clinical background is important to interpret the nature of WMC during the evaluation of PSD.

### *3. Brain Atrophy*

Method in assessing cerebral atrophy for PSD is similar to that in assessing for any dementia. Cortical, subcortical, general, or regional atrophy can be assessed qualitatively and quantitatively by CT using various methods [89, 90]. Widening of cortical sulci and fissures with relatively normal ventricular size reflect predominant cortical atrophy. Ventricular enlargement with relatively normal cortical sulci and fissures reflect predominant subcortical atrophy. Pattern of regional atrophy may also provide diagnostic clue for PSD. For example, severe predominant frontal lobe atrophy in PSD may suggest concurrent frontotemporal dementia. Ventricular enlargement of temporal horn and sylvian fissure enlargement may support concurrent AD in a demented patient with stroke and progressive prestroke cognitive impairment.

Various CT based visual rating scales on enlargement of sulci /fissures and ventricles are available [90, 93]. As in visual rating for WMC, standard template has been used as reference in grading cortical and subcortical atrophy. Linear measurements on the width of sulci /fissures and various regions of the ventricle may provide a more objective measure than visual scales. Linear measurements for the ventricle commonly include maximal distance between the lateral borders of the frontal horns, the sum of the shortest distances between the caudate and the anterior end of the septum pellucidum, the maximal width of the third ventricle, or the width of the bodies of the lateral ventricles at their waist. Apart from using the actual width of the ventricles, it is also common to divide the ventricular width by the width of the brain at the same level so as to take into account for the individual variation of the brain or head size. This gives the ventricular brain ratio (VBR), [99] which is more of an index for general cerebral atrophy and is probably a more relevant index to cognitive impairment than the actual ventricular width [100]. Some had used the summation of various ventricular measures and divide it by the brain width to represent cerebral atrophy [101].

Planimetric measurement (cross sectional area) of the inter-hemispheric fissure, the brain surface area, or ventricular size, at a particular level can be determined quantitatively via the CT workstation [102, 103]. Finally, volumetric measurement for CSF space, intracranial or brain volume is also possible with various CT automated techniques [90, 92]. Area based VBR, volume based VBR or ventricular cranial ratio (VCR) can be calculated accordingly. Volumetric method is probably the best CT related measurement for assessing cerebral atrophy in terms of sensitivity, specificity, and reliability both for cross-sectional study or longitudinal study that evaluates progression of atrophy [90, 103] Although quantitative CT density has been used as a measurement for cerebral atrophy in the past, this method is now considered to be obsolete due to its invalidity in reflecting cerebral atrophy [90]. The limitation of CT in the assessment of atrophy of the medial temporal or hippocampal region has been discussed.

## T1-, T2- and PD Weighted and FLAIR Magnetic Resonance Imaging

T1-, T2-, PD, and/or FLAIR that are based on spin echo (SE) techniques have become standard MRI protocols for the evaluation of ischemic PSD for many centers. Relative to CT, MRI in general has better differentiation between anatomical structures (e.g. gray matter, white matter and CSF), greater ease of imaging at different planes, e.g. coronal or sagittal, greater sensitivity in detecting infarcts, lacunar infarcts, or WMC, and better visualization of structures at the temporal region and posterior fossa given the absence of bone-hardening artifact and availability of coronal plan. Furthermore, different sequence that yields unique or complementary information can be obtained at a single scanning session, although a longer scanning time relative to CT is required. All these advantages of MRI make it the preferred imaging modality over CT in the evaluation of PSD.

### *1. Brain Lesions*

Cerebral infarct is usually assessed by axial T1-weighted MRI and is seen as hypointense area. Principles of evaluation are similar to that used for CT. Site, laterality, pattern of infarct are determined. Coronal and/or sagittal section may help to better visualize the extent of infarct. As in CT, size of infarct on MRI can be represented by simple linear measurements of the widest diameter of the infarct. Areas and volumes of infarcts can be determined by various formulas or computerized program. Special caution is given to differentiate between lacunar infarct and perivascular space on MRI. Perivascular space is more visible on MRI than on CT given the better resolution of the former modality. Perivascular spaces are commonly located in the basal ganglia and centrum ovale. It may be punctate or linear. As with lacunar infarct, it is hypointense on T1-weighted imaging. In general, perivascular space is smaller than lacunar infarct. Pathological study with MRI correlation found that size of <3mm in diameter was highly predictive of perivascular space, [104] except around the anterior commissure, where perivascular spaces could be large. This criterion has been used in most studies for its differentiation. Methods of T1- and T2-weighted MRI in evaluation of ICH for PSD follow that of evaluation for stroke and will not be discussed in this review.

### *2. White Matter Changes*

Relative to CT, MRI is superior in the detection of WMC. Traditionally, SE axial PD weighted and T2-weighted MRI imaging is used in the evaluation of WMC. In general, T1-weighted imaging is insensitive to detection of WMC (figure 2b) [105]. On PD weighted image, WMC are hyperintense but signal intensity is lower for CSF. Evaluation of periventricular WMC is hence best performed by PD weighted image because delineation between CSF and WMC is easier with PD weighted image, while it may sometimes be difficult with T2-weighted imaging as both appear bright on T2-weighted. Some center prefers using T2-weighted imaging over PD weighted in the evaluation of deep WMC as better contrast is exhibited between lesions and white matter with the former image [100] Note that recently fast SE has been increasingly used to acquire T2- and PD weighted imaging in view of time consideration. However, the CSF signal is brighter than that in a conventional SE, making differentiation between periventricular WMC and ventricle slightly more difficult. Hence, a "true" PD weighted image cannot be obtained with fast SE. A more recent technique in the evaluation of WMC is the use of FLAIR, where the CSF signal is attenuated by the use of a long inversion time that nullifies the signal of water (figure 2d). Periventricular WMC is hence easily differentiated from the ventricular CSF. Some studies have suggested that FLAIR is more sensitive and accurate in detection of periventricular and subcortical lesions than that of PD/T2-weighted imaging [94, 106] However, sensitivity of

FLAIR is reduced at the posterior fossa and diencephalon region. It is as yet uncertain whether FLAIR can replace T2/PD weighted imaging in the evaluation of WMC.

Several descriptions on WMC related hyperintense signals on T2/PD-weighted or FLAIR have been used.

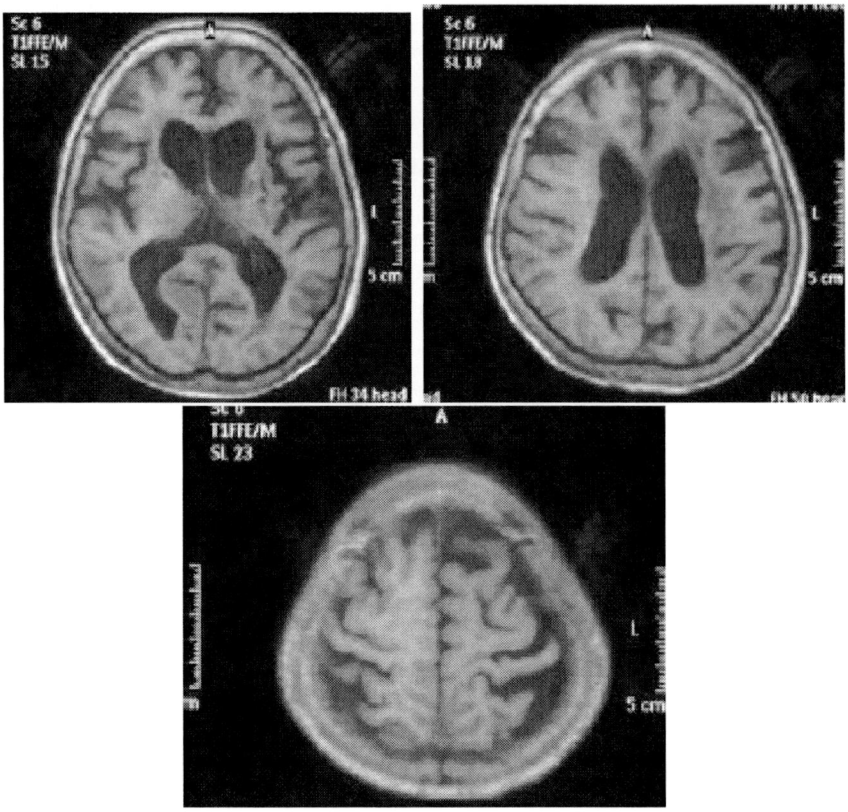

Figure 2b. T1-weighted

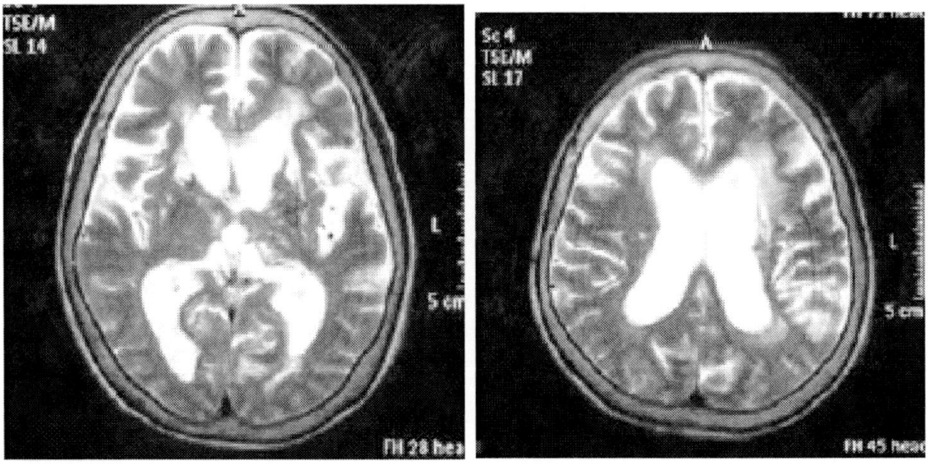

Figure 2c. Continued on next page

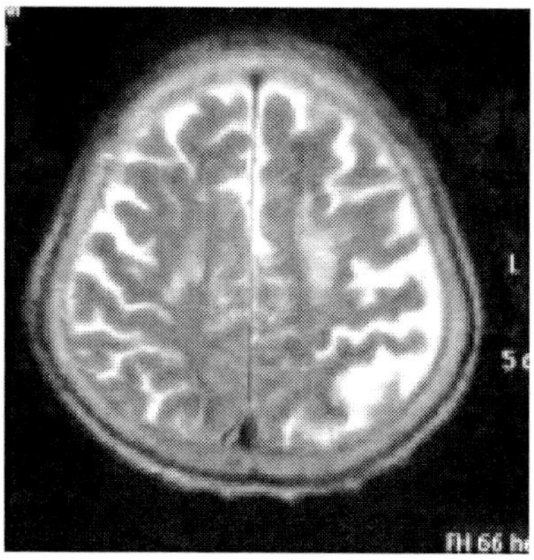


Figure 2c. T2-weighted

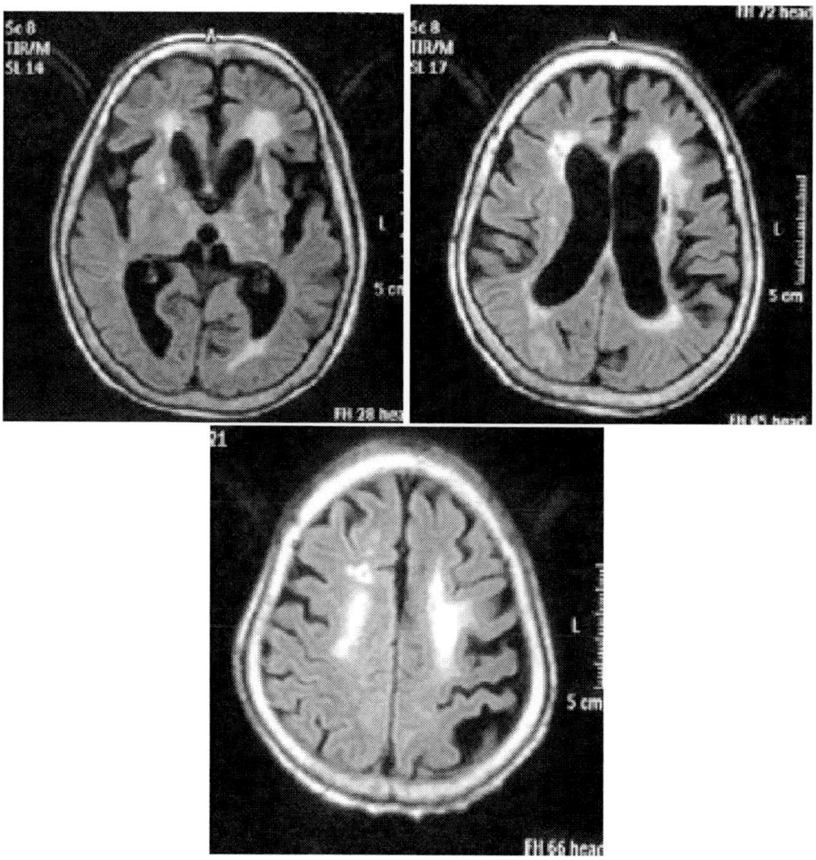


Figure 2d. FLAIR

MRI was performed 6 months after the event. T1-weighted (figure 2b) reveals multiple small hypointensities (lacunar infarcts). WMC are not well-visualized on T1weighted relative to T2-weighted (figure 2c) or FLAIR (figure 2d). Cortical atrophy of the frontal and parietal lobe (widening of Sylvian fissures and sulci, more prominent on the left) is present. Note that delineation between WMC and CSF is much more easier on FLAIR than that on T2-weighted.

Hyperintensities around frontal and occipital horns are called "caps" and those around the lateral ventricles are described as "bands", "rims", "linings", "smooth halo", or "irregular" hyperintensities extending into the deep white matter. "Punctate", "focal", "patchy", and "confluent" have been used to describe extent of WMC, mostly at the deep white matter region.

On T2- weighted, PD weighted, or FLAIR imaging, WMC need to be distinguished from perviascular space. Perivascular space is hyperintense on T2-weighted, hypointense on FLAIR and relative hypointense or poorly visible on PD weighted, while WMC are hyperintense on all 3 imaging.

Both visual and quantitative volumetric methods have been used to assess the severity of WMC on MRI. Multitude of MRI based visual rating scales are available [94, 96, 100, 107-110] and many of it have been summarized by Mantyla et al (see appendix) [111, 112]. The scales are in general more sophisticated than that based on CT given the better visualization of WMC by MRI over CT. Most of the scales rate periventricular and deep white matter region separately because pathology and relevance to cognition may vary with the location [67, 109]. Some scales only rate WMC at either periventricular or deep white matter region, while some scales give a combined rating of both regions [111] Standard templates are commonly used for reference [100, 107]. The Wahlund's scale is applicable for both MRI and CT. [94]. In general, inter-rater agreement of the visual scales are acceptable and few of these scales, e.g. Manolio, Fazekas and Schmidt, and Sheltens and Wahlund, have good correlations with volumetric measures [107, 108, 110, 113]. However, comparative studies have demonstrated that different visual scales probably measure different aspects of WMC. This may explain the inconsistent findings regarding the frequency, extent, and clinical correlates of WMC [111]. Furthermore, for assessment of progression of WMC, studies found that visual scales showed little correlation with volumetrics and low inter-rater agreement [112, 114]. On this regard, a new "white matter lesion change scale" was recently proposed, showing better correlation with volumetric measure over time [112].

Volume of WMC can be determined quantitatively with MRI workstation using various automated methods [112-114]. Although volumetric measurement is probably the best method for both cross-sectional and longitudinal studies of WMC and its progression, the assessment time is longer and level of expertise is greater than that required with visual methods. Note that the volume of WMC can be represented as ratio over total brain or cranial volume too [115].

### *3. Brain Atrophy*

Evaluation of brain atrophy with MRI provides more information with greater accuracy than that with CT because different planes and better visualization are possible with MRI. The usual protocol for atrophy measures includes axial and 3 dimensional coronal T1-weighted imaging. Global cortical atrophy can be assessed qualitatively by evaluation of size of sulci/fissures on axial T1-weighted imaging [107]. Qualitative regional cortical atrophy is also possible with frontal lobe (axial), [100] parietal lobe (coronal), [100] and medial temporal lobe (coronal) [100, 116]. Model templates for reference are commonly used [100, 107] Most of these visual methods have acceptable inter-rater agreement. Surface area of the corpus callosum can also be quantified via software program, yet a mid-sagittal plane is needed for its assessment [117]. Note that if the detection of hippocampal sclerosis is important, additional coronal T2-weighted or FLAIR image is also needed, which may demonstrate hippocampal hyperintensity in the presence of sclerosis. Recently, sophisticated quantitative volumetric method for assessing atrophy of cortical gray matter, both global and regional cortical atrophy, had been applied for study of PSD [115].

Apart from cortical atrophy, total brain, hemispheric and regional volumes including hippocampal volume can all be quantified by MRI techniques [115, 118, 119]. Longitudinal evaluation of change in cerebral atrophy can be done either serially, or more recently, by the registration plus subtraction technique [120].

Qualitative ratings of ventricular size using MRI have been used [107, 119]. Similar to CT, linear and planimetric measurements of the ventricle can be obtained via MRI and the data is usually represented as ratio over the respective brain measures to give the VBR [100, 121]. Absolute ventricular volume, volume based VBR or VCR can all be obtained by MRI and are relevant to study of dementia [115, 118].

## PET, SPECT, and Xenon CT

While CT and above MRI sequences provide structural information, PET, SPECT, and xenon CT provide information on cerebral perfusion and/or metabolism, which reflect pathological process that is undetectable by structural imaging [36, 87, 92, 122-129]. These functional imaging techniques have been used in the study of PSD for over 2 decades.

### *1. Positron Emission Tomography*

Positron emission tomography is the most sensitive and comprehensive, yet expensive functional imaging. It is able to determine quantitatively regional cerebral blood flow (CBF), oxygen metabolism ($CMRO_2$), oxygen extraction fraction (OEF), and /or glucose metabolism (CMRgl). $^{15}$Oxygen steady state technique is commonly used for the determination of CBF, $CMRO_2$, and OEF, while flurodeoxyglucose tagged with $^{18}$Fluroine (18 FDG) is the most commonly used isotope for determination of CMRgl in study of PSD. Strength of PET is that viability or metabolic reserve of brain tissue can be reflected by the pattern of metabolic parameters. For instance, increased OEF associated with reduced CBF and reduced/preserved $CMRO_2$ suggests misery perfusion and pending infarction.

### *2. Single Photon Emission Computed Tomography*

Single photon emission computed tomography is less sensitive, yet less costly, and can provide regional cerebral semi-quantitative assessment on CBF. However, oxygen metabolism cannot be measured by SPECT. Furthermore, different to PET, it provides only ratios of perfusion at region of interest relative to another brain region and absolute CBF cannot be provided. $^{99}Tc^{m}$ labeled derivative of hexamethyl propylene amine oxime (MHPAO) has been the most frequently used tracer for study of PSD.

Since spatial resolution of PET and SPECT is poor, techniques in co-registering PET and SPECT images to CT or MRI have been used recently.

### 3. Xenon CT

Similar to SPECT, xenon CT only measures CBF. Although the intravenous $^{133}$xenon method had been used to study PSD, [130] it has been replaced by stable xenon inhalation method. The later method permits differentiated measurement of cortical and subcortical structures. Although as in PET, absolute CBF can be determined, the potential side effects of inhaled xenon and its associated motion artifacts related to patient's movements, and the need of meticulous monitoring during the procedure, (e.g. electroencephalogram, electrocardiogram, blood pressure, arterial oxygen saturation, and/or end tidal carbon dioxide concentration), make use of xenon CT relatively limited.

### 4. Cerebral Vasoreactivity

Apart from cerebral perfusion and metabolism, cerebral vasoreactivity can also be assessed using above modalities. Use of inhaled carbon dioxide in the study of cerebral vasoreactivity has now been mostly replaced by acetazolamide due to patient's discomfort associated with the former agent. Intravenous injection of acetazolamide increases CBF by 30-40% in a patient with intact cerebral vasoreactivity. The inability to increase CBF following acetazolamide challenge suggests impaired cerebral vasoreactivity. The change in CBF from baseline can be determined by PET, SPECT, or xenon CT.

### 5. Functions and Findings of PET, SPECT, and Xenon CT in Poststroke Dementia

#### *a. Pathophysiology of White Matter Changes*

To date, studies in PSD using PET, SPECT, or xenon CT have served important functions in the study of PSD. First, it helps to elucidate the pathogenesis of WMC, which is an important substrate in PSD. An early study using $^{15}$oxygen steady state PET technique among patients with subcortical VaD found that CBF was reduced at subcortical white matter region [127]. This further lends support to the ischemic origin for WMC and is consistent with the pathological findings and clinical association between WMC and vascular risk factors [131]. Although this same study failed to demonstrate an increase in OEF at any cerebral region, a later study by De Reuck et al had shown that OEF was significantly increased at all cerebral regions, including the white matter, among patients with lacunar dementia who had reduced CBF and $CMRO_2$. [87] This finding suggests that at least in some patients with subcortical VaD, chronic misery perfusion at the white matter region occurs. This provides insight and opportunity for potential therapeutic intervention. Furthermore, the same group had demonstrated that cerebral vasoreactivity was severely impaired at all cerebral regions using PET study with acetazolamide challenge [132]. Hence, apart from narrowed small arteries, ischemia may be further compounded by impaired regulatory reserve, which is particularly detrimental to the white matter in the presence of postural hypotensive change, low output cardiac failure, or aggressive anti-hypertensive treatment. Note that although, reduced subcortical CBF and CMRgl among patients with severe SVD have been demonstrated by most studies, Sabri et al failed to demonstrate such an association [126].

*b. Mechanisms of Poststroke Dementia*

More importantly, the various functional imaging have helped to elucidate the mechanisms of dementia in PSD, especially for PSD associated with subcortical brain lesions. Studies have consistently demonstrated that subcortical lesions, either single strategic lesion or diffuse ischemic lesions, are associated with cortical hypometabolism and/or hypoperfusion despite absence of structural cortical lesions, [36, 87, 123, 124, 127] and that these metabolic or perfusional abnormalities correlate with cognitive performances [123, 124, 129] and even predict cognitive progression [125]. These findings support that disconnection of subcortical white matter fiber tracts or specific circuits may be responsible for the PSD. An earlier study found that the correlation between hypoperfusion and cognitive impairment was particularly strong among stroke patients (mostly lacunar stroke) with mild dementia (mini-mental state examination [MMSE] of >15), whereas this correlation was weak among severely demented patients with larger infarcts [92]. In the later group, infarct volume was found to be more relevant than hypoperfusion in determining cognitive performance. Though it must be emphasized that in another study, the hypoperfusion was found to extend beyond the infracted areas among those with large infarct, and hence hypoperfusion may also affect cognitive performances independent of volume of infarct even among those with large infarct [87].

*c. Differentiation between Etiologies of Dementia*

Given that unique pattern of hypometabolism and hypoperfusion exists in AD and subcortical ischemic lesions, functional imaging may help to delineate the contribution of each disease in accounting for the dementia poststroke. This is particularly useful in case where such delineation is difficult, e.g. progressive cognitive decline occurs after a small lacunar stroke. Using 18 FDG PET, Reed et al demonstrated that among cognitive impaired stroke patient with subcortical lacunar infarct, memory loss correlated with prefrontal lobe hypometabolism, whereas in AD (but not in subcortical lacunar infarct), memory correlated with hippocampal and temporal lobe hypometabolism [129].

In general, irrespective of subtypes of VaD, pattern of hypometabolism will be more focal, patchy and variable affecting cortical and subcortical areas, compared with typical hypometabolism affecting the parietotemporal association areas seen in AD.

*d. Monitoring Effects of Therapy*

Positron emission tomography has also been utilized in monitoring the effect of drug therapy. An early study demonstrated that CBF as measured by PET could be increased by certain drug (e.g. propentofylline) and this improvement correlated with clinical stabilization [133]. A recent study also evaluated the effect of cholinesterase inhibitor on regional CBF among patients with poststroke VaD [134]. This study shown that the drug increased CBF, which was more significant in the frontal region among the treated patients, and suggested that cholinesterase inhibitor might regulate CBF and such effects were more pronounced in the more affected brain region.

In summary, the value of PET, SPECT, and xenon CT in study of PSD cannot be underestimated. Yet, its cost, complexity and/or the potential problems associated with the availability and use of radioactive tracer, have limited its use mainly for research purpose.

# I. Imaging Determinants for Ischemic Poststroke Dementia

## Poststroke Dementia at 3 Months

Few recent large hospital-based prospective studies have yielded various imaging determinants for PSD based on multivariate regression analyses. Imaging determinants based on studies that evaluated PSD (i.e. including those with prestroke dementia and prior stroke) 3 months poststroke include [17, 48, 50, 70] volume of infarcts in any superior middle cerebral artery, [17] any [48, 70] or number (mostly lacunar infarcts) of left sided infarcts, [17] lacunar infarct, [70] extent of WMC, [17] and medial temporal lobe atrophy [17]. Note that for studies demonstrating the relevance of left sided infarcts, patients with severe aphasia were excluded, [17, 48, 70] hence suggesting that left sided lesions can also be associated with global cognitive impairment. Findings of our recent study are similar to previous studies in that extent of WMC, MCA territorial infarct, and cerebral atrophy measure were found to predict PSD. [50]. It appears that large infarct along MCA territory, lacunar infarcts and its frequency, left sided laterality, extent of WMC, general cerebral atrophy, and medial temporal lobe atrophy all correlate with PSD in general.

Two of the above studies had performed sub-analyses upon those with new onset dementia at 3 months poststroke [17, 50]. Number of relevant imaging features decreased after excluding those with prestroke dementia. Volume of left anterior corona radiata infarct, which is probably a strategic site, became the only determinant in one study [17]. Extent of WMC remained a strong determinant in our study [50]. In general, influence of general cerebral atrophy or medial temporal lobe atrophy decrease when patients with prestroke dementia were excluded. A large proportion of these excluded patients might probably have underlying AD. While vascular factors, such as volume of left sided anterior corona radiata infarct or extent of WMC, play more important role in new onset dementia at 3 months poststroke.

Two recent studies evaluated dementia at 3 months poststroke among those with first stroke (excluding prior stroke). [73, 135]. Volume of left sided anterior corona radiata infarct, [135] large MCA territory infarction, [73] frontal lobe lesion, [73] extent of WMC, [135] and medial temporal lobe atrophy [135] were found to predict dementia. These determinants are similar to studies including patients with any dementia in that the relevance of left sided anterior infarct, extent of WMC, and medial temporal lobe atrophy were demonstrated.

## Delayed Poststroke Dementia

Few studies also evaluated the imaging determinants of delayed PSD at mean follow up of 3-4 years [18, 19, 136]. These studies had excluded those with prestroke dementia. Baseline imaging features that were found to predict delayed PSD were extent of WMC, [19, 136] silent infarct, [19] multiple ischemic lesions (mostly lacunar infarcts), [18] and cortical atrophy [18]. Only one of these studies evaluated the influence of medial temporal lobe atrophy on delayed PSD, but failed to demonstrate such an association [136]. An interesting finding noted by 2 separate studies is that etiology for incident dementia shifted from Alzheimer' type in the first year to VaD type in later years [18, 19]. This suggests that vascular lesions may unmask an underlying asymptomatic AD early on poststroke, while the cerebral vascular load predisposes development of VaD in later years.

The above findings are derived from hospital-based studies, which may not represent the general population. To our knowledge, community study that investigates imaging determinants for PSD is lacking. Yet, the consistent pattern observed in the above hospital-based studies increases the validity of their findings.

## Lacunar Infarct, Cognitive Impairment, and Dementia

Imaging determinants for dementia or cognitive impairment among stroke associated with lacunar infarct have been particularly studied given that SVD is probably the most prevalent form of VaD [14, 86, 95, 115, 126, 137-142]. Although some of these studies investigated imaging correlates among patients with varying severity levels of cognitive impairment, from normal, mild to severe cognitive impairment (dementia) [86, 140-142] and some studies included random sample of patients with lacunar infarcts who might or might not suffer from overt stroke, [86, 115, 141] these studies will also be included given its potential relevance of PSD among lacunar stroke.

Miyao et al found that among those with WMC, more patients developed dementia over a period of 2 years poststroke than those without it [139]. However, influence of cerebral atrophy was not assessed in that study. In another study by Loeb et al, cerebral atrophy, rather than WMC, was found to predict dementia 4 years after lacunar stroke [95]. We demonstrated that WMC correlated with performance in executive tests and not in MMSE, [138] yet its severity did not predict dementia at 3 months after lacunar stroke [14]. Furthermore, when atrophy measures and site of lacunar infarct were added into the analyses, significance of WMC disappeared, whereas left frontal lobe atrophy and presence of thalamic lacune became significant predictors of cognitive performances [142]. Studies by Fein et al and Mungas et al demonstrated that atrophy of cortical gray matter and hippocampus, rather than WMC and lacunar infarcts, was the strongest determinant for dementia and cognitive performances in those with lacunar infarcts; and that WMC mainly correlated with performance on executive measure [115, 137]. Furthermore, baseline cortical atrophy, rather than ischemic measures (WMC and lacunes), was found to predict cognitive decline over a period of 3 years [86]. Sabri et al also noted similar findings in that cerebral atrophy, rather than ischemic measures, predicted cognitive impairment in those with lacunar stroke [126]. The importance of cerebral or cortical atrophy is consistent with findings based on functional imaging studies in that cortical, cerebral or frontal lobe hypometabolism and hypoperfusion were found to correlate with cognitive performances [123, 124, 129].

Yamauchi et al particularly investigated influence of corpus callosal atrophy in patients with lacunar infarcts and WMC and noted that the former predicted performance in MMSE while the later predicted performance in executive task [117].

Based on the above findings, it appears that in patients with lacunar stroke, various measures of brain atrophy, including cerebral, cortical, or regional (frontal lobe, hippocampus, corpus callosum) atrophy, are stronger determinants for cognitive performances and dementia over WMC. White matter changes affect mainly executive function and its association with severe cognitive impairment or dementia is less definitive.

The mechanisms for brain atrophy in patients with lacunar stroke deserve further remarks as one may argue that the atrophy is due to concurrent AD, which may also account for the cognitive impairment. Yet, pattern of cortical atrophy based on structural and functional studies in those with lacunar stroke is different to those with AD [115, 129]. Hypotheses for this atrophy include secondary axonal and trans-synaptic degeneration following primary subcortical ischemic injury and subclinical microinfarcts not visible by neuroimaging. In fact, cortical and callosal atrophy were found to correlate with extent of ischemic WMC [115, 140] The mechanisms for hippocampal atrophy in patients with lacunar infarcts are probably more variable, which include concurrent AD, hippocampal sclerosis, secondary degeneration, subclinical ischemia, or other unknown pathogenic processes [115].

## White Matter Changes and Cognitive Impairment

As mentioned above, WMC are important imaging determinant for PSD and for executive dysfunction. There are certain factors that need also to be considered in the evaluation of the relationship between WMC and cognitive impairment. First, the relationship between WMC and cognitive impairment may not be linear and that a certain severity threshold of WMC may need to be exceeded before significant cognitive decline is induced. Our recent study suggested that the correlation of WMC with executive dysfunction might only be significant for marked WMC [138]. Second, cognitive impact of WMC may vary with its location. Periventricular lesion may induce greater cognitive impairment than deep WMC [109]. Hence studies that evaluated total WMC might dilute the cognitive influence of region specific WMC. Third, cognitive effect of WMC was recently shown to vary with educational level [143]. Those who are highly educated may have normal cognition despite having severe WMC. Fourth, the conventional imaging techniques may be either too sensitive or non- specific in detecting actual ischemic white matter lesions, given that radiological WMC may represent varying pathological changes as discussed previously [67]. Last, traditional criteria were used in many studies to define dementia. These criteria place less emphasis on executive dysfunction. Furthermore, psychometric batteries used in studies might not be comprehensive for the assessment of executive dysfunction. Hence, the impact of WMC might be underestimated.

## Strategic Infarct Dementia (Figure 1)

Over the years, small case series reported the occurrence of new onset persistent dementia after a single stroke involving certain strategic areas in the absence of other relevant brain lesions such as severe WMC or atrophy that might account for the dementia. These areas include thalamus, angular gyrus, genu of the left internal capsule, anterior corpus callosum, inferior medial temporal lobe, hippocampus, frontal lobe, and caudate nucleus [34-

37]. Strategic single infarct dementia accounts less than 10% of VaD [35]. Although, exact data regarding concomitant WMC and brain atrophy are lacking in most of these case series, most authorities accept this concept.

## Cerebellar Infarct and Cognitive Impairment

Although risk of PSD after cerebellar infarct is lower relative to hemispheric infarct and association between cerebellar stroke and dementia has not been emphasized, [48] case series on infratentorial infarct (mostly cerebellar infarct) based on MRI demonstrated that executive function and visuospatial skills were impaired in cerebellar infarct, furthermore, global intelligence decline or dementia might result if large areas are involved. This study suggested the existence of certain cerebrocerebellar circuits that may be relevant to both motor and cognitive functions [144].

## CADASIL and Imaging Features

CADASIL is an inhereditary disease affecting small arteries secondary to mutations within the *Notch3* gene and is associated with young stroke, dementia, migraine-like headaches, seizures, and other behavioral and motor features similar to that of subcortical VaD. Although in general it is uncommon, it is the commonest form of genetic form of PSD. Imaging features are similar to that of subcortical VaD, in that diffuse WMC and multiple lacunar infarcts are present. Yet certain imaging features help to differentiate between the two. Auer et al demonstrated with MRI (T2-weighted and FLAIR) that CADASIL patients had more extensive bilateral temporal, temporopolar and superior frontal WMC and bilateral signal reductions within the dentate nucleus, deep cerebellar white matter, crus cerebri, and thalamus [145]. Imaging determinants of cognitive impairment in CADASIL include quantitative volume of WMC on MRI [146] and cerebral hypometabolism on PET [147].

### *Perivascular Space and Cognitive Impairment*

Although perivascular space is associated with ageing, SVD, and cerebral atrophy, it is considered to be clinically silent and is not routinely evaluated in PSD. However, dilated and multiple perivascular space (état criblé) may rarely associate with dementia in the absence of other pathologies [148]. Hence, perviascular space must be noted during imaging study if it is particularly severe.

## Imaging Criteria for Poststroke Vascular Dementia (Table 4)

As mentioned earlier in this review, several clinical diagnostic criteria have been proposed to aid in diagnosing VaD and its subtypes [16, 20, 23, 26]. Imaging criteria have been incorporated into few of these criteria as objective evidence for the presence and relevance of CVD [16, 23, 26]. Most of the imaging criteria were developed more than 10 years ago, which were based on studies and case series on PSD that preceded the development of the criteria. Imaging criteria differ from imaging determinants of PSD. The former helps to determine the vascular contribution in PSD while the later predicts whether dementia will develop poststroke. Among the various diagnostic criteria for VaD, the NINDS-AIREN has the most specific imaging criteria and this set of imaging criteria will be discussed first.

**Table 4. Imaging criteria for poststroke dementia**

**4a. Operationalized imaging criteria of NINDS-AIREN criteria**

| |
|---|
| *Topography*<br>- Large-vessel stroke – Large-vessel stroke is an infarction defined as a parenchymal defect in an arterial territory involving the cortical gray matter<br>- ACA – only bilateral ACA infarcts are sufficient to meet the NINDS-AIREN criteria<br>- PCA – infarcts in the PCA territory can be included only when they involve the following regions: Paramedian thalamic infarction: the infarct includes the cortical gray matter of the temporal/occipital lobe and extends into the paramedian part (defined as extending to the third ventricle) of the thalamus; the extension may be limited to the gliotic rim of the infarct that surrounds the parenchymal defect<br>- Inferior medical temporal lobe lesions<br>Association areas – an MCA infarction needs to involve the following regions:<br>- Parietotemporal: the infarct involves both the parietal and temporal lobe (e.g, angular gyrus)<br>- Temporo-occipital: the infarct involves both the temporal and occipital lobe<br>Watershed carotid territories – a watershed infarction is defined as an infarct in the watershed area between the MCA and PCA or the MCA and ACA in the following regions:<br>- Superior frontal region<br>- Parietal region<br>Small-vessel disease<br>Ischemic pathology resulting from occlusion of small perforating arteries may manifest itself as lacunes or white matter lesions. Lacune is defined as a lesion with CSF-like intensity on all sequences on MRI (water density on CT) surrounded by white matter or subcortical gray matter > 2mm. Care should be taken not to include Virchow-Robin spaces, which typically occur at the vertex and around the anterior commisure near the substantia perforata. |
| Ischemic white matter lesions are defined as circumscribed abnormalities with high signal on T2-weighted images not following CSF signal (mildly hypodense compared with surrounding tissue on CT) with a minimum diameter of 2 mm.<br>Multiple basal ganglia and frontal white matter lacunes – criteria are met when at lest 2 lacunes in the basal ganglia region (including thalamus and internal capsule) and at lest 2 lacunes in the frontal white matter are present.<br>Extensive periventricular white matter lesions in the white matter abutting the ventricles and extending irregularly into the deep white matter, or deep/subcortical white matter lesions. Smooth caps and bands by themselves are not sufficient. Gliotic areas surrounding large-vessel strokes should not be included here.<br>Bilateral thalamic lesion – to meet the criteria, at least 1 lesion in each thalamus should be present. |

| |
|---|
| *Severity*<br>Large-vessel disease of the dominant hemisphere – if there is a large-vessel infarct as defined above, to meet the criteria it has to be in the dominant hemisphere. In the absence of clinical information, the left hemisphere is considered dominant.<br>Bilateral large-vessel hemispheric strokes – 1 of the infarcts should involve an area listed under topography but is in the nondominant hemisphere, while the infarct in the dominant hemisphere does not meet the topography criteria.<br>Leukoencephalopathy involving at lest ¼ of the total white matter when they are confluent (grade 3 in the ARWMC scale) in at least 2 regions of the ARWMC scale and beginning confluent (grade 2 in the ARWMC scale) in 2 other regions. A lesion is considered confluent when >20 mm or consists of ≥2 smaller lesions fused by more than connecting bridges.<br><br>*Fulfillment of radiological criteria for probable VaD*<br>Large-vessel disease – both the topography and severity criteria should be met (a lesion must be scored in at least 1 subsection of both topography and severity).<br>Small-vessel disease – for white matter lesions, both the topography and severity criteria should be met (a lesion must be scored in at least 1 subsection of both topography and severity); for multiple lacunes and bilateral thalamic lesions, only the topography criterion is sufficient. |

ACA indicates anterior cerebral artery; PCA, posterior cerebral artery; MCA, middle cerebral artery; CSF, cerebrospinal fluid; and ARWMC, age-related white matter changes.

**4b. Imaging criteria for subcortical VaD**

| |
|---|
| *A. Computed tomography*<br>Extending periventricular and deep white matter lesions: patchy or diffuse symmetrical areas of low attenuation (intermediate density between that of normal white matter and that of intraventricular cerebrospinal fluid) with ill defined margins extending to the centrum semiovale, and at least one lacunar infarct.<br>AND<br>Absence of cortical and/or cortico-subcortical non-lacunar territorial infarcts and watershed infarcts, haemorrhages indicating large vessel disease, signs of normal pressure hydrocephalus, and specific causes of white matter lesions (e.g. multiple sclerosis, sarcoidosis, brain irradiation).<br>*B. Magnetic resonance imaging*<br>- To include predominantly "white matter cases"; extending periventricular and deep white matter lesions: extending caps (>10 mm as measured parallel to ventricle) or irregular halo (>10 mm broad, irregular margins and extending into deep white matter) and diffusely confluent hyperintensities (>25 mm, irregular shape) or extensive white matter change (diffuse hyperintensity without focal lesions), and lacune(s) in the deep gray matter.<br>OR<br>- To include predominantly "lacunar cases": multiple lacunes (e.g. >5) in the deep gray matter and at least moderate white matter lesions: extending caps or irregular halo or diffusely confluent hyperintensities or extensive white matter changes.<br>AND<br>- Absence of cortical and/or cortico-subcortical non-lacunar territorial infarcts and watershed infarcts, haemorrhages, signs of normal pressure hydrocephalus, and specific causes of white matter lesions (e.g. multiple sclerosis, sarcoidosis, brain irradiation). |

**4c. Pullicino's imaging criteria**

| Grade | Description | Criteria† |
|---|---|---|
| 0 | VaD absent | No infarcts; WMS, <3; VI, any dimension |
| 1 | VaD unlikely | Single infarct; VOL, <100 mL; Vl, any dimension |
| 2 | VaD possible | Multiple infarcts; VOL, <100 mL; Vl, ≥60 |
| | | Infarct(s); VOL, ≥100 mL; Vl, <60 |
| | | WMS, 3; Vl, ≥60 |
| | | WMS, 4; Vl, <60 |
| 3 | VaD probable | Infarct(s); VOL, ≥100 mL; Vl, ≥60 |
| | | WMS, 4; Vl, ≥60 |

VOL, infarct volume; Vl, ventricular index; and WMS, white matter scale. †Each line gives a different allowable combination for that particular grade.

## NINDS-AIREN Imaging Criteria (Tables 1b and 4a)

The NINDS-AIREN task force emphasized that probable VaD could not be made without imaging abnormality in vivo irrespective of any stroke like clinical or physical features [16]. Although recognizing there are no pathognomonic brain CT or MRI images for VaD, they proposed a list of radiological findings describing both "topography" and "severity" of the lesions that favor diagnosis of VaD. The strength of the NINDS-AIREN criteria is its high specificity in diagnosing VaD, [149] hence it has been the most widely used criteria in clinical studies. However, its sensitivity is low [25]. Patients with genuine poststroke VaD may be excluded from the study and hence findings from studies may not be generalized (figure 3). Furthermore, van Straaten et al found that the inter-rater agreement on its imaging criteria was low [150]. Part of the reason they noted was that specifications on certain items are lacking in the original criteria. For examples, the original criteria did not specify the exact number that is needed to be qualified as "multiple" lacunar infarcts, or the methods in approximating 25% of the total white matter for defining extensive WMC. In the same study, they discussed areas of uncertainties and then they operationalized it by adding relevant specifications, yet without changing the key contents of the criteria (table 4a). Inter-rater agreement improved slightly afterwards, mainly among the experienced raters.

Note that although the NINDS-AIREN criteria may help to determine the vascular contribution in a stroke patient with dementia, it may not predict the development of dementia poststroke. Ballard et al recently shown that among 125 consecutive stroke patients without prestroke dementia, no significant differences were noted between patients with and without PSD on any criteria of the imaging parameters within the NINDS-AIREN criteria [151]. The only different imaging feature was that hippocampal atrophy was more severe in those with PSD over those without PSD. Note that the average age of that cohort was about 10 years older than that of other studies on PSD. Hence, the predictive power of the NINDS-AIREN criteria for development of dementia is low, which may be particularly true among older stroke patients where hippocampal atrophy may have greater cognitive influence.

In summary, we propose that modification is needed for the NINDS-AIREN imaging criteria to improve its sensitivity and the criteria should preferably be operationalized to improve its inter-rater agreement.

## Imaging Criteria for Subcortical VaD (Table 4b)

As mentioned earlier, research criteria have been recently proposed for diagnosis of subcortical VaD [26]. Imaging criteria based on both CT and MRI have been incorporated into this set of criteria. The extent of WMC and number of lacunar infarcts has been specified. Similar to NINDS-AIREN imaging criteria, it serves not to predict dementia among stroke patients. Yet, applying this set of imaging criteria among stroke patients, significantly more demented patients were noted among those with MRI fulfilling the criteria (40.7%) than patients with MRI not fulfilling the criteria (28.7%). Furthermore, those with MRI-defined severe SVD had less severe stroke but greater functional dependence, more depression, and apraxic gait disorders than those with other stroke subtypes. Albeit the imaging criteria have not been subjected to pathological validation study, it appears that the criteria are able to select a unique group of patients.

## ADDTC (Table 1c)

Overall, the ADDTC is more conservative in linking particular type and pattern of vascular related brain lesions with dementia [23]. Hence, the imaging criteria are less stringent and specific than the NINDS-AIREN. To qualify a demented case as probable ischemic VaD, the criteria only require evidence of at least one infarct outside the cerebellum by CT or T1-weighted MRI. Presence of multiple infarcts in brain regions known to affect cognition is considered as supportive of probable VaD. However, the exact number and sites of brain infarcts have not been specified. Although periventricular and deep WMC on T2-weighted MRI that are excessive for age are mentioned to be potentially related with VaD, the criteria suggest that further research is needed before defining its relevance. Overall, given the less restrictions, the ADDTC has higher sensitivity than the NINDS-AIREN criteria, yet its specificity is lower [24, 25].

## Imaging Criteria by Pullicino et al. [84] (Table 4c)

Pullicino et al proposed imaging criteria that could be used to predict the certainty of VaD [84]. The design of the criteria was based on the assumption that severity of vascular related brain damage correlates with the proportion of vascular component that contributes to the dementia syndrome and to the severity of dementia. The severity of vascular brain damage is reflected by the number and volume of infarcts (estimation by formula), severity of WMC (visual rating), and atrophy index[101] based on CT. Certainty of VaD is divided into four grades. Using these criteria with NINDS-AIREN as the reference, 78% of patients with grade 3 severity were classified correctly as having probable VaD, while 7% of those with grade 0 severity were classified correctly as no VaD. Intermediate grades (1 or 2) probably reflected mixed dementia. Furthermore, imaging grading was found to correlate with severity of cognitive impairment among those with CVD. The limitations of these criteria however are that small strategic infarcts may be misclassified as having no VaD and that severe WMC may not always associate with severe cognitive impairment. Although further modification and validation against pathology study is needed before its clinical application, this study highlights the potential utility of incorporating qualitative and/or quantitative assessment of multiple measures of vascular related brain lesions into the imaging criteria for VaD.

### Other Imaging Criteria

The lack of imaging criteria in HIS probably affects is sensitivity in detecting vascular components. Loeb and Gandolfo proposed a simplified version of HIS that incorporated imaging features 2 decades ago [152]. They assigned score of 2 and 3 for those with isolated and multiple CT hypodensity respectively. However, its application in recent studies is scarce. In DSM IV [21] and ICD-10 [22] criteria for VaD, need of imaging evidence for CVD is only optional.

## J. Recent Imaging Applications in PSD

Recent imaging applications in PSD include using either advanced techniques or techniques that have been well established in other areas but have recently been applied also in PSD. Most of these techniques revolve around MRI.

### Diffusion Weighted Imaging

In brief, DWI measures the self-diffusion of water. In conventional MRI, diffusion effects are negligible. Application of a strong magnetic field gradient to an imaging pulse sequence allows diffusion sensitivity to be measurable. Strength and deviation of the gradient pulse determine the degree of diffusion weighting, which is expressed by the "b-value" of the sequence in s/mm$^2$. Higher b values of up to 1000 s/mm$^2$ are required to obtain a good contrast. Diffusion gradients are applied in at least 3 orthogonal directions. These images are usually combined to give the "trace" image, which represents the geometric mean of the individual images. In regions of acute cerebral infarcts where diffusion of water is restricted, the lesions appear hyperintense on DWI (figure 2f). Apparent diffusion coefficients (ADC) map can also be calculated from acquisitions with different b-values. In infarcted tissues with restricted water mobility, ADC maps appear dark and the regional ADC value is lower (figure 2f). Its superiority in detection of acute cerebral infarct over that of conventional MRI has been well established. In PSD, DWI may help to determine the site of acute infarct accurately during the first few days poststroke and to differentiate between acute and old/silent infarcts with reference to conventional MRI.

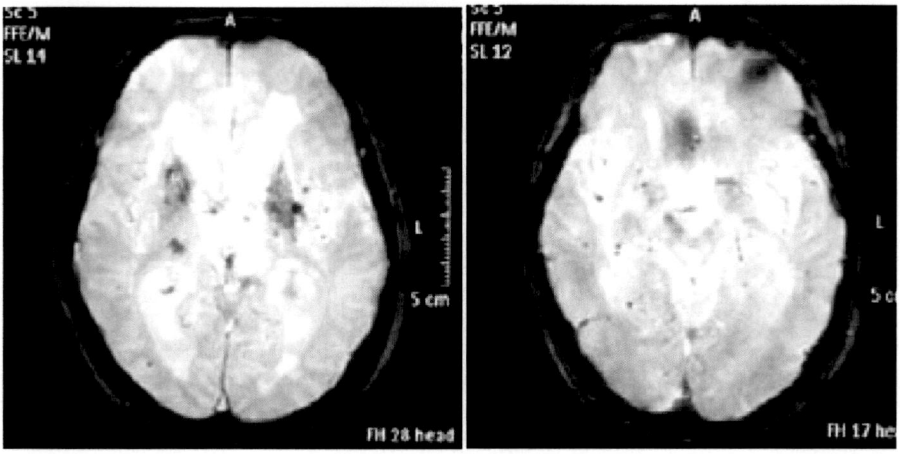


Figure 2e. T2*GE

Recent studies have suggested the potential of using DWI in assessing disease activity in those with SVD, subcortical VaD, or CADASIL [153, 154]. These studies demonstrated the occasional presence of "subclinical" recent lacunar infarcts based on DWI among patients with lacunar infarcts (8%), subcortical VaD (20%), and CADASIL (10.5%) who had no recent overt stroke event. The authors suggested that that presence of recent subclinical infarcts might reflect active disease. Further study is needed to assess whether it predicts rate of cognitive decline and whether it can be used as a surrogate marker in clinical trials.

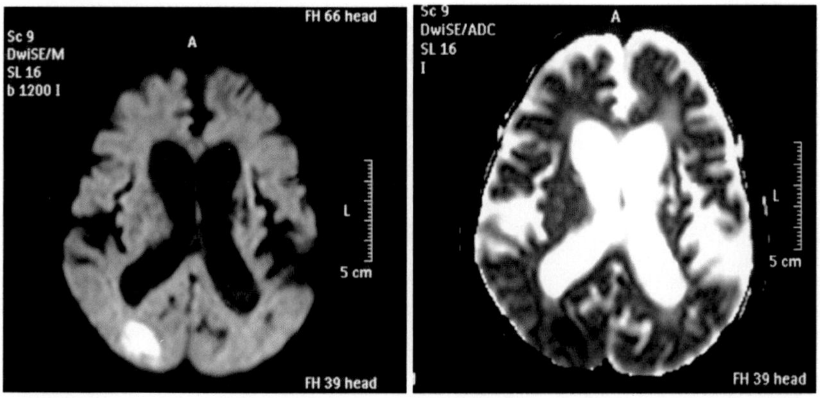


Figure 2f. DWI (left) and ADC map (right)

T2* GE MRI (figure 2e) of the same patient showing scattered small round hyointensities of varying size, which represent microbleeds. DWI at b=1200 s/mm$^2$ (figure 2f, left) reveals a "subclinical" acute infarct (hyperintense) at right occipital area that corresponds with hypointensity on the ADC maps (figure 2f, right). The patient was clinically stable at time of MRI. Note that the size of the acute infarct is relatively large and is located near the surface. MRA (not shown here) revealed severe stenosis of the posterior cerebral artery. This patient had mixed large and small artery disease.

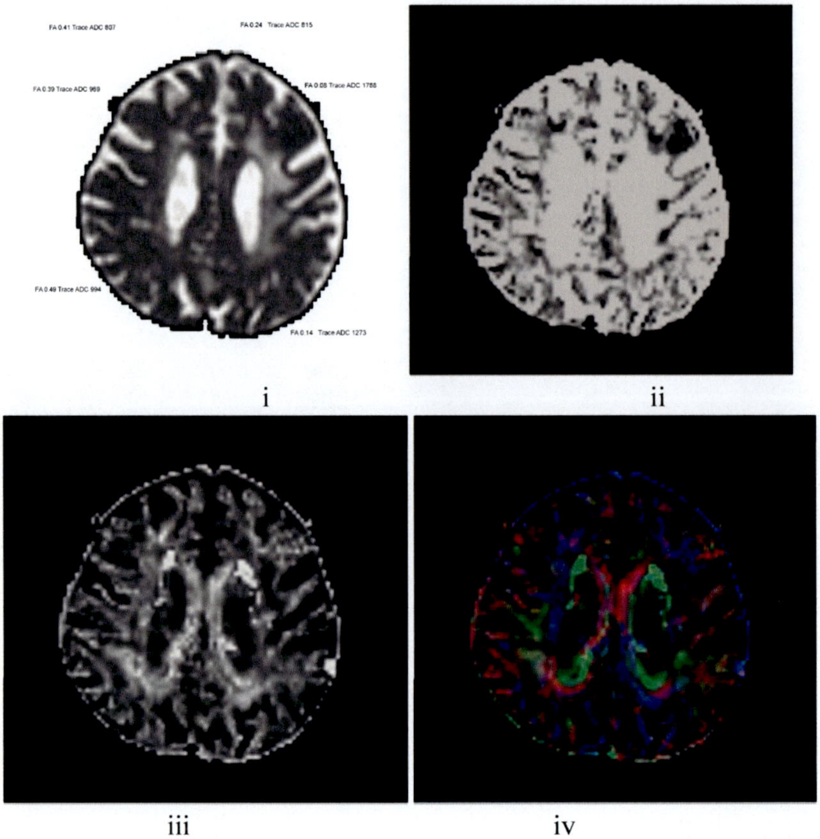


Figure 2g. i. B0; ii. Diffusion trace; iii. FA; iv. Color FA

Regions of interest were placed at normal appearing white matter on right (yellow cross) and left side (red cross) (figure 2g I, B0 image). The diffusion trace (figure 2g ii, x$10^9$ s/mm$^2$) at the left red cross (0.615) was slightly higher than that on the right yellow cross (0.607), while the FA (figure 2g iii) at the left (0.24) was lower than that at the right (0.41). This is suggestive of more severe damage of white matter fibre on the left than on the right side. The trace was higher and FA was lower at regions of WMC than that at normal appearing white matter (values not shown). In the color FA (figure 2g iv), each color represents fibres running at different direction (green=anterior-posterior, blue=caudal-cephalic, red=right-left).

## Diffusion Tensor Imaging

Perhaps more important to the study of PSD is the recently developed MR technique of DTI, which is a further development of DWI. In the CSF or gray matter, diffusion is "isotropic", i.e. water can diffuse equally and easily in each direction, while in white matter myelinated fiber, diffusion is restricted in a sense that water molecules move preferentially along a fiber rather than perpendicular to it. This type of diffusion behavior is called "anisotropic" diffusion and the ADC at a point varies according to the direction in which it is measured. Determination of the complete diffusion information requires DWI with at least six diffusion-encoding gradient directions and the diffusion properties are described mathematically by a tensor. A tensor is a matrix of values; each corresponds to a gradient orientation and a cell orientation. The diffusion tensor MRI can provide information about the integrity of white matter tracts by estimation of the diffusion trace (i.e. averaged ADC) and the directionality. The later is commonly expressed as the fractional anisotropy (FA).

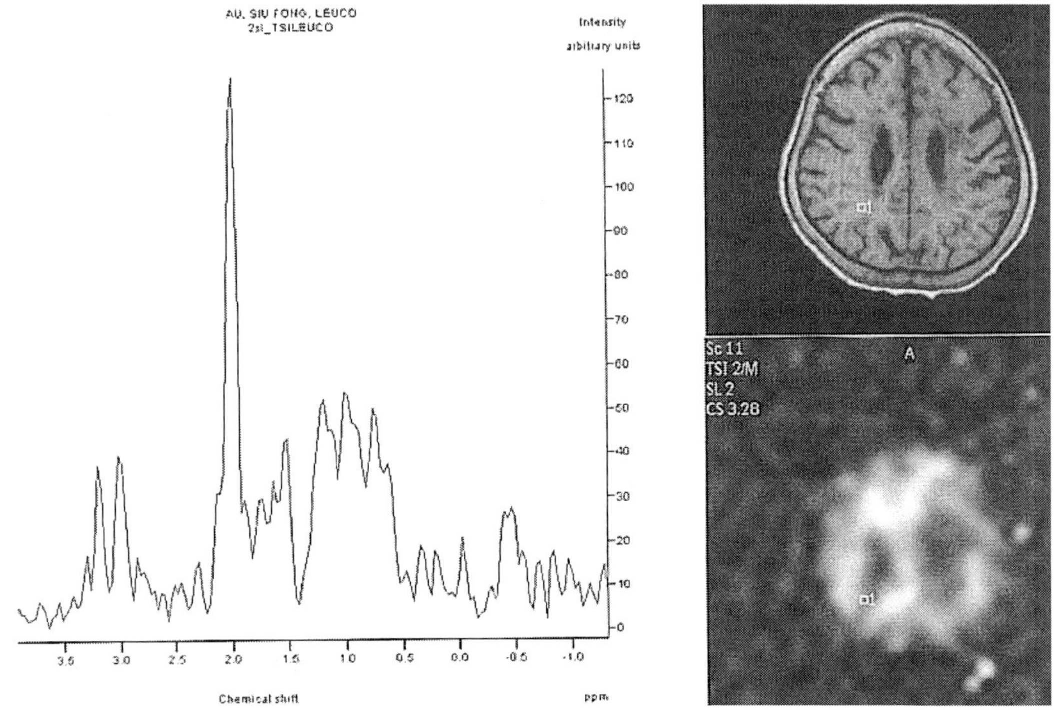


Figure 2h. $^{1}H$ MRS

A single voxel MRS study at right posterior white matter region. The spectrum with various peaks of the metabolites is shown on the right. MRS study at different regions may help to elucidate the mechanism of dementia in subcortical VaD and differentiate it from other types of dementing illnesses (see text).

As mentioned before that WMC as shown on conventional MRI may represent heterogeneous pathologies, DTI can now provide a more specific measure for ischemic pathological WMC, i.e. loss of axons and myelins and gliosis. Jones et al found that in region of WMC, diffusion trace was elevated and FA was reduced, and that the elevation of trace was less than that found in large mature infarcts.[155] These changes are consistent with axonal loss and gliosis as loss of axons will result in increased diffusion, but the extent of this increase is probably limited by the accompanying gliosis, while in infracted areas, the diffusion trace approaches that of free water and may hence be higher than that in areas of WMC. Furthermore, loss of ordered axonal tracts and the accompanying non-directionally orientated gliosis result in marked loss of FA.

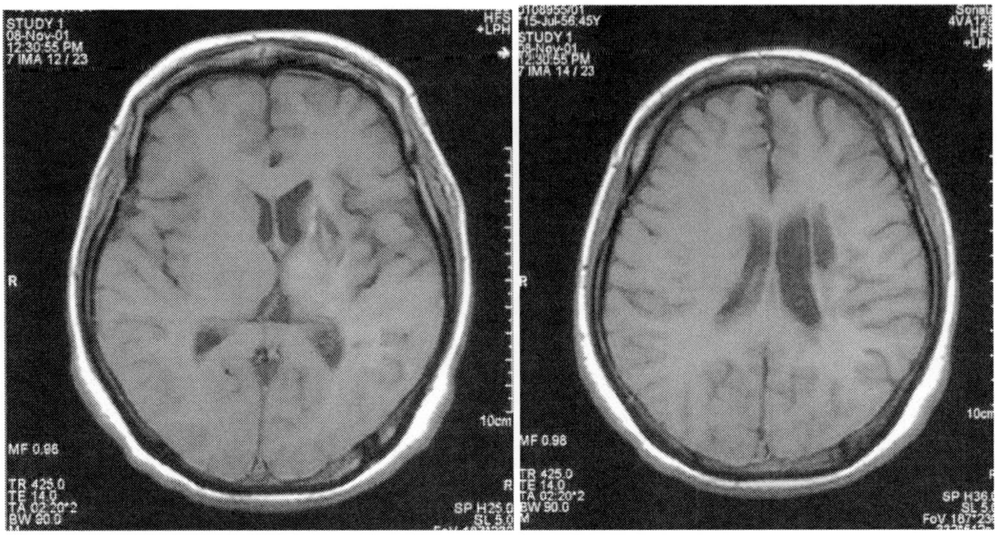


Figure 3. A case of poststroke vascular dementia not fulfilling NINDS-AIREN imaging criteria

> The patient is a 45-year-old woman with poststroke dementia. Her dementia developed within 3 months after the stroke episode. At 1 year poststroke, she had residual mild expressive aphasia, poor attention span, anterograde memory loss, emotional lability, and depression. Her MMSE was 19/30. T1-weighted MRI shows left lentiform nucleus infarct (left) extending to the left corona radiata (right) with compensatory dilation of the lateral ventricle. MRA (not shown) showed severe stenosis of the left MCA. Even though the patient clearly had poststroke VaD, she was excluded from a multi-center drug trial, as her imaging features do not fulfill the imaging criteria of NINDS-AIREN.

O'Sullivan demonstrated recently that diffusion tensor measures (mean diffusivity and FA) on normal appearing white matter among patients with lacunar stroke correlated significantly with executive dysfunction, while measures of lesions (WMC and lacunar infarcts) volume on conventional T1-weighted and FLAIR did not correlate with executive dysfunction [156]. These findings probably suggest that DTI measure for white matter structural abnormality is more sensitive and at the same time more specific than conventional MRI. Interestingly, DTI measures in region of WMC as demonstrated by conventional MRI did not correlate with cognitive measures. Similar findings were also noted in patients with CADASIL by the same group of investigators [157]. A recent longitudinal study using DTI techniques (diffusion trace histograms analyses for the whole brain) also demonstrated its usefulness in monitoring progression of tissue damage among CADASIL patients [158]. Further study is needed to evaluate the correlation between cognitive deterioration and changes in DTI measures over time and its role as a surrogate marker in clinical trials [88]. Note that recent advances in DTI techniques have made fiber-tracking possible and 3 dimensional anatomical details of white matter fibers can be reconstructed via appropriate software programs. Yet its role in the evaluation of PSD needs further research.

## Magnetization Transfer Imaging

Similar to DTI, MTI technique aims also to measure tissue integrity with greater specificity than conventional MRI. Contrast on MTI is based upon interactions between "free" water protons and protons "bound" to macromolecules, e.g. myelin. By using a special off-resonance pulse, which saturates the magnetization of bound protons, magnetization will also be transferred from the free to the bound protons, thus reducing the magnetic resonance signal. Tissue integrity is related to measure of the bound protons. The magnetization transfer data are commonly quantified as the magnetization transfer ratio (MTR), which is obtained by dividing the signal intensities in the region of interest without a magnetization transfer prepulse by those with such a prepulse and multiply by 100. Tissue damage (e.g. ischemic WMC) is reflected by a low MTR, which implies the incapability of macromolecules to exchange magnetization with free water protons.

Although MTI has been used mainly in the study of WMC associated with multiple sclerosis, it has also been recently applied in those with cerebral SVD and CADASIL.[159, 160] Among patients with SVD and normal subjects, although MTR of total MRI visible WMC and non-periventricular WMC were similar between the two groups, MTR of periventricular WMC were significantly lower in patients than that in controls.[160] This suggested that myelin loss might probably be more severe in periventricular WMC relative to other regions of WMC. In another recent study among CADASIL patients, MTR was not only lower in the MRI visible WMC, but was also lower in the normal appearing white and gray matter. Moreover, MTR from all tissues (apart from normal appearing gray matter) were found to correlate with age, physical disability, and cognitive impairment [159]. Overall, these initial findings suggest that similar to DTI, MTI and MTR may be more specific for pathological white matter damage and more sensitive for detection of early disease changes.

## T2$^*$-Weighted GE (Figure 2e)

The superiority of T2$^*$-weighted GE sequence over basic SE sequence in detection of microbleeds has been established. Microbleed is associated with ICH, SVD, stroke patients, hypertensive elderly, CADASIL, or CAA. Microbleed is currently believed to be a manifestation of small arterial damage, in which minimal blood leaks through damaged small artery. Its presence may not only reflect severity of SVD, [161] more importantly, it may predict development of intracerebral bleeding with use of antithrombotic and thrombolytic treatments. Werring et al recently demonstrated that among stroke patients, number and location (basal ganglia and frontal lobes) of microbleeds visible on T2$^*$-weighted GE images correlated significantly with executive dysfunction independent of the extent of WMC.[68] Further study is needed to confirm its relevance to PSD.

### Magnetic Resonance Perfusion

In previous section, the role of PET, SPECT, and xenon CT in elucidating the ischemic origin of WMC by demonstrating reduced CBF at regions of subcortical ischemic lesions had been mentioned. However, there are certain limitations with these standard functional imaging modalities. First, such techniques require exposure to radioactive substance. Second, only semi-quantitative measurements can be obtained by SPECT. Third, poor spatial resolution with these modalities and need of co-registration of PET or SPECT images to MRI/CT, hence making delineation between normal appearing white matter and WMC overall difficult. Recent advance in MRI has now made it possible to perform quantification of CBF using exogenous contrast-based perfusion MRI along with high spatial resolution. This technique was recently applied in the evaluation of WMC among patients with lacunar stroke by O'Sullivan et al. [162]. This study demonstrated clearly that not only CBF was reduced in WMC relative to normal appearing white matter, it was also reduced in normal appearing periventricular white matter among stroke patients relative to that in controls. It will be of paramount importance to investigate whether presence of reduced CBF at normal appearing white matter predicts development of actual WMC, and if that occurs, to further explore therapy that can reverse this perfusion deficit and /or development of WMC.

### Magnetic Resonance Spectroscopy (Figure 2h)

In vivo MRS measures the regional distribution of important metabolites (e.g. N-acetylaspartate [NAA], myo-inositol, creatine [Cr], choline [Cho]-containing compounds) in the brain. Similar to standard functional studies, it can reveal abnormalities that are not visible on structural imaging, and hence can help to understand the mechanisms of cognitive impairment in stroke or differentiation between dementias. It has been increasingly used particularly in the evaluation of cognitive impairment associated with cerebral SVD in recent years [163, 164]. Using proton ($^1$H) MRS, Capizzano et el demonstrated that patients with dementia and lacunaes had reduced NAA not only in white matter region, but also in gray matter region relative to healthy controls [163]. In another study, Schuff et al also demonstrated that patients with SVD had lower NAA in frontal cortex and left parietal cortex relative to that in AD patients and cortical NAA was noted to decrease with increasing WMC and number of lacunes. In the same study, adding parietal NAA to MRI-derived hippocampal atrophy improved separation between SVD and AD from 79% to 89%. This study with MRS confirms the importance of cortical dysfunction associated with subcortical ischemic lesions and suggests a characteristic pattern of metabolite change that may serve as a basis for improved diagnosis.

## L. Take-Home-Messages

Poststroke dementia has been a neglected area although it is common, disabling, and potentially preventable. Different to AD, which is a homogeneous entity, PSD is heterogeneous with complexity far exceeds that of AD or the traditional concept of multi-infarct dementia. Findings from imaging studies have contributed significantly to our present understanding and management of PSD. It is currently believed that PSD may involve complex interactions between vascular etiologies, vascular related brain lesions, brain atrophy, co-existing dementing diseases, host factors, and vascular risk factors. At present, potential treatments depend on its underlying vascular etiology and etiology of dementia; hence, we propose to classify PSD according to these two factors. Basic imaging modalities for the evaluation of PSD are CT and MRI (T1-, T2-, and PD weighted and FLAIR), which can provide relevant imaging variables including vascular related brain lesions (e.g. size, site, laterality, multiplicity, pattern), extent of WMC, and brain atrophy (cortical, subcortical, general, regional). Common imaging variables that predict poststroke VaD include size of left sided anterior corona radiata infarct and extent of WMC. Lesions at other strategic sites (e.g. thalamus, genu of internal capsule, angular gyrus) causing poststroke VaD are generally less common. Although atrophy measures appear to affect cognition more than ischemic measures (WMC and lacunar infarcts) in lacunar stroke, cortical and callosal atrophy correlates with extent of WMC. Findings from xenon CT, PET, and SPECT have also contributed to our understanding of the pathophysiology of WMC and mechanisms of dementia in PSD. Although it is also able to differentiate between different etiologies of dementia, its cost, complexity, and inconvenience have limited its clinical utility. The NINDS-AIREN criteria incorporate the most detailed imaging criteria to aid the diagnosis of VaD, yet modification is needed to improve its sensitivity and inter-rater agreement. Recent applications of more advanced MRI techniques including DWI, DTI, MTI, MR perfusion, and MRS, have enhanced early detection of ischemic brain tissue with increased specificity, better understanding on the pathophysiology of WMC, and/or our ability to differentiate between various etiologies of dementia in PSD. Further study is warranted to evaluate the usefulness of imaging variables (e.g. progression of WMC and cerebral perfusion and metabolism) as surrogate markers in clinical trials.

# Appendix

## Commonly Used Visual Scales for Rating Severity of WMC

*1. Fazekas and Schmidt Scale* [109]

White matter hyperintensity (WMH)

(0) Absent
(1) Punctate
(2) Beginning confluent
(3) Confluent or irregular periventricular hyperintensities

*2. The Scheltens Scale* [111]

| | | |
|---|---|---|
| Periventricular hyperintensities (PVH 0-6) | | |
| Caps: occipital | 0 /1 /2 | 0 = absent |
| Frontal | 0 /1 /2 | 1 = ≤ 5mm |
| Bands: lat. Ventricles | 0 /1 /2 | 2 = > 5mm and < 10 mm |
| White matter hyperintensities (WMH 0-24) | | |
| Frontal | 0 /1 /2 /3 /4 /5 /6 | 0 = n.a. |
| Parietal | 0 /1 /2 /3 /4 /5 /6 | 1 = < 3 mm; n ≤ 5 |
| Occipital | 0 /1 /2 /3 /4 /5 /6 | 2 = < 3 mm; n > 6 |
| Temporal | 0 /1 /2 /3 /4 /5 /6 | 3 = 4-10 mm; n ≤ 5 |
| | | 4 = 4 mm, n > 6 |
| | | 5 = > 11 mm; n > 1 |
| | | 6 = confluent |
| Basal ganglia hyperintensities (BG 0-30) | | |
| Caudate Nucleus | 0 /1 /2 /3 /4 /5 /6 | |
| Putamen | 0 /1 /2 /3 /4 /5 /6 | |
| Globus Pallidus | 0 /1 /2 /3 /4 /5 /6 | |
| Thalamus | 0 /1 /2 /3 /4 /5 /6 | |
| Internal capsule | 0 /1 /2 /3 /4 /5 /6 | |
| Infra-tentorial foci of hyperintensity (ITF 0-24) | | |
| Cerebellum | 0 /1 /2 /3 /4 /5 /6 | |
| Mesencephalon | 0 /1 /2 /3 /4 /5 /6 | |
| Pons | 0 /1 /2 /3 /4 /5 /6 | |
| Medulla | 0 /1 /2 /3 /4 /5 /6 | |

Semiquantative rating of signal hyperintensities in separate regions, with the range of the scale, between brackets. n = number of lesions; n.a. = no abnormalities.

*3. The Age Related WMC Rating Scale for MRI or CT* [95]

| | |
|---|---|
| *White matter lesions* | |
| 0 | No lesions (including symmetrical, well-defined caps or bands) |
| 1 | Focal lesions |
| 2 | Beginning confluence of lesions |
| 3 | Without involvement of U fibers |
| *Basal ganglia lesions* | |
| 0 | No lesions |
| 1 | 1 focal lesion (≥5mm) |
| 2 | >1 focal lesion |
| 3 | Confluent lesions |

White matter changes on MRI were defined as bright lesions ≥5mm on T2, PD, or FLAIR images. Lesions on CT were defined as hypodense areas of ≥5mm; left and right hemispheres were rated separately. The following brain areas were used for rating: frontal, parieto-occipital, temporal, infratentorial/cerebellum, and basal ganglia (striatum, globus pallidus, thalamus, internal/external capsule, and insula).

# Reference


[1] Ivan CS, Seshadri S, Beiser A, et al. Dementia after stroke: the Framingham Study. *Stroke* 2004; 35:1264-8.

[2] Tatemichi TK, Desmond DW, Mayeux R, et al. Dementia after stroke: baseline frequency, risks, and clinical features in a hospitalized cohort. *Neurology* 1992; 42:1185-93.

[3] Tatemichi TK, Paik M, Bagiella E, et al. Risk of dementia after stroke in a hospitalized cohort: results of a longitudinal study. *Neurology* 1994; 44:1885-91.

[4] Desmond DW, Moroney JT, Sano M, et al. Incidence of dementia after ischemic stroke: results of a longitudinal study. *Stroke* 2002; 33:2254-60.

[5] Zhou DH, Wang JY, Li J, et al. Study on frequency and predictors of dementia after ischemic strokeThe Chongqing Stroke Study. *J. Neurol.* 2004; 251:421-7.

[6] Chiu HF, Lam LC, Chi I, et al. Prevalence of dementia in Chinese elderly in Hong Kong. *Neurology* 1998; 50:1002-9.

[7] Lobo A, Launer LJ, Fratiglioni L, et al. Prevalence of dementia and major subtypes in Europe: A collaborative study of population-based cohorts. Neurologic Diseases in the Elderly Research Group. *Neurology* 2000; 54:S4-9.

[8] Moroney JT, Bagiella E, Tatemichi TK, et al. Dementia after stroke increases the risk of long-term stroke recurrence. *Neurology* 1997; 48:1317-25.

[9] Desmond DW, Moroney JT, Sano M, et al. Mortality in patients with dementia after ischemic stroke. *Neurology* 2002; 59:537-43.

[10] Barba R, Morin MD, Cemillan C, et al. Previous and incident dementia as risk factors for mortality in stroke patients. *Stroke* 2002; 33:1993-8.

[11] Sachdev PS, Brodaty H, Valenzuela MJ, et al. The neuropsychological profile of vascular cognitive impairment in stroke and TIA patients. *Neurology* 2004; 62:912-9.

[12] Pohjasvaara T, Leskela M, Vataja R, et al. Post-stroke depression, executive dysfunction and functional outcome. *Eur. J. Neurol.* 2002; 9:269-75.

[13] Tatemichi TK, Desmond DW, Stern Y, et al. Cognitive impairment after stroke: frequency, patterns, and relationship to functional abilities. *J. Neurol. Neurosurg. Psychiatry* 1994; 57:202-7.

[14] Mok VCT, Wong A, Lam WWM, et al. Cognitive impairment and functional outcome after stroke associated with small vessel disease. *J. Neurol. Neurosurg. Psychiatry* 2004:560-566.

[15] Hachinski VC, Lassen NA, Marshall J. Multi-infarct dementia. A cause of mental deterioration in the elderly. *Lancet* 1974; 2:207-10.

[16] Roman GC, Tatemichi TK, Erkinjuntti T, et al. Vascular dementia: diagnostic criteria for research studies. Report of the NINDS-AIREN International Workshop. *Neurology* 1993; 43:250-60.

[17] Pohjasvaara T, Mantyla R, Salonen O, et al. How complex interactions of ischemic brain infarcts, white matter lesions, and atrophy relate to poststroke dementia. *Arch. Neurol.* 2000; 57:1295-300.

[18] Altieri M, Di Piero V, Pasquini M, et al. Delayed poststroke dementia: a 4-year follow-up study. *Neurology* 2004; 62:2193-7.

[19] Henon H, Durieu I, Guerouaou D, et al. Poststroke dementia: incidence and relationship to prestroke cognitive decline. *Neurology* 2001; 57:1216-22.
[20] Hachinski VC, Iliff LD, Zilhka E, et al. Cerebral blood flow in dementia. *Arch. Neurol.* 1975; 32:632-7.
[21] Association AP. *Diagnostic and statistical manual disorders*: Washington, DC, 1994.
[22] Organization. WH. ICD-10 Classification of Mental and Behavioural Disorders: *Diagnostic Criteria for Research*. Geneva; WHO, 1993.
[23] Chui HC, Victoroff JI, Margolin D, et al. Criteria for the diagnosis of ischemic vascular dementia proposed by the State of California Alzheimer's Disease Diagnostic and Treatment Centers. *Neurology* 1992; 42:473-80.
[24] Pohjasvaara T, Mantyla R, Ylikoski R, et al. Comparison of different clinical criteria (DSM-III, ADDTC, ICD-10, NINDS-AIREN, DSM-IV) for the diagnosis of vascular dementia. National Institute of Neurological Disorders and Stroke-Association Internationale pour la Recherche et l'Enseignement en Neurosciences. *Stroke* 2000; 31:2952-7.
[25] Gold G, Giannakopoulos P, Montes-Paixao Junior C, et al. Sensitivity and specificity of newly proposed clinical criteria for possible vascular dementia. *Neurology* 1997; 49:690-4.
[26] Erkinjuntti T, Inzitari D, Pantoni L, et al. Research criteria for subcortical vascular dementia in clinical trials. *J. Neural. Transm. Suppl.* 2000; 59:23-30.
[27] Meyer JS, Xu G, Thornby J, et al. Is mild cognitive impairment prodromal for vascular dementia like Alzheimer's disease? *Stroke* 2002; 33:1981-5.
[28] Feinberg TE, Rothi LJ, Heilman KM. Multimodal agnosia after unilateral left hemisphere lesion. *Neurology* 1986; 36:864-7.
[29] Kertesz A, Ferro JM, Shewan CM. Apraxia and aphasia: the functional-anatomical basis for their dissociation. *Neurology* 1984; 34:40-7.
[30] Van Zandvoort MJ, Kappelle LJ, Algra A, et al. Decreased capacity for mental effort after single supratentorial lacunar infarct may affect performance in everyday life. *J. Neurol. Neurosurg. Psychiatry* 1998; 65:697-702.
[31] Rockwood K, Wentzel C, Hachinski V, et al. Prevalence and outcomes of vascular cognitive impairment. Vascular Cognitive Impairment Investigators of the Canadian Study of Health and Aging. *Neurology* 2000; 54:447-51.
[32] Mok VC, Fan YH, Lam WW, et al. Small subcortical infarct and intracranial large artery disease in Chinese. *J. Neurol. Sci.* 2003; 216:55-9.
[33] Wong KS, Gao S, Chan YL, et al. Mechanisms of acute cerebral infarctions in patients with middle cerebral artery stenosis: a diffusion-weighted imaging and microemboli monitoring study. *Ann. Neurol.* 2002; 52:74-81.
[34] Mendez MF, Adams NL, Lewandowski KS. Neurobehavioral changes associated with caudate lesions. *Neurology* 1989; 39:349-54.
[35] Auchus AP, Chen CP, Sodagar SN, et al. Single stroke dementia: insights from 12 cases in Singapore. *J. Neurol. Sci.* 2002; 203-204:85-9.
[36] Tatemichi TK, Desmond DW, Prohovnik I, et al. Confusion and memory loss from capsular genu infarction: a thalamocortical disconnection syndrome? *Neurology* 1992; 42:1966-79.

[37] Bhatia KP, Marsden CD. The behavioural and motor consequences of focal lesions of the basal ganglia in man. *Brain* 1994; 117 ( Pt 4):859-76.
[38] Babikian V, Ropper AH. Binswanger's disease: a review. *Stroke* 1987; 18:2-12.
[39] Ishii N, Nishihara Y, Imamura T. Why do frontal lobe symptoms predominate in vascular dementia with lacunes? *Neurology* 1986; 36:340-5.
[40] Roman GC, Erkinjuntti T, Wallin A, et al. Subcortical ischaemic vascular dementia. *Lancet Neurol.* 2002; 1:426-36.
[41] Mori S, Sadoshima S, Ibayashi S, et al. Impact of thalamic hematoma on six-month mortality and motor and cognitive functional outcome. *Stroke* 1995; 26:620-6.
[42] Szirmai I, Vastagh I, Szombathelyi E, et al. Strategic infarcts of the thalamus in vascular dementia. *J. Neurol. Sci.* 2002; 203-204:91-7.
[43] Bugiani O. A beta-related cerebral amyloid angiopathy. *Neurol. Sci.* 2004; 25 Suppl 1:S1-2.
[44] Gray F, Dubas F, Roullet E, Escourolle R. Leukoencephalopathy in diffuse hemorrhagic cerebral amyloid angiopathy. *Ann. Neurol.* 1985; 18:54-9.
[45] Olichney JM, Hansen LA, Hofstetter CR, et al. Association between severe cerebral amyloid angiopathy and cerebrovascular lesions in Alzheimer disease is not a spurious one attributable to apolipoprotein E4. *Arch. Neurol.* 2000; 57:869-74.
[46] Dichgans M. Cerebral autosomal dominant arteriopathy with subcortical infarcts and leukoencephalopathy: phenotypic and mutational spectrum. *J. Neurol. Sc*i. 2002; 203-204:77-80.
[47] Tatemichi TK, Foulkes MA, Mohr JP, et al. Dementia in stroke survivors in the Stroke Data Bank cohort. Prevalence, incidence, risk factors, and computed tomographic findings. *Stroke* 1990; 21:858-66.
[48] Desmond DW, Moroney JT, Paik MC, et al. Frequency and clinical determinants of dementia after ischemic stroke. *Neurology* 2000; 54:1124-31.
[49] Pohjasvaara T, Erkinjuntti T, Ylikoski R, et al. Clinical determinants of poststroke dementia. *Stroke* 1998; 29:75-81.
[50] Tang WK, Chan SS, Chiu HF, et al. Frequency and determinants of poststroke dementia in Chinese. *Stroke* 2004; 35:930-5.
[51] Henon H, Pasquier F, Durieu I, et al. Preexisting dementia in stroke patients. Baseline frequency, associated factors, and outcome. *Stroke* 1997; 28:2429-36.
[52] Barba R, Castro MD, del Mar Morin M, et al. Prestroke dementia. *Cerebrovasc. Dis.* 2001; 11:216-24.
[53] Snowdon DA, Greiner LH, Mortimer JA, et al. Brain infarction and the clinical expression of Alzheimer disease. The Nun Study. *Jama* 1997; 277:813-7.
[54] Esiri MM, Nagy Z, Smith MZ, et al. Cerebrovascular disease and threshold for dementia in the early stages of Alzheimer's disease. *Lancet* 1999; 354:919-20.
[55] Mobius HJ, Stoffler A. New approaches to clinical trials in vascular dementia: memantine in small vessel disease. *Cerebrovasc. Dis*. 2002; 13 Suppl 2:61-6.
[56] Pantoni L, Rossi R, Inzitari D, et al. Efficacy and safety of nimodipine in subcortical vascular dementia: a subgroup analysis of the Scandinavian Multi-Infarct Dementia Trial. *J. Neurol. Sci.* 2000; 175:124-34.

[57] Erkinjuntti T, Kurz A, Gauthier S, et al. Efficacy of galantamine in probable vascular dementia and Alzheimer's disease combined with cerebrovascular disease: a randomised trial. *Lancet* 2002; 359:1283-90.

[58] Mirra SS, Heyman A, McKeel D, et al. The Consortium to Establish a Registry for Alzheimer's Disease (CERAD). Part II. Standardization of the neuropathologic assessment of Alzheimer's disease. *Neurology* 1991; 41:479-86.

[59] Jellinger KA. The pathology of ischemic-vascular dementia: an update. *J. Neurol. Sci.* 2002; 203-204:153-7.

[60] Erkinjuntti T, Haltia M, Palo J, et al. Accuracy of the clinical diagnosis of vascular dementia: a prospective clinical and post-mortem neuropathological study. *J. Neurol. Neurosurg. Psychiatry* 1988; 51:1037-44.

[61] White L, Petrovitch H, Hardman J, et al. Cerebrovascular pathology and dementia in autopsied Honolulu-Asia Aging Study participants. *Ann. NY Acad. Sci.* 2002; 977:9-23.

[62] Fazekas F, Kleinert R, Roob G, et al. Histopathologic analysis of foci of signal loss on gradient-echo T2*-weighted MR images in patients with spontaneous intracerebral hemorrhage: evidence of microangiopathy-related microbleeds. *AJNR Am. J. Neuroradiol.* 1999; 20:637-42.

[63] Kalaria RN, Kenny RA, Ballard CG, et al. Towards defining the neuropathological substrates of vascular dementia. *J. Neurol. Sci.* 2004; 226:75-80.

[64] Lammie GA. Pathology of lacunar infarction. In: Donnan GA, Norrving, B., Bamford, J.M., Bogousslavsky, J., ed. *Subcortical stroke*. Oxford: Oxford University Press, 2002:37-46.

[65] Wardlaw JM, Sandercock PA, Dennis MS, et al. Is breakdown of the blood-brain barrier responsible for lacunar stroke, leukoaraiosis, and dementia? *Stroke* 2003; 34:806-12.

[66] Moody DM, Brown WR, Challa VR, et al. Periventricular venous collagenosis: association with leukoaraiosis. *Radiology* 1995; 194:469-76.

[67] Fazekas F, Kleinert R, Offenbacher H, et al. Pathologic correlates of incidental MRI white matter signal hyperintensities. *Neurology* 1993; 43:1683-9.

[68] Werring DJ, Frazer DW, Coward LJ, et al. Cognitive dysfunction in patients with cerebral microbleeds on T2*-weighted gradient-echo MRI. *Brain* 2004; 127:2265-75.

[69] Barba R, Martinez-Espinosa S, Rodriguez-Garcia E, et al. Poststroke dementia : clinical features and risk factors. *Stroke* 2000; 31:1494-501.

[70] Tatemichi TK, Desmond DW, Paik M, et al. Clinical determinants of dementia related to stroke. *Ann. Neurol.* 1993; 33:568-75.

[71] Klimkowicz A, Dziedzic T, Slowik A, et al. Incidence of pre- and poststroke dementia: cracow stroke registry. *Dement. Geriatr. Cogn. Disord.* 2002; 14:137-40.

[72] Lin JH, Lin RT, Tai CT, et al. Prediction of poststroke dementia. *Neurology* 2003; 61:343-8.

[73] Censori B, Manara O, Agostinis C, et al. Dementia after first stroke. *Stroke* 1996; 27:1205-10.

[74] Pohjasvaara T, Erkinjuntti T, Vataja R, et al. Dementia three months after stroke. Baseline frequency and effect of different definitions of dementia in the Helsinki Stroke Aging Memory Study (SAM) cohort. *Stroke* 1997; 28:785-92.

[75] Inzitari D, Di Carlo A, Pracucci G, et al. Incidence and determinants of poststroke dementia as defined by an informant interview method in a hospital-based stroke registry. *Stroke* 1998; 29:2087-93.
[76] Kokmen E, Whisnant JP, O'Fallon WM, et al. Dementia after ischemic stroke: a population-based study in Rochester, Minnesota (1960-1984). Neurology 1996; 46:154-9.
[77] Moroney JT, Tang MX, Berglund L, et al. Low-density lipoprotein cholesterol and the risk of dementia with stroke. *Jama* 1999; 282:254-60.
[78] Cummings JL. Frontal-subcortical circuits and human behavior. *Arch. Neurol.* 1993; 50:873-80.
[79] Royall DR, Lauterbach EC, Cummings JL, et al. Executive control function: a review of its promise and challenges for clinical research. A report from the Committee on Research of the American Neuropsychiatric Association. *J. Neuropsychiatry. Clin. Neurosci.* 2002; 14:377-405.
[80] Tierney MC, Black SE, Szalai JP, et al. Recognition memory and verbal fluency differentiate probable Alzheimer disease from subcortical ischemic vascular dementia. *Arch. Neurol.* 2001; 58:1654-9.
[81] Ballard C, Rowan E, Stephens S, et al. Prospective follow-up study between 3 and 15 months after stroke: improvements and decline in cognitive function among dementia-free stroke survivors >75 years of age. *Stroke* 2003; 34:2440-4.
[82] Sachdev PS, Brodaty H, Valenzuela MJ, et al. Progression of cognitive impairment in stroke patients. *Neurology* 2004; 63:1618-23.
[83] Nyenhuis DL, Gorelick PB, Freels S, et al. Cognitive and functional decline in African Americans with VaD, AD, and stroke without dementia. *Neurology* 2002; 58:56-61.
[84] Pullicino P, Benedict RH, Capruso DX, et al. Neuroimaging criteria for vascular dementia. *Arch. Neurol.* 1996; 53:723-8.
[85] Auchus AP, Brashear HR, Titusville NJ, et al. Results of a trial of galantamine in subjects with vascular dementia confirmed by central MRI reading. *56th Annual Meeting of the American Academy of Neurology* (abstract) 2004.
[86] Mungas D, Reed BR, Jagust WJ, et al. Volumetric MRI predicts rate of cognitive decline related to AD and cerebrovascular disease. *Neurology* 2002; 59:867-73.
[87] De Reuck J, Decoo D, Marchau M, et al. Positron emission tomography in vascular dementia. *J. Neurol. Sci.* 1998; 154:55-61.
[88] Schmidt R, Scheltens P, Erkinjuntti T, et al. White matter lesion progression: a surrogate endpoint for trials in cerebral small-vessel disease. *Neurology* 2004; 63:139-44.
[89] Jobst KA, Smith AD, Szatmari M, et al. Detection in life of confirmed Alzheimer's disease using a simple measurement of medial temporal lobe atrophy by computed tomography. *Lancet* 1992; 340:1179-83.
[90] DeCarli C, Kaye JA, Horwitz B, et al. Critical analysis of the use of computer-assisted transverse axial tomography to study human brain in aging and dementia of the Alzheimer type. *Neurology* 1990; 40:872-83.
[91] Broderick JP, Brott TG, Grotta JC. Intracerebral hemorrhage volume measurement. *Stroke* 1994; 25:1081.

[92] Kawamura J, Meyer JS, Terayama Y, et al. Cerebral hypoperfusion correlates with mild and parenchymal loss with severe multi-infarct dementia. J Neurol Sci 1991; 102:32-8.

[93] Gorelick PB, Chatterjee A, Patel D, et al. Cranial computed tomographic observations in multi-infarct dementia. A controlled study. *Stroke* 1992; 23:804-11.

[94] Wahlund LO, Barkhof F, Fazekas F, et al. A new rating scale for age-related white matter changes applicable to MRI and CT. Stroke 2001; 32:1318-22.

[95] Loeb C, Gandolfo C, Croce R, et al. Dementia associated with lacunar infarction. *Stroke* 1992; 23:1225-9.

[96] van Swieten JC, Hijdra A, Koudstaal PJ, et al. Grading white matter lesions on CT and MRI: a simple scale. *J. Neurol. Neurosurg. Psychiatry* 1990; 53:1080-3.

[97] Pantoni L, Garcia JH. The significance of cerebral white matter abnormalities 100 years after Binswanger's report. A review. *Stroke* 1995; 26:1293-301.

[98] Geroldi C, Galluzzi S, Testa C, et al. Validation study of a CT-based weighted rating scale for subcortical ischemic vascular disease in patients with mild cognitive deterioration. *Eur. Neurol.* 2003; 49:193-209.

[99] Albert M, Naeser MA, Levine HL, et al. Ventricular size in patients with presenile dementia of the Alzheimer's type. *Arch. Neurol.* 1984; 41:1258-63.

[100] Victoroff J, Mack WJ, Grafton ST, et al. A method to improve interrater reliability of visual inspection of brain MRI scans in dementia. *Neurology* 1994; 44:2267-76.

[101] Hughes CP, Gado M. Computed tomography and aging of the brain. *Radiology* 1981; 139:391-6.

[102] Damasio H, Eslinger P, Damasio AR, et al. Quantitative computed tomographic analysis in the diagnosis of dementia. *Arch. Neurol.* 1983; 40:715-9.

[103] Turkheimer E, Cullum CM, Hubler DW, et al. Quantifying cortical atrophy. *J. Neurol. Neurosurg. Psychiatry* 1984; 47:1314-8.

[104] Bokura H, Kobayashi S, Yamaguchi S. Distinguishing silent lacunar infarction from enlarged Virchow-Robin spaces: a magnetic resonance imaging and pathological study. *J. Neurol.* 1998; 245:116-22.

[105] Mantyla R, Aronen HJ, Salonen O, et al. The prevalence and distribution of white-matter changes on different MRI pulse sequences in a post-stroke cohort. *Neuroradiology* 1999; 41:657-65.

[106] Herskovits EH, Itoh R, Melhem ER. Accuracy for detection of simulated lesions: comparison of fluid-attenuated inversion-recovery, proton density--weighted, and T2-weighted synthetic brain MR imaging. *AJR Am. J. Roentgenol.* 2001; 176:1313-8.

[107] Manolio TA, Kronmal RA, Burke GL, et al. Magnetic resonance abnormalities and cardiovascular disease in older adults. The Cardiovascular Health Study. *Stroke* 1994; 25:318-27.

[108] Schmidt R, Fazekas F, Kleinert G, et al. Magnetic resonance imaging signal hyperintensities in the deep and subcortical white matter. A comparative study between stroke patients and normal volunteers. *Arch. Neurol.* 1992; 49:825-7.

[109] de Groot JC, de Leeuw FE, Oudkerk M, et al. Cerebral white matter lesions and cognitive function: the Rotterdam Scan Study. *Ann. Neurol.* 2000; 47:145-51.

[110] Scheltens P, Barkhof F, Leys D, et al. A semiquantative rating scale for the assessment of signal hyperintensities on magnetic resonance imaging. *J. Neurol. Sci.* 1993; 114:7-12.

[111] Mantyla R, Erkinjuntti T, Salonen O, et al. Variable agreement between visual rating scales for white matter hyperintensities on MRI. Comparison of 13 rating scales in a poststroke cohort. *Stroke* 1997; 28:1614-23.

[112] Prins ND, van Straaten EC, van Dijk EJ, et al. Measuring progression of cerebral white matter lesions on MRI: visual rating and volumetrics. *Neurology* 2004; 62:1533-9.

[113] Fan YH, Lam WW, Mok VC, et al. Variability and validity of a simple visual rating scale in grading white matter changes on magnetic resonance imaging. *J. Neuroimaging*. 2003; 13:255-8.

[114] Kapeller P, Barber R, Vermeulen RJ, et al. Visual rating of age-related white matter changes on magnetic resonance imaging: scale comparison, interrater agreement, and correlations with quantitative measurements. *Stroke* 2003; 34:441-5.

[115] Fein G, Di Sclafani V, Tanabe J, et al. Hippocampal and cortical atrophy predict dementia in subcortical ischemic vascular disease. *Neurology* 2000; 55:1626-35.

[116] Scheltens P, Leys D, Barkhof F, et al. Atrophy of medial temporal lobes on MRI in "probable" Alzheimer's disease and normal ageing: diagnostic value and neuropsychological correlates. *J. Neurol. Neurosurg. Psychiatry* 1992; 55:967-72.

[117] Yamauchi H, Fukuyama H, Shio H. Corpus callosum atrophy in patients with leukoaraiosis may indicate global cognitive impairment. *Stroke* 2000; 31:1515-20.

[118] Bigler ED, Neeley ES, Miller MJ, et al. Cerebral volume loss, cognitive deficit and neuropsychological performance: comparative measures of brain atrophy: I. Dementia. *J. Int. Neuropsychol. Soc.* 2004; 10:442-52.

[119] Coffey CE, Wilkinson WE, Parashos IA, et al. Quantitative cerebral anatomy of the aging human brain: a cross-sectional study using magnetic resonance imaging. *Neurology* 1992; 42:527-36.

[120] O'Brien JT, Paling S, Barber R, et al. Progressive brain atrophy on serial MRI in dementia with Lewy bodies, AD, and vascular dementia. *Neurology* 2001; 56:1386-8.

[121] Liu CK, Miller BL, Cummings JL, et al. A quantitative MRI study of vascular dementia. *Neurology* 1992; 42:138-43.

[122] Starkstein SE, Sabe L, Vazquez S, et al. Neuropsychological, psychiatric, and cerebral blood flow findings in vascular dementia and Alzheimer's disease. *Stroke* 1996; 27:408-14.

[123] Kwan LT, Reed BR, Eberling JL, et al. Effects of subcortical cerebral infarction on cortical glucose metabolism and cognitive function. *Arch. Neurol.* 1999; 56:809-14.

[124] Pappata S, Mazoyer B, Tran Dinh S, et al. Effects of capsular or thalamic stroke on metabolism in the cortex and cerebellum: a positron tomography study. *Stroke* 1990; 21:519-24.

[125] Reed BR, Eberling JL, Mungas D, et al. Frontal lobe hypometabolism predicts cognitive decline in patients with lacunar infarcts. *Arch. Neurol.* 2001; 58:493-7.

[126] Sabri O RE, Hellwig D, Schneider R, et al. Neuropsychological impairment correlates with hypoperfusion and hypometabolism but not with severity of white matter lesions on MRI in patients with cerebral microangiopathy. *Stroke* 1999; 30:556-66.

[127] Yao H, Sadoshima S, Kuwabara Y, et al. Cerebral blood flow and oxygen metabolism in patients with vascular dementia of the Binswanger type. *Stroke* 1990; 21:1694-9.
[128] Rogers RL, Meyer JS, Mortel KF, et al. Decreased cerebral blood flow precedes multi-infarct dementia, but follows senile dementia of Alzheimer type. *Neurology* 1986; 36:1-6.
[129] Reed BR, Eberling JL, Mungas D, et al. Memory failure has different mechanisms in subcortical stroke and Alzheimer's disease. *Ann. Neurol.* 2000; 48:275-84.
[130] Loizou LA, Kendall BE, Marshall J. Subcortical arteriosclerotic encephalopathy: a clinical and radiological investigation. *J. Neurol. Neurosurg. Psychiatry* 1981; 44:294-304.
[131] Pantoni L, Garcia JH. Pathogenesis of leukoaraiosis: a review. *Stroke* 1997; 28:652-9.
[132] De Reuck J, Decoo D, Hasenbroekx MC, et al. Acetazolamide vasoreactivity in vascular dementia: a positron emission tomographic study. *Eur. Neurol.* 1999; 41:31-6.
[133] Mielke R, Kessler J, Szelies B, et al. Vascular dementia: perfusional and metabolic disturbances and effects of therapy. *J. Neural. Transm. Suppl.* 1996; 47:183-91.
[134] Lojkowska W, Ryglewicz D, Jedrzejczak T, et al. The effect of cholinesterase inhibitors on the regional blood flow in patients with Alzheimer's disease and vascular dementia. *J. Neurol. Sci.* 2003; 216:119-26.
[135] Pohjasvaara T, Mantyla R, Salonen O, et al. MRI correlates of dementia after first clinical ischemic stroke. *J. Neurol. Sci.* 2000; 181:111-7.
[136] Cordoliani-Mackowiak MA, Henon H, Pruvo JP, et al. Poststroke dementia: influence of hippocampal atrophy. *Arch. Neurol.* 2003; 60:585-90.
[137] Mungas D, Jagust WJ, Reed BR, et al. MRI predictors of cognition in subcortical ischemic vascular disease and Alzheimer's disease. *Neurology* 2001; 57:2229-35.
[138] Wen HM, Mok VC, Fan YH, et al. Effect of white matter changes on cognitive impairment in patients with lacunar infarcts. *Stroke* 2004; 35:1826-30.
[139] Miyao S, Takano A, Teramoto J, et al. Leukoaraiosis in relation to prognosis for patients with lacunar infarction. *Stroke* 1992; 23:1434-8.
[140] Yamauchi H, Fukuyama H, Ogawa M, et al. Callosal atrophy in patients with lacunar infarction and extensive leukoaraiosis. An indicator of cognitive impairment. *Stroke* 1994; 25:1788-93.
[141] Corbett A, Bennett H, Kos S. Cognitive dysfunction following subcortical infarction. *Arch. Neurol.* 1994; 51:999-1007.
[142] Mok V, Chang C, Wong A, et al. Neuroimaging determinants of cognitive performances in stroke associated with small vessel disease. *Journal of Neuroimaging* 2005; In press.
[143] Dufouil C, Alperovitch A, Tzourio C. Influence of education on the relationship between white matter lesions and cognition. *Neurology* 2003; 60:831-6.
[144] Malm J, Kristensen B, Karlsson T, et al. Cognitive impairment in young adults with infratentorial infarcts. *Neurology* 1998; 51:433-40.
[145] Auer DP, Putz B, Gossl C, et al. Differential lesion patterns in CADASIL and sporadic subcortical arteriosclerotic encephalopathy: MR imaging study with statistical parametric group comparison. *Radiology* 2001; 218:443-51.

[146] Dichgans M, Filippi M, Bruning R, et al. Quantitative MRI in CADASIL: correlation with disability and cognitive performance. *Neurology* 1999; 52:1361-7.

[147] Tatsch K, Koch W, Linke R, et al. Cortical hypometabolism and crossed cerebellar diaschisis suggest subcortically induced disconnection in CADASIL: an 18F-FDG PET study. *J. Nucl. Med.* 2003; 44:862-9.

[148] Vital C, Julien J. Widespread dilatation of perivascular spaces: a leukoencephalopathy causing dementia. *Neurology* 1997; 48:1310-3.

[149] Wetterling T, Kanitz RD, Borgis KJ. Comparison of different diagnostic criteria for vascular dementia (ADDTC, DSM-IV, ICD-10, NINDS-AIREN). *Stroke* 1996; 27:30-6.

[150] van Straaten EC, Scheltens P, Knol DL, et al. Operational definitions for the NINDS-AIREN criteria for vascular dementia: an interobserver study. *Stroke* 2003; 34:1907-12.

[151] Ballard CG, Burton EJ, Barber R, et al. NINDS AIREN neuroimaging criteria do not distinguish stroke patients with and without dementia. *Neurology* 2004; 63:983-8.

[152] Loeb C, Gandolfo C. Diagnostic evaluation of degenerative and vascular dementia. *Stroke* 1983; 14:399-401.

[153] Choi SH, Na DL, Chung CS, et al. Diffusion-weighted MRI in vascular dementia. *Neurology* 2000; 54:83-9.

[154] O'Sullivan M, Rich PM, Barrick TR, et al. Frequency of subclinical lacunar infarcts in ischemic leukoaraiosis and cerebral autosomal dominant arteriopathy with subcortical infarcts and leukoencephalopathy. *AJNR Am. J. Neuroradiol.* 2003; 24:1348-54.

[155] Jones DK, Lythgoe D, Horsfield MA, et al. Characterization of white matter damage in ischemic leukoaraiosis with diffusion tensor MRI. *Stroke* 1999; 30:393-7.

[156] O'Sullivan M, Morris RG, Huckstep B, et al. Diffusion tensor MRI correlates with executive dysfunction in patients with ischaemic leukoaraiosis. *J. Neurol. Neurosurg. Psychiatry* 2004; 75:441-7.

[157] O'Sullivan M, Singhal S, Charlton R, et al. Diffusion tensor imaging of thalamus correlates with cognition in CADASIL without dementia. *Neurology* 2004; 62:702-7.

[158] Molko N, Pappata S, Mangin JF, et al. Monitoring disease progression in CADASIL with diffusion magnetic resonance imaging: a study with whole brain histogram analysis. *Stroke* 2002; 33:2902-8.

[159] Iannucci G, Dichgans M, Rovaris M, et al. Correlations between clinical findings and magnetization transfer imaging metrics of tissue damage in individuals with cerebral autosomal dominant arteriopathy with subcortical infarcts and leukoencephalopathy. *Stroke* 2001; 32:643-8.

[160] Tanabe JL, Ezekiel F, Jagust WJ, et al. Magnetization transfer ratio of white matter hyperintensities in subcortical ischemic vascular dementia. *AJNR Am. J. Neuroradiol.* 1999; 20:839-44.

[161] Fan YH, Mok VC, Lam WW, et al. Cerebral microbleeds and white matter changes in patients hospitalized with lacunar infarcts. *J. Neurol.* 2004; 251:537-41.

[162] O'Sullivan M, Lythgoe DJ, Pereira AC, et al. Patterns of cerebral blood flow reduction in patients with ischemic leukoaraiosis. *Neurology* 2002; 59:321-6.

[163] Capizzano AA, Schuff N, Amend DL, et al. Subcortical ischemic vascular dementia: assessment with quantitative MR imaging and 1H MR spectroscopy. *AJNR Am. J. Neuroradiol*. 2000; 21:621-30.

[164] Schuff N, Capizzano AA, Du AT, et al. Different patterns of N-acetylaspartate loss in subcortical ischemic vascular dementia and AD. *Neurology* 2003; 61:358-64.

In: State-of-the-Art Imaging in Stroke, Volume 2
Editor: Bernhard Schaller, pp. 143-162
ISBN 978-1-60021-499-8


*Chapter V*

# Imaging Post-Stroke Aphasia

***Argye E. Hillis***
The Johns Hopkins University School of Medicine,
Baltimore, MD, U.S.A.

## A. Contributions to Experimental/ Theoretical Knowledge

### Imaging Studies of Aphasia Syndromes

*CT Scans.* Imaging studies of aphasia began as soon as CT scans of the brain were available to reliably demonstrate the site of lesion in patients following chronic stroke. These early studies largely confirmed lesion/syndrome associations based on earlier autopsy studies. For example, a number of investigators obtained CT scans of patients with Broca's aphasia, characterized by nonfluent, agrammatic speech and writing, better naming of nouns than verbs or function words, impaired speech articulation, spelling impairments, and relatively intact auditory comprehension except for syntactically complex sentences. These patients were often, although not always (see [1]) found to have infarcts involving the distribution of the superior division of the left middle cerebral artery, involving left posterior inferior frontal cortex (including Broca's area, or Brodmann's area, or BA, 44 and 45 [2]; see also [3]). At that time there was a theoretical debate concerning whether or not Broca's Aphasia (or any other aphasia syndrome) was a theoretically coherent syndrome; imaging studies contributed to resolving this issue. The controversy concerned whether or not a single underlying deficit could account for the various features of the syndrome, such as agrammatic speech production and asyntactic comprehension (see [4]; [5] for discussion). Agrammatic speech production refers to telegraphic speech, often devoid of function words such as "the" and "of". Asyntactic comprehension refers to misunderstanding the syntactic structure of sentences, while understanding the content words. For example, a patient may misunderstand the sentence, "The man was kissed by the woman" as "The man kissed the woman." Although some authors believed that these two deficits reflected damage to a single underlying syntactic processing mechanism [4, 6, 7], others argued that impaired production and comprehension were dissociable deficits that frequently co-occur because they are subserved by adjacent brain regions [8-11]. Imaging studies confirmed that small lesions affecting only part of the distribution of the superior division of the left MCA result in only one or two of the clinical features of Broca's aphasia. For example, from CT scan studies it was observed that damage to Broca's area alone resulted in non-fluent, effortful speech with impaired articulation due to impaired motor planning of speech production, but did not result in the entire syndrome of Broca's aphasia [12]. Rather, the complete syndrome of Broca's aphasia, including agrammatic speech and asyntactic comprehension, required a more extensive damage in the distribution of the superior division of the left MCA [12, 13].

Likewise, CT scan studies showed that Wernicke's Aphasia, characterized by fluent, jargon speech with impaired comprehension of both spoken and written words resulted from extensive damage in the territory of the inferior division of the left MCA [2, 14, 15]. More discrete damage affecting only a small part of that distribution was found, mostly with later MRI studies that could reveal smaller lesions, to result in individual components of the syndrome, such as impaired naming [16] or jargon speech with intact comprehension of written words [17]. Transcortical motor aphasia is a syndrome that is very similar to Broca's aphasia, except that the individual is able to repeat fluently and accurately. Evidence from CT studies indicate that transcortical motor aphasia is typically associated with infarcts in the territory of the left anterior cerebral artery (ACA) territory [18] or "watershed" territory between the left ACA and left MCA [19]. "Watershed" territory refers to the borders between two territories, which can become infarcted when there is a drop in blood flow, such that blood does not reach the distal part of the vascular territory. Transcortical sensory aphasia, which is similar to Wernicke's aphasia, except that repetition is preserved, is associated with infarcts in the watershed territory between the left MCA and posterior cerebral artery (PCA) [20], as illustrated by Figure 1. Mixed transcortical aphasia, characterized by preserved repetition, but impairment in all other language functions, is associated with lesions involving both watershed territories between the left ACA and MCA, and between left PCA and MCA, preserving Broca's and Wernicke's area, but cutting these important language areas off from the remainder of the brain [21]. To illustrate, Maeshima, et al. [21] reported a case of mixed transcortical aphasia caused by cerebral embolism. MRI showed left frontal and parieto-occipital infarcts, but single photon emission CT (SPECT) revealed a larger area of hypoperfusion involving all of the left hemisphere except for a portion of the left perisylvian language areas (Broca's and Wernicke's areas). Results were consistent with the hypothesis that mixed transcortical aphasia is due to isolation of perisylvian speech areas, disconnecting them from surrounding areas. This combination of watershed lesions, sometimes referred to as "isolation of the speech area" often occurs when there is a sudden drop in blood pressure, such blood flow is insufficient to reach the distal vascular territories. However, damage from other causes that happens to isolate Broca's and Wernicke's areas from other parts of the brain can also cause Mixed Transcortical Aphasia, as illustrated in Figure 2.

Another well described language syndrome, alexia without agraphia (also called pure alexia or "letter-by-letter reading") is characterized by impaired reading, but preserved recognition of words spelled aloud and preserved writing. Often patients can read very slowly, by naming individual letters, although letter identification is typically at least mildly impaired. Autopsy studies from the 1800's provide evidence that this clinical syndrome is associated with co-occurrence of two lesions – one in the left occipital lobe (causing right homonymous hemianopia) and one in the splenium of the corpus collosum.

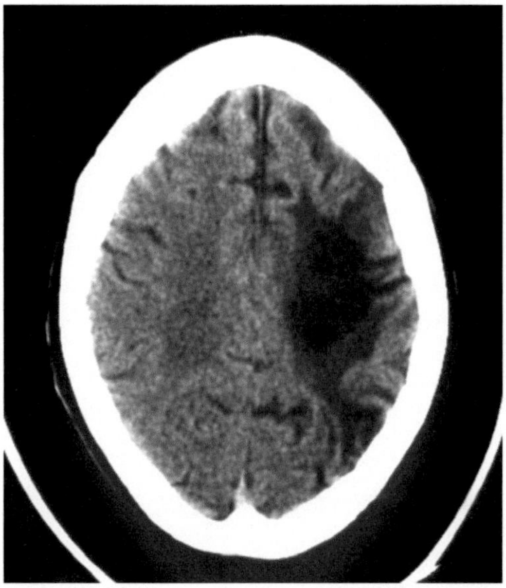

Figure 1. CT scan of a patient with a posterior "watershed" lesion between left PCA and left MCA territory and associated transcortical sensory aphasia (fluent, jargon speech and impaired comprehension, but intact repetition).

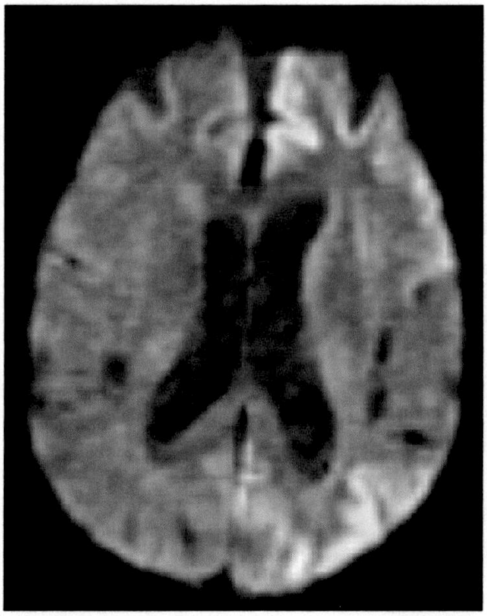

Figure 2. DWI of a patient with mixed transcortical aphasia associated with "isolation of the speech area" associated with subtle cortical signal abnormalities on DWI caused by Creutzfeldt Jakob Disease.

Both of these lesions are caused by occlusion of the left PCA. Dejerine [22] accounted for the syndrome by postulating that the patient would process visual information (printed words) in the right occipital lobe only (because of the lesion in the left occipital lobe), but the visual information could not be transferred to the left hemisphere to be understood or named due to the lesion in the splenium. The same combination of lesions can account for patients with "Optic Aphasia" -- impaired naming of visually presented objects, with intact naming of the same objects to definition or tactile exploration, but some preserved "recognition" of the visual stimulus by performing an appropriate gesture. Again, the deficit is ascribed to the fact that all visual information must be first processed in the right hemisphere but "recognition" of the stimulus cannot be transferred to the left hemisphere to support naming [23]. This lesion/syndrome association for Alexia without Agraphia and Optic Aphasia has been confirmed with CT and MRI scans of patients with alexia without agraphia and/or Optic Aphasia [24-26]. Occasional patients with Alexia without Agraphia (and Optic Aphasia) have had damage to the left occipital lobe and/or fusiform gyrus without damage to the splenium [24]. However, one such patient was found to have hypoperfusion of the splenium, using magnetic resonance perfusion weighted imaging, which reveals dysfunctional as well as structurally damaged tissue [27]; see Figure 3). When the splenium was reperfused, reading and picture naming improved.

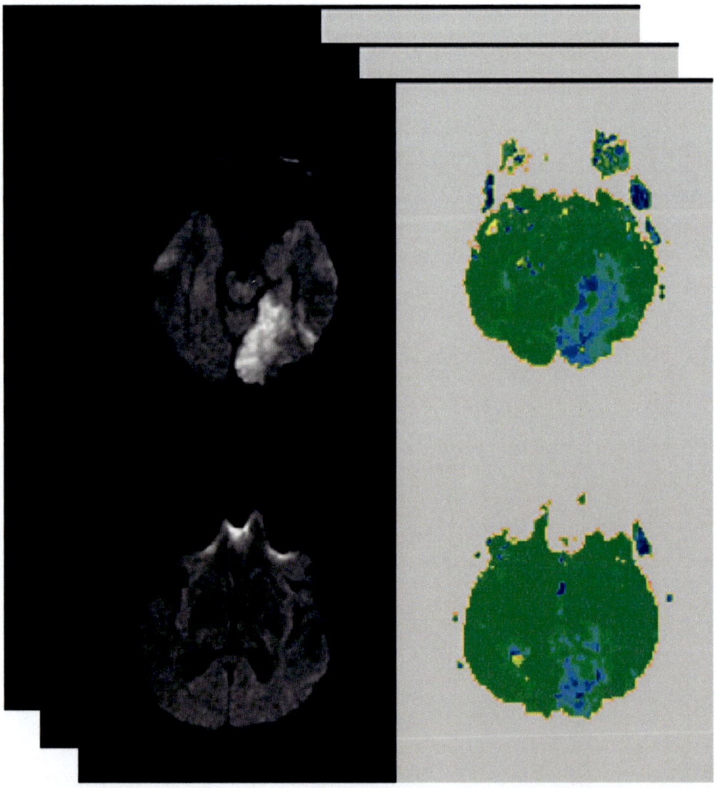

Figure 3. DWI (left) and PWI (right) of a patient with Pure Alexia and Optic Aphasia, associated with infarct in the left occipital lobe, but hypoperfusion of the entire left PCA territory, including the splenium.

*Functional Imaging.* Post-stroke aphasia syndromes have also been studied using FDG-Positron emission tomography (PET) to determine areas of altered metabolism associated with some task; $O^{15}$ PET, SPECT, or arterial spin labeling perfusion MRI to determined areas of altered blood flow; bolus-tracking PWI to determine areas of altered arrival and clearance of a bolus of contrast (closely related to blood flow); and fMRI to determine areas where a hemodynamic response is temporally linked to an event or task.

For example, PET studies by Metter and colleagues demonstrated that the area of altered cerebral glucose metabolism in aphasic patients consistently extends beyond brain regions that are structurally damaged. In their studies, all right-handed patients with left hemisphere structural lesions and aphasia had altered metabolism in left temporoparietal cortex [28, 29; see 30 for review]. The aphasic patients inconsistently had metabolic abnormalities in undamaged, left prefrontal lobe and thalamus that could account for variations in their clinical deficits.

MRI studies that reveal areas of dysfunctional tissue have largely confirmed the relationships between clinical aphasia syndromes and particular vascular territories as described above. To illustrate, many studies employing only structural imaging studies had led to the conclusion that purely subcortical lesions (particularly lesions in the caudate nucleus) can cause nearly any of the aphasia syndromes described above [1,31; see [32] for review). However, a recent study of patients with left caudate lesions and no cortical damage on structural MRI demonstrated with PWI that the presence of a particular aphasia syndrome could be explained by hypoperfusion in commonly associated cortical vascular territory [33]. For example, Broca's aphasia was observed after left caudate stroke only when there was concomitant hypoperfusion in territory of the superior division of the left MCA, including Broca's area. Likewise, Wernicke's aphasia occurred only in cases with hypoperfusion of Wernicke's area.

### *Subcortical Aphasia*

The study of aphasia syndromes in patients with caudate stroke indicates that aphasia after subcortical stroke may be due to cortical dysfunction rather than the subcortical infarct itself. This possibility was also indicated by earlier studies of aphasia following subcortical stroke (identified on CT scan), that demonstrated cortical dysfunction using SPECT [34] or PET [28, 35, 36]. However, it was unclear from these studies whether the cortical dysfunction was secondary to the subcortical lesion (due to loss of input from the subcortical structure to the cortex; i.e., diaschisis) or independent of the subcortical lesion. In the latter case, severe stenosis/plaque of the left MCA could cause both occlusion of a lenticulostriate artery (causing a subcortical infarct) and hypoperfusion of language cortex. In this case, cortical hypoperfusion would not be due to the infarct. A study of patients with aphasia after acute, nonthalamic subcortical stroke who underwent treatment to improve cortical perfusion provided evidence for the latter account. That is, a series of patients with aphasia after infarcts restricted to the subcortical tissue showed hypoperfusion of the left MCA cortex before intervention and showed immediate resolution of the aphasia when blood flow was restored to the cortex (with urgent endarterectomy, internal carotid artery stenting, or induced blood pressure elevation). Reperfusion was demonstrated by PWI before and after treatment [37]. If the aphasia had been due to diaschisis or directly due to the subcortical damage, it would not have resolved with reperfusion of the cortex, since the subcortical infarct was still present after intervention.

### *Evidence for the Neural Substrates Underlying Specific Cognitive Processes Underlying Language*

So far, we have discussed language deficits primarily in terms of clinical syndromes. As pointed out above, each syndrome is a collection of deficits in relatively independent language functions that depend on areas of the brain that are supplied by a single major artery or branch. For instance, Broca's aphasia includes impaired planning and programming of speech articulation, impaired naming of verbs and functors, and asyntactic comprehension (impaired processing of complex syntactic forms). These component features commonly co-occur not because they have a shared underlying cognitive process, but because they both depend on areas of brain supplied by the anterior division of the left MCA. But there is accumulating evidence that each of these language tasks (e.g., naming of verbs) is also complex, requiring a number of cognitive processes that can be independently disrupted by brain damage. To illustrate, oral naming of a picture of an action (say, "running"), requires: (i) recognizing the picture as a familiar action; (ii) accessing a semantic representation of [running] that distinguishes it from other actions such as [walking] or [swimming]; (iii) accessing a modality-independent lexical representation, or lemma, that specifies its grammatical class; (iv) selecting a particular morphological form ("running" versus run, ran, runs); (v) accessing a modality-specific lexical phonological representation that specifies the learned pronunciation; (vi) accessing motor plans and programs for articulating the phonological form; and (vii) implementing these motor plans with a complex sequence of movements of the jaw, lips, palate, tongue, vocal cords, and respiratory system. These various components of verb naming could each take place in separate regions of the brain, such that an entire network of brain regions is necessary to perform the task. Functional imaging (PET and fMRI) have confirmed that overt naming of pictures results in "activation" in numerous brain regions, predominantly -- but not exclusively -- in the left hemisphere (e.g., [38]; see [39] for review). These regions, including Broca's area and Wernicke's area, overlap with regions of activation during related tasks, such as oral reading or naming verbs associated with aurally presented nouns [40]. Some studies have attempted to identify the neural substrates of individual components of such complex processes, primarily through "subtraction" of activation of a task that involves all of the same components of processing except the one of interest. For example, to identify the area of brain responsible for accessing the lexical phonological representation (the phonological lexicon) for word recognition, Howard and colleagues [41] subtracted activation associated with hearing spoken words presented backwards and saying the word, "crime" from activation associated with word repetition, and found a significant increase in regional cerebral blood flow in left superior and middle temporal gyri [41].

More recent PET studies have identified an area in the left midfusiform gyrus that appears to be engaged in all lexical tasks, irrespective of the modality [42-44]. However, fMRI studies have shown that this region (or an adjacent region) is reliably engaged in prelexical orthographic processing required for reading words or pseudowords [25, 45]. To evaluate these potential roles of left midfusiform gyrus in reading versus naming, we recently carried out a study of reading, naming, and magnetic resonance diffusion weighted imaging (DWI, which is highly sensitive to ischemia within minutes to hours of onset) and perfusion weighted imaging (PWI, which reveals areas of low blood flow corresponding to dysfunction) in a series of 80 patients with acute, let hemisphere stroke. We found that lesions or hypoperfusion in left midfusiform gyrus were associated with acute disruption of oral and written naming, but did not reliably cause impaired reading comprehension [46]. These findings were consistent with the proposal that the left midfusiform gyrus is essential for modality-independent lexical processing, but not essential for reading comprehension. However, the available data from functional imaging showing reliable activation in left midfusiform gyrus during reading and related tasks could be reconciled with the lesion data indicating that damage to this region does not reliably disrupt reading by proposing that either the left or the right midfusiform gyrus is necessary for computing a prelexical location- and font-independent representation of the visual word or pseudoword for reading [46].

Other components of the complex process of naming verbs have also been identified with functional imaging studies or MRI. For example, access to modality-specific lexical representations of verbs, but not nouns, is impaired by acute dysfunction of left, posterior frontal regions shown on DWI and/or PWI [37]. Furthermore, two patients with impaired written naming of verbs (but relatively intact written naming of nouns and oral naming of both nouns and verbs) associated with hypoperfusion of left Broca's area showed recovery of written naming of verbs when blood flow was restored to Broca's area, providing further evidence that this region is critical for accessing orthographic representations of verbs [47]. The proposal that left posterior frontal regions are particularly important for producing verbs (perhaps because verbs require selection of a particular morphological form; e.g., run, runs, running) has been supported by evidence from repetitive transcranial magnetic stimulation (rTMS; 48), as well as PET and lesion studies [49,50].

Planning and orchestrating speech articulation in order to produce names of verbs as well as nouns also seem to depend on Broca's area. In a recent study of 80 patients with acute left hemisphere stroke, hypoperfusion and/or infarction of Broca's area (demonstrated with DWI and PWI within 24 hours of onset) was strongly associated with impaired motor planning and programming of speech articulation (a deficit sometimes known as apraxia of speech) [51]. This study confirmed some earlier CT scan studies indicating that lesions in Broca's area were associated with apraxia of speech [13, 52]. However, this study did not confirm a previous conclusion that lesions involving the left anterior insula cause apraxia of speech [53]. This conclusion was based on the finding among 25 patients with chronic apraxia of speech, the most common (and universal) area of overlap in their lesions on MRI or CT scan was the anterior insula.

However, this result might have resulted from the combined facts that (i) patients with chronic apraxia of speech have large left MCA lesions and (ii) the insula is the most common area of overlap in large left MCA lesions (see [51] for discussion).

A

B

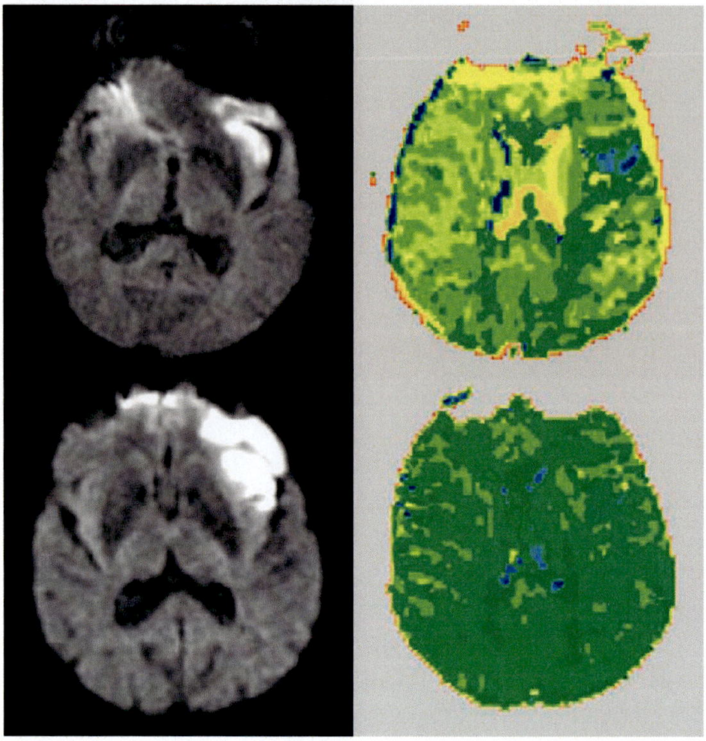

Figure 4. Panel A. DWI (left) and PWI (right) scans of a patient with selective impairment in oral naming of verbs < 24 hours from stroke onset, showing hypoperfusion of left premotor cortex (and infarct involving more inferior and anteriomedial frontal lobe and insula). Panel B. DWI (left) and PWI (right) in the same patient, one day later, when oral verb naming had recovered in association with restored perfusion of left premotor area. Results indicate that the left premotor regions is essential for oral naming, particularly of verbs.

As illustrated by the preceding examples, two advantages of MRI over CT for identifying lesions associated with discrete processes are that (i) MRI has much better resolution for identifying small infarcts, which are likely to cause selective deficits, and (ii) MRI can show deficits at the acute stage of stroke, before reorganization or recovery. Although many studies of aphasia have included only patients in the chronic stage of aphasia (6 months or more after stroke), such patients typically have large strokes, since patients with small strokes generally recover quickly. Furthermore, it is often difficult to determine what part of a large lesion is responsible for the residual deficit, since the patient may have undergone substantial recovery and reorganization. As noted above, one method that has commonly been employed to determine the region most likely to be responsible for a chronic deficit is lesion overlap. The assumption is that the area of damage shared by the most patients with the deficit is likely to be responsible for the function that failed to recover. However, this method might simply reveal the area most vulnerable to infarct, since some regions are commonly involved in stroke lesions [54]. For instance, the insula is involved in nearly all infarcts caused by occlusion of the left MCA [55]. As noted, this observation may account for the finding that the insula (or part of the insula) is the area of greatest overlap among patients with chronic apraxia of speech, which only persists in patients with large left MCA strokes. One way to avoid the bias toward identifying areas that are most vulnerable to infarct is to "subtract out" lesions of patients without the deficit. The problem with this method in chronic aphasia is that there is an important risk of "subtracting out" lesions that did cause the deficit of interest, but the deficit resolved before the study. A related method of identifying an area of lesion most strongly associated with a quantified deficit involves a voxel-based approach using SPM [56]. The voxel-based approach allows one to examine the entire brain for lesion/deficit associations, without biasing the results by examining specific regions of interest. However, there are limitations of this methodology as well. For example, if the study includes patients who initially had the deficit of interest after an acute lesion (say, in a particular cluster of voxels) but whose deficit has recovered due to cortical plasticity, the study may underestimate the importance of that cluster of voxels in causing the deficit. This voxel-based approach requires registering the brains of patients to an atlas. This registration allows comparison to functional imaging studies (that typically involve such registration). However, it must be kept in mind that the voxels in one patient may not correspond to the same cytoarchitectural field as the "same" voxels in another patient. This problem cannot be avoided by any region of interest method, either, since the cytoarchitectural fields within specific gyral locations are variable across individuals [57]. Given this variability, it is not clear that voxel-based approaches have a significant advantage over region of interest approaches, except that the former does not require any predetermined hypothesis about what areas may be associated with a deficit. Voxel-based approaches require a large number of patients with and without damage to any area that might be of interest. That is, it is not possible to determine the relationship between any cluster of voxels and a deficit unless there are a substantial number of patients with lesions involving that cluster and a substantial number of patients without lesions involving that cluster (as well as a substantial number of patients showing a wide range of severities of the deficit being studied).

Several recent developed imaging methods can reveal the entire area of dysfunctional tissue, including areas of low blood flow that may contribute to acute language deficits (and perhaps chronic deficits; see [58]. We have noted that abnormalities on PWI (also called dynamic contrast perfusion MRI, or bolus-tracking perfusion MRI), which shows areas of delayed arrival and clearance of a bolus of contrast, have been associated with particular language deficits. This method is particularly useful in acute stroke, since it is acquired in less than two minutes, is not particularly sensitive to motion artifact, and has good spatial resolution over the entire brain. It can be repeated serially over the course of recovery, to determine areas where hypoperfusion is associated with a particular deficit, and where reperfusion results in recovery of the deficit. For example, the patient in Figure 4 had a selective impairment in oral naming of verbs when PWI showed hypoperfusion of left premotor cortex, and showed recovery of oral verb naming when PWI showed restored perfusion of left premotor area, indicating that this region is crucial for oral naming, particularly of verbs.

Other methods for demonstrating focal hypoperfusion associated with particular aphasic deficits include arterial spin labeling (ASL) perfusion, CT perfusion, SPECT, and PET. ASL has the advantages that it can show absolute blood flow (whereas PWI shows relative blood flow), and can be used repeatedly to show areas of increased blood flow associated with activation as well as areas of decreased blood flow associated with dysfunction and arterial stenosis. However, it requires more time, is more sensitive to motion artifact than PWI, and loses information in areas of extremely low blood flow. Neither PWI nor ASL involve ionizing radiation; ASL also requires no intravenous injection. ASL has been used to identify areas of hypoperfusion associated with language deficits in patients with dementias [59] and chronic stroke [58]. CT perfusion also measures absolute blood flow, and can be used easily in acute stroke. Currently, most methods of ASL and CT perfusion do not provide whole brain coverage. Nevertheless, they can be useful for quantifying blood flow changes in selected areas that are associated with language performance. A recent study of acute aphasia using CT perfusion [60] is described under contributions to clinical knowledge.

## Imaging Mechanisms of Language Recovery after Post-Stroke Aphasia

Among the earliest and longstanding hypotheses about how patients recover from aphasia after stroke is that the intact right hemisphere assumes the functions of the damaged left hemisphere. One observation that provided evidence for this hypothesis is that patients who recover language after extensive strokes in the left hemisphere can show recurrence of aphasia after a second stroke in the right hemisphere, indicating that language functions had been "taken over" by the right hemisphere during recovery [61, 62]. A second line of evidence for this proposal came from sodium amytal injection (Wada testing) of the carotid artery, which temporarily renders much of the ipsilateral hemisphere dysfunctional. Injection of the right carotid in recovered aphasic patients caused re-occurrence of aphasia in some patients, again indicating that language had been assumed by the right [63, 64]. More recently, supportive evidence has come from functional imaging studies (fMRI and PET) that show more right hemisphere activation during language tasks in recovered aphasic patients than in normal subjects [65-71]. Other functional imaging studies reveal activation in non-infarcted regions of the left hemisphere during language tasks that is greater in recovered aphasic patients than normal subjects [72-75]. Together, these studies indicate that both right hemisphere regions (particularly regions homologous to Wernicke's and Broca's areas) and prei-lesional regions of the left hemisphere contribute to reorganization and recovery. What areas assume the functions of the damaged region likely depends on the extent of perisylvian left hemisphere damage, the time since onset of lesion, and the language functions that were affected [76]. It is likely that the right hemisphere is capable of assuming some language functions (e.g., word meaning) more than others (e.g., converting from print to sound to read unfamiliar words). In functional imaging studies of patients with post-stroke aphasia, some of the activation may be related to retrieval effort more than retrieval success [77]. Furthermore, reorganization of structure/function relationships is likely to be dynamic. That is, some language functions may initially be taken over by homologous regions in the right hemisphere and later cross back to perilesional left hemisphere areas. In fact, the highest degree of language recovery is seen in patients who show this transfer of language back to the left hemisphere [78].

However, reorganization is not the only mechanism of aphasia recovery demonstrated with imaging. At least early recovery may reflect restoration of tissue function, through reperfusion of ischemic but non-infarcted regions or through stabilization of ionic balance and membrane integrity. To illustrate, in a series of 80 acute stroke patients, all patients who showed impaired word comprehension at Day 1 and recovered word comprehension at Day 3 to 5 showed initial hypoperfusion of Wernicke's area, followed by reperfusion of this area at Day 3 to 5 [79]. These results confirmed the essential role of Wernicke's area in word comprehension and showed that recovery of word comprehension in the first five days did not occur through reorganization, but only occurred if Wernicke's area was salvaged through restored blood flow. However, later recovery of word comprehension in cases of infarct to Wernicke's area likely occurs through reorganization [65]. Other studies have shown that reperfusion of other left perisylvian regions results in recovery of other language functions in acute stroke [80].

# B. Contributions to Clinical Knowledge

## Diagnosis of the Etiology of Aphasia

Clearly the greatest usefulness of brain imaging in stroke is making an accurate diagnosis to guide appropriate treatment, as reviewed in previous chapters. Imaging reveals the nature of the brain injury (hemorrhage, infarct, hypoperfusion) causing aphasia in individual cases. In some cases, even though the diagnosis may be clear (e.g., a subcortical infarct on CT), the cause of aphasia may not be clear without additional imaging (e.g., associated cortical hypoperfusion revealed by PWI, CT perfusion, SPECT, or PET, as described earlier). In other cases of aphasia the CT or conventional MRI may be relatively benign, but blood flow studies can account for the language deficits.

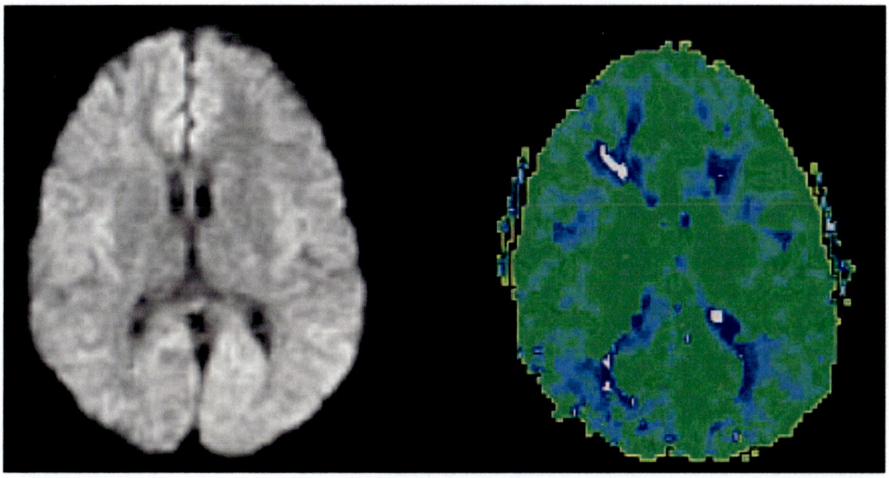

Figure 5. DWI (left) and PWI (right) of a patient with a benign CT scan but profound impairment in reading and naming associated with severe hypoperfusion in bilateral inferior temporal and occipital cortex and frontal cortex, relative to subcortical areas, due to moyamoya syndrome.

For example, the patient whose scans are shown in Figure 5 had a benign CT scan, but PWI showed areas of severe hypoperfusion that explained her profound impairment in reading and naming. Cerebral angiogram confirmed the diagnosis of moyamoya syndrome. This patient underwent encephalomyosynagniosis to improve perfusion of the left temporal and occipital regions (confirmed with repeat PWI), which resulted in recovery of reading and naming [81].

## Prognosis for Recovery from Aphasia

The above case illustrates that when the lesion seen on CT or structural MRI is smaller than what would be expected for the degree or type of aphasia, some sort of blood flow imaging is warranted to determine the cause of the aphasia. Further, since the severity of aphasia is strongly correlated with the volume of hypoperfusion seen on PWI [47, 82], an aphasia severity score might be used to predict the volume of hypoperfusion. This prediction would make it possible to estimate the degree of "diffusion-perfusion mismatch", or volume of dysfunctional, but potentially salvageable tissue. This concept of calculating a "diffusion-clinical mismatch" to determine the amount of tissue that might be salvaged with reperfusion was evaluated in a recent study of aphasia [83]. First, it was shown that either of two simple, bedside tests of language (oral naming of pictures or word repetition) could be used to predict the volume of hypoperfusion on PWI. The regression equation was used to predict perfusion abnormality with either clinical aphasia score for each patient; then the volume of infarct on DWI for that patient was subtracted, to determine the diffusion-clinical mismatch. It was then demonstrated that larger diffusion-clinical mismatch was associated with better language recovery, consistent with the hypothesis that the volume of diffusion-clinical mismatch was related to the volume of potentially salvageable tissue (in terms of functional recovery). The only patient with a >20% diffusion-clinical mismatch who failed to show language improvement showed no reperfusion on repeat PWI.

Another recent study demonstrated that perfusion CT (P-CT) can reveal the volume of dysfunctional tissue that correlates with aphasia severity [60]. Patients were evaluated with P-CT and language testing within six hours of symptom onset, then serially over one week. In the first six hours, 13/24 patient had deficits in all language domains; all 13 had large areas of hypoperfusion in thc lcft MCA cortex revealed by P-CT. Language scores were associated with hypoperfusion in specific areas within the MCA territory. Furthermore, aphasia improved significantly more when the hypoperfused tissue showed restored blood flow, than when it evolved toward infarct. These results provide additional evidence that changes in aphasia in the acute stage reflect changes in perfusion documented with imaging (and might be used as a substitute for imaging when the latter is not possible).

## Treatment

Knowing the location of a stroke or volume of a stroke does not directly guide treatment decisions. However, the combination of DWI and PWI (or the combination of DWI and language testing) can identify which patients might benefit from aggressive intervention to restore blood flow to improve speech or language, as noted above. To illustrate, a patient with sudden onset severe aphasia whose MRI shows a small infarct on DWI but a large area of hypoperfusion in left perisylvian ("language") cortex would likely show improved language if blood flow can be restored to left perisylvian cortex. Such improvements were demonstrated in a series of patients with left subcortical stroke, as noted earlier. Moreover, reperfusion of specific regions of the brain improved specific language functions [84]. In many of these cases, the patients had worsening aphasia over several days, before imaging revealed a large DWI-PWI mismatch, with mismatch territory involving language cortex. Since these patients were not candidates for thrombolyisis days after symptom onset, investigational treatment to restore perfusion was necessary.

Investigation treatment was based on the following reported observations. In ischemic tissue, unlike normal tissue, there is a loss of autoregulation, such that increasing systemic blood pressure results in improved regional blood flow in the ischemic areas of brain [85]. Based on this observation, several groups have studied temporary blood pressure elevation to improve blood flow and function [86-88]. Since this intervention should be most effective in patients with large area of hypoperfusion that is not yet infracted, we conducted a small, randomized trial of pharmacologically induced blood pressure elevation in patients selected on the basis of a large, persistent DWI-PWI mismatch up to one week post onset of symptoms. Since many of these patients had subcortical infarct and cortical hypoperfusion, we measured response to treatment by evaluating cortical function (language skills in patients with left hemisphere stroke, spatial attention in patients with right hemisphere stroke) and repeat PWI. Patients who were randomized to blood pressure elevation showed significantly more improvement on language or spatial attention testing, and greater reductions in volume of hypoperfusion, than patients randomized to conventional management [47]. Even though this study was small, the effect size was large enough to demonstrate a benefit of treatment for improving aphasia or neglect in patients selected on the basis of a large DWI-PWI mismatch up to one week post onset. Results illustrated the potential of perfusion imaging to help select patients for specific interventions to improve aphasia.

Urakawa, et al. [89] reported successful treatment to restore perfusion that resulted in resolution of aphasia and other neurological deficits with local thrombolytic therapy given to a patient 24 hours after onset of left middle cerebral artery (MCA) occlusion. In this patient a Xenon CT cerebral blood flow study revealed hypoperfusion in the left MCA territory, which showed negative cerebrovascular reactivity, while FLAIR only showed only a smaller area of slight hyperintensity in the left frontal white matter. Angiogram revealed left MCA occlusion. Intra-arterial thrombolysis with urokinase, done 24 hours after onset of symptoms resulted in immediate improvement of aphasia and motor symptoms. This study illustrates again how imaging evidence of an area of symptomatic hypoperfusion beyond the infarct is likely to indicate the potential usefulness of restoring blood flow, and may therefore be useful for identifying candidates for specific interventions to improve aphasia.

Functional imaging studies (PET and fMRI) have also been used to evaluate effects of language therapy on degree and location of neural activation measured with these techniques. For example, Thompson and colleagues (e.g. [70] performed fMRI before and after treatment of sentence comprehension deficits in patients with chronic Broca's aphasia. They found increased activation of right hemisphere regions homologous to language cortex (Wernicke's area in all patients, Broca's area in two patients) after treatment, indicating that treatment may have induced reorganization of structure/function relationships. Similarly, Musso and colleagues, [69] demonstrated that treatment of auditory comprehension in patients with Wernicke's aphasia resulted in improved performance on a test of following spoken directions, that correlated with increased activation in the right hemisphere homologue of Wernicke's area and left precuneous (using PET). Therapy for reading impairment has also been associated with changes in areas of activation on fMRI [90]

## C. Future Directions

As new imaging techniques become available, investigators are beginning to combine complementary methods to address questions about brain/behavioral relationships. For example, several groups have combined rTMS with PET or fMRI, to determine if regions of "activation" on functional imaging indicate adaptive or maladaptive neural activity. In some cases in which rTMS is used to suppress neural activity in tissue that showed activation on fMRI, there is actually improvement, rather than reduction, in ability to carry out a language task (indicating that the activation on fMRI did not reflect activity ctitical to the task). For example, Naeser, et al. [91, 92] reported that nonfluent aphasic patients whose scans show activation in the right hemisphere homologue of Broca's area showed improved naming performance after rTMS that suppressed part of this area (BA 44). However, rTMS suppression of the cortex contralateral to stroke can also impair language function (92). Others have used PET to identify areas to target with rTMS or have used PET and TMS together to demonstrate connectivity [93]. The latter is done by applying TMS to an area of interest, and then evaluating the areas where the TMS results in changes in blood flow (inhibitory or excitory connections). This methodology may help identify networks of connected cortical regions underlying specific language functions.

PET studies of particular receptors or transporters, or molecular MRI using markers of plasticity, may also be useful in identifying areas of metabolic changes associated with specific aphasic deficits or associated with reorganization (due to treatment and/or spontaneous recovery). Diffusion Tensor Imaging (DTI) can reveal damage to white matter tracks that may explain deficits due to "disconnection" of cortical regions underlying language. For example, a recent white matter tractography study using DTI demonstrated two white matter tracts connecting Broca's and Wernicke's area, one of which connected these areas via the angular gyrus [94]. The authors argued that the two tracts can account for variations in Conduction aphasia. Another study using voxel-based statistical analyses of DTI showed an asymmetry of the arcuate fasciculus, with higher fractional anisotropy in the left hemisphere, consistent with a role of this tract in language [95]. However, still another DTI study of a patient with mixed transcortical sensory aphasia revealed a lesion in the arcuate fasciculus, a finding that did not support the necessary role of this tract in repetition, as proposed by Geschwind [20], since repetition was intact from the onset of stroke in this patient [96]. Finally, results from DTI in patients with pure alexia are consistent with the hypothesize role of the splenium in transferring visual information from the right occipital lobe to the left inferior temporal cortex in reading [97, 98]. Another recent study showed how DTI fiber tracking and intraoperative cortical stimulation could be used together to delineate subcortical pathways between various cortical regions critical for speech and language [99]. This combination of techniques may be useful clinically (to allow sparing of eloquent regions and their connections during neurosurgery) as well as useful in terms of demonstrating connectivity between brain regions critical for language. These cases illustrate how the study of language and aphasia will be enhanced with DTI and with combined methodologies.

## D. Take Home Message

Both structural and functional neuroimaging are rapidly evolving. Neuroimaging has been critical to demonstrating that classic aphasia syndromes arise after stroke because areas of the brain necessary for particular language functions predictably fall in the territory of the same artery. Such syndromes can reflect either permanent damage to the vascular territory or hypoperfusion caused by stenosis or occlusion of the artery. More selective deficits (components of aphasic syndromes) arise when acute damage or hypoperfusion involves only a small part of the vascular territory; or as a result of reorganization after chronic brain damage, such that other components of the aphasia syndrome are assumed by other parts of the brain.

## E. Acknowledgements

The research reported in this chapter from the author's laboratory was supported by as by an NIDCD grant, RO1 DC05375.

## References

[1] Kirk A, Kertesz A. Cortical and subcortical aphasias compared. *Aphasiology* 1994; 8: 65-82.

[2] Naeser MA, Hayward RW. Lesion localization in aphasia with cranial computed tomography and Boston Diagnostic Aphasia Examination. *Neurology* 1978; 28:545-551.

[3] Alexander MP, Naeser MA, Palumbo C. Broca's area aphasia: Aphasia after lesions including frontal opeculum. *Neurology* 1990; 40:353-362.

[4] Zurif EB. Psycholinguistic interpretations of the aphasias. In: *Biological Perspectives on Language* (Caplan D, Lecours AR, Smith A, eds). Cambridge, MA: MIT Press. 1984.

[5] Berndt RS. Symptom co-occurrence and dissociation in the interpretation of agrammatism. In: *The Cognitive Neuropsychology of Language* (Coltheart M, Sartori G, Job R, eds). New Jersey: Lawrence Erlbaum Associates, 1987.

[6] Caramazza A, Zurif E. Dissociation of algorithmic and heuristic processes in language comprehension. *Brain Lang* 1976; 3:572-582.

[7] Grodzinsky J. The syntactic characterization of agrammatism. *Cognition* 1984; 16:99-120.

[8] Nespoulous J-L, Dordain M, Peron C, et al. Agrammatism in sentence production without comprehension deficits: Reduced availability of syntactic structures and/or grammatical morphemes? *Brain Lang* 1988; 33:273-295.

[9] Caramazza A, Hillis AE. The disruption of sentence production: some dissociations. *Brain Lang* 1989; 35: 625-650.

[10] Berndt R, Caramazza A. How "regular" is sentence compehension in Broca's aphasia? It depends on how you select your patients. *Brain Lang* 1999; 67:242-247.

[11] Caramazza A, Capitani E, Rey A, et al. Agrammatic Broca's aphasia is not associated with a single pattern of coprehension performance. *Brain Lang* 2001; 76:158-184.

[12] Mohr JP. Broca's area and Broca's aphasia. In: *Studies in Neurolinguistics*, Vol 1 (Whitaker H, ed), New York: Academic Press; 1976.

[13] Mohr JP, Pessin Ms, Finkelstein S, et al. Broca Aphasia: pathological and clinical. *Neurology* 1978; 28:311-324.

[14] Selnes OA, Niccum N, Knopman DS, et al. Recovery of Single Word Comprehension: CT-scan Correlates. *Brain Lang* 1984 21:72-84.

[15] Alexander MP. Aphasia: clinical and anatomical aspects. In: *Behavioral Neurology and Neuropsychology* (Feinberg TE, Farah MJ, eds), pp133-150. New York: McGraw Hill; 1977.

[16] Raymer A, Foundas AL, Maher LM, et al. Cognitive neuropsychological analysis and neuroanatomical correlates in a case of acute anomia. *Brain Lang* 1997; 58:137-156.

[17] Hillis AE, Boatman D, Hart J, et al. Making sense out of jargon: a neurolinguistic and computational account of jargon aphasia. *Neurology* 1999; 53:1813-1824.

[18] Kumral E, Bayulkem G, Evyapan D, et al. Spectrum of anterior cerebral artery territory infarction: clinical and MRI findings. *Eur. J. Neurol.* 2002; 9:615-624.

[19] Evrard S, Woimant F, Le Coz P, et al. Watershed cerebral infarcts: retrospective study of 24 cases. *Neurol. Res.* 1992; 14:97-99.

[20] Geschwind N. Disconnexion syndromes in animals and man. *Brain* 1965; 88:237-294, 585-644.

[21] Maeshima S, Toshiro H, Sekiguchi E, et al. Transcortical mixed aphasia duc to cerebral infarction in left inferior frontal love and temporo-parietal lobe. *Neuroradiology* 2002; 44:133-137.

[22] Dejerine J. Sur un cas de cécité verbale avec agraphie, suivi d'autopsie. *Comptes Rendus Hebdomadaires des Séances et Mémoires de la Société de Biologie*. Ninth series 1891; 3:197-201.

[23] Freund CS. Über optische Aphasia and Seelenblindheit. *Archiv Psychiatrie und Nervenkrankheiten* 1889; 20:276-297.

[24] Binder JR, Mohr JP. The topography of callosal reading pathways: a case-control analysis. *Brain* 1992; 115:1807-1826.

[25] Cohen L, Dehaene S, Naccache L, et al. The visual word form area: spatial and temporal characterization of an initial stage of reading in normal subjects and posterior split-brain patients. *Brain* 2000 ; 123:291-307.

[26] Hillis AE, Caramazza A. Cognitive and neural mechanisms underlying visual and semantic processing. *J. Cogn. Neurosci.* 1995; 7:457-478.

[27] Marshall RS. Neuroimaging correlates of stroke recovery. Paper presented at the 28th International Stroke Meeting. Phoenix, AZ; 2003.

[28] Metter EJ, Kempler D, Hanson WR, et al. Cerebral glucose metabolism: differences in Wernicke's, Broca's and Conduction aphasia. In: *Clinical Aphasiology*, Vol. 16 (Brookshire RH, ed), pp97-104. Minneapolis: BRK Publishers; 1986.

[29] Metter EJ, Wasterlain CG, Kuhl DE, et al. FDG positron emission tomography to a study of aphasia. *Ann. Neurol.*1983; 10:173-183.

[30] Metter EJ. Brain-behavior relationships in aphasia studied by positron emission tomography. *Ann. NY Acad. Sci.* 1991; 620:153-164.

[31] Naeser MA, Alexander MP, Helms-Estabrook N, et al. Aphasia with predominantly subcortical lesion sites. *Arch. Neurol.* 1982; 39:2-14.

[32] Nadeau S, Crosson B. Subcortical aphasia. Brain Lang 1997; 58:355-402.

[33] Hillis AE, Barker PB, Wityk RJ, et al. Variability in subcortical aphasia is due to variable sites of cortical hypoperfusion. *Brain Lang* 2004; 89:524-530.

[34] Vallar G, Perani D, Cappa SF, et al. Recovery of aphasia and neglect after subcortical stroke: neuropsychological and cerebral perfusion study. *J. Neurol. Neurosurg. Psychiatry* 1988; 51:1269-1276.

[35] Skyhøj-Olsen T, Bruhn P, Oberg RG. Cortical hypoperfusion as a possible cause of "subcortical aphasia." *Brain* 1986; 106:393-410.

[36] Baron JC, D'Antona R, Pantano P, et al. Effects of thalamic stroke on energy metabolism in the cerebral cortex. *Brain* 1986; 109:1243-1259.

[37] Hillis AE, Kane A, Tuffiash E, et al. Reperfusion of specific brain regions by raising blood pressure restores selective language functions in subacute stroke. *Brain Lang* 2002; 79:495-510.

[38] Warburton E, Wise RJS, Price CJ, et al. Noun and verb retrieval by normal subjects: Studies with PET. *Brain* 1996; 119:159-179.

[39] Price C. An overview of speech comprehension and production. In: *Human Brain Function* (Frackowiak RSJ, Friston KJ, Frith CD, Dolan RJ, Price CJ, Zeki S, Ashburner J, Penny W (eds), pp517-532. London: Elsevier; 2004.

[40] Peterson SE, Fox PT, Posner MI, et al. Positron emission tomography studies of the cortical anatomy of single word processing. *Nature* 1988; 331:585-589.

[41] Howard D, Patterson K, Wise R, et al. The cortical localization of the lexicons. *Brain* 1992; 115:1769-1782.

[42] Buchel C, Raedler T, Sommer M, et al. White matter asymmetry in the human brain: a diffusion tensor MRI study. *Cereb Cortex* 2004; 14:945-951.

[43] Price CJ, Devlin JT. The myth of the visual word form area. *Neuroimage* 2003;19:473-481.

[44] Price CJ, Winterburn D, Giraud AL, et al. Cortical localization of the visual and auditory word form areas: A reconsideration of the evidence. *Brain Lang* 2003;86:272-286.

[45] Cohen L, Lehericy S, Chochon F, et al. Language-specific tuning of visual cortex? Functional properties of the visual word form area. *Brain* 2002; 125:1054-1069.

[46] Hillis AE, Newhart M, Heidler J, et al. The roles of the "visual word form area" in reading. *Neuroimage* 2005; 24:548-559.

[47] Hillis AE, Wityk R, Barker PB, et al. Neural regions essential for writing verbs. *Nat. Neurosci.* 2003; 6:19-20.

[48] Shapiro KA, Pascual-Leone A, Mottaghy FM, et al. Grammatical distinctions in the left frontal cortex. *J. Cogn. Neurosci.* 2001; 13:713-720.

[49] Tranel D, Damasio H, Damasio A. On the neurology of naming. In: *Anomia* (Goodglass H, ed), London: Academic Press; 1997.

[50] Tranel D, Adolphs R, Demasio AR. A neural basis for the retrieval of words for actions. *Cogn. Neuropsych.* 2001; 18:655-670.

[51] Hillis AE, Work M, Breese EL, et al. Re-examining the brain regions crucial for orchestrating speech articulation. *Brain* 2004; 127:1479-1487.

[52] Schiff HB, Alexander MP, Naeser MA, et al. Aphemia. Clinical-anatomic correlations. *Arch. Neurol.* 1983; 40:720-727.

[53] Dronkers NF. A new brain region for coordinating speech articulation. *Nature* 1996; 384:159-161.

[54] Caviness V, Makris N, Montinaro E, et al. Anatomy of stroke, Part I: An MRI-based topographic and volumetric system of analysis. *Stroke* 2002; 22:2549-2556.

[55] Finley A, Saver J, Alger J, et al. Diffusion weighted imaging assesment of insular vulnerability in acute middle cerebral artery infarction [abstract]. *Stroke* 2003; 34:259.

[56] Bates E, Wilson SM, Saygin AP, et al. Voxel-based lesion-symptom mapping. Nature *Neurosci* 2003; 6:448-450.

[57] Whitaker HA, Selnes O. Anatomic variations in the cortex: individual differences and the problem of the localization of language functions. *Ann. NY Acad. Sci.* 1976 ; 280:844-854.

[58] Love T, Swinney D, Wong E, et al. Perfusion imaging and stroke: A more sensitive measure of the brain bases of cognitive deficits. *Aphasiology* 2002; 16:873-883.

[59] Cooke A, DeVita C, Gee J, et al. Neural basis for sentence comprehension deficits in frontotemporal dementia. *Brain Lang* 2003; 85:211-221.

[60] Croquelois A, Wintermark M, Reichart M, et al. Aphasia in hyperacute stroke: language follow brain penumbra dynamics. *Ann. Neurol.* 2003; 54:321-329.

[61] Nielson JM Agnosia, *Apraxia, and Aphasia*. New York: Hoeber, 1946.

[62] Levine DM, Mohr JP. Language after bilateral cerebral infarctions: role of the minor hemisphere. *Neurology* 1979; 29:927-938.

[63] *Kinsbourne M. The minor cerebral hemisphere as a source of aphasic speech. Arch.* Neurol. 1971; 25:302-306.

[64] Czopf J. Role of the non-dominant hemisphere in the restitution of speech in aphasia. *Archiv für Psychiatrie und Nervenkrankheiten* 1972; 216:162-171.

[65] Weiller C, Isensee C, Rijntjes M, et al. Recovery of Wernicke's aphasia: a positron emission tomographic study. A*nn. Neurol.* 1995; 37:723-732.

[66] Ohyama M, Senda M, Kitamura S, et al. Role of the nondominant hemisphere and undamaged area during word repetition in poststroke aphasics. A PET activation study. *Stroke* 1996; 27:897-903.

[67] Cappa SF, Perani D, Grassi F, et al. A PET follow-up study of recovery after stroke in acute aphasics. *Brain Lang* 1997; 56:55-67.

[68] Thulborn KR, Carpenter PA, Just MA. Plasticity of language-related brain function during recovery from stroke. *Stroke* 1999; 30:749-754.

[69] Musso M, Weiller C, Kiebel S, et al. Training-induced brain-plasticity in aphasia. *Brain* 1999; 122:1781-1790.

[70] Thompson CK, Fix SC, Gitelman DR, et al. fMRI studies of agrammatic sentence comprehension before and after treatment. *Brain Lang* 2000; 74:387-391.

[71] Leff A, Crinion J, Scott S, et al. A physiological change in homotopic cortex following left posterior temporal lobe infarction. *Ann. Neurol.* 2002; 51:533-558.

[72] Karbe H, Kessler J, Herholz K, et al. Long-term prognosis of poststroke aphasia studied with positron emission tomography. *Arch. Neurol.* 1995; 52:186-190.

[73] Heiss WD, Kessler J, Thiel A, et al. Differential capacity of left and right hemispheric areas for compensation of poststroke aphasia. *Ann. Neurol.* 1999; 45:430-438.

[74] Warburton E, Swinburn K, Price CJ, et al. Mechanisms of recovery from aphasia: evidence from positron emission tomographic studies. *J. Neurol. Neurosurg. Psychiatry* 1999; 66:155-161.

[75] Thiel A, Herholz K, Koyuncu A, et al. Plasticity of language networks in patients with brain tumors: a positron emission tomography activation study. *Ann. Neurol.* 2001; 50:620-629.

[76] Hillis AE, Wityk RJ, Barker PB, et al. (2002) Subcortical asphasia and neglect in acute stroke: the role of cortical hypoperfusion. *Brain* 2002; 125:1094-1104.

[77] Perani D, Cappa SF, Tettamanti M, et al. A fMRI study of word retrieval in aphasia. *Brain Lang* 2003; 85:357-368.

[78] Metter EJ, Reige WR, Hanson WR, et al. Comparisons of metabolic rates, language and memory in subcortical aphasia. *Brain Lang* 1983; 19:33-47.

[79] Hillis AE, Heidler J. Mechanisms of early aphasia recovery: evidence from MR perfusion imaging. *Aphasiology* 2002; 16:885-896.

[80] Hillis AE, Tuffiash E, Wityk RJ, et al. Regions of neural dysfunction associated with impaired naming of actions and objects in acute stroke. *Cogn. Neuropsych.* 2002; 19:523-534.

[81] Wityk R, Hillis AE, Beauchamp N, et al. Perfusion-weighted MRI in adult moyamoya syndrome: characteristic patterns and change after surgical intervention: case report. *Neurosurgery* 2002; 51:1499-1506.

[82] Hillis AE, Barker P, Beauchamp N, et al. MR perfusion imaging reveals regions of hypoperfusion associated with aphasia and neglect. *Neurology* 2000; 55:782-788.

[83] Reineck L, Agarwal S, Hillis AE. The "diffusion-clinical mismatch" predicts early language recovery in acute stroke. *Neurology;* in press.

[84] Hillis AE, Wityk RJ, Barker PB, et al. Change in perfusion in acute nondominant hemisphere stroke may be better estimated by tests of hemispatial neglect than by the NIHSS. *Stroke* 2003; 34:2392-2398.

[85] Astrup J, Symon L, Branston NM, et al. Cortical evoked potential and extracellular K+ and H+ at critical levels of brain ischemia. *Stroke* 1977; 8:51-57.

[86] Wise G, Sutter R, Burkholder J. The treatment of brain ischemia with vasopressor drugs. *Stroke* 1972; 3:135-140.

[87] Rordorf G, Cramer SC, Efird JT, et al. Pharmacological elevation of blood pressure in acute stroke. *Stroke* 1997; 28:2133-2138.

[88] Rordorf G, Koroshetz W., Ezzeddine MA, et al. A pilot study of drug-induced hypertension for treatment of acute stroke. *Neurology* 2001; 56:1210-1213.

[89] Urakawa M, Ueda Y, Yamashita T. Successful local thrombolytic therapy for atherosclerotic middle cerebral artery occlusion 24 hours after onset: case report. No *Shinkei Geka* 2003; 31:195-199.

[90] Small SL, Flores D, Noll DC. Grapheme to phoneme conversion in acquired dyslexia: Neurobiological changes accompany therapy. *Brain Lang* 1997; 60:127-131.

[91] Naeser MA, Martin PI, Baker EH, et al. Overt propositional in chronic nonfluent aphasia with the dynamic susceptiblity constrast fMRI method. *Neuroimage* 2004; 22:29-41.

[92] Naser MA, Baker EH, Palumbo CL, et al. Lesion site patterns in severe, nonverbal aphasia to predict outcome with a computer-assisted treatment program. *Arch. Neurol.* 1998; 55:1438-48.

[93] Fox P, Ingham R, George MS, et al. Imaging human intra-cerebral connectivity by PET during TMS. *Neuroreport* 1997; 8:2787-2791.

[94] Catani M, Jones DK, Fytche DH. Perisylvian language networks of the human brain. *Ann. Neurol.* 2005; 57:8-16.

[95] Buchel C, Price C, Friston K. A multimodal language region in the ventral visual pathway. *Nature* 1998; 394:274-277.

[96] Selnes OA, van Zijl P, Barker PB, et al. MR Diffusion Tensor Imaging documented Arcuate Fasciculus lesion in a patient with normal repetition performance. *Aphasiology* 2002; 16:897-902.

[97] Molko N, Cohen L, Mangin JF, et al. Visualizing the neural bases of a disconnection syndrome with diffusion tensor imaging. *J. Cogn. Neurosci.* 2002; 14:629-36.

[98] Le TH, Mukherjee P, Henry RG, et al. Diffusion tensor imaging with three-dimensional fiber tractography of traumatic axonal shearing injury: an imaging correlate for the posterior callosal "disconnection" syndrome: case report. Neurosurgery 2005; 56:189.

[99] Henry RG, Berman JI, Nagarajan SS, et al. Subcortical pathways serving cortical language sites: initial experience with diffusion tensor imaging fiber tracking combined with intraoperative language mapping. *Neuroimage* 2004; 21:616-622.

In: State-of-the-Art Imaging in Stroke, Volume 2
Editor: Bernhard Schaller, pp. 163-194
ISBN 978-1-60021-499-8


*Chapter VI*

# Poststroke Swallowing Difficulties and Imaging

***Samantha Jefferson and Shaheen Hamdy***
Univeristy of Manchester, Department of Gastrointestinal Sciences,
Hope Hospital, Manchester, UK

## Abstract

Swallowing problems are very common following stroke and may lead to a variety of serious complications. Although the majority of patients spontaneously recover there are a number who are left with residual swallowing difficulties. This chapter will first examine what is known about the physiology and imaging of normal deglutition, as a background to the pathophysiology and imaging of dysphagia following stroke. Imaging with computed tomography and magnetic resonance imaging and the effect of lesion location on the different aspects of swallowing function will then be considered, followed by a discussion of videofluoroscopy and other ways of imaging swallowing. This chapter will conclude by discussing the possible future uses of functional imaging in the study of dysphagia following stroke.

## Swallowing Physiology

Before describing the changes that can occur following stroke it is important to consider what happens during a normal physiological swallow. The action of swallowing occurs approximately 580 times every day, it is a complex and coordinated action requiring the intact function of a large number of muscles in the oral cavity, pharynx, larynx and oesophagus. It has evolved in order to transport food from the mouth to the stomach whilst, at the same time, protecting the airway. Disruption of control to any one of these structures or functions may result in swallowing difficulties.

The normal physiological swallow is traditionally divided into 4 distinct phases, an oral preparatory phase, oral transit phase, pharyngeal phase and oesophageal phase. The duration and characteristics of each phase may vary depending on the consistency and volume of food ingested and the amount of voluntary control exerted. Saliva swallows do not usually involve an oral phase, but trigger a more reflexive pharyngeal swallow directly.

## Oral Preparatory Phase

During this phase food is mixed with saliva, manipulated within the mouth and masticated as necessary in order to prepare a bolus ready for swallowing. A labial seal is maintained to prevent spillage and therefore nasal breathing is required. The soft palate is pulled down to seal off the pharynx, unless active mastication is occurring. The prepared bolus is held either between the tongue and the anterior hard palate or on the floor of the mouth in front of the tongue until the oral transit phase commences.

## Oral Transit Phase

The tongue begins transit by cupping the bolus in the midline, then pushing up against the hard palate in a coordinated rolling wave from anterior to posterior and thus propelling the bolus posteriorly. The soft palate is raised to close off the nasopharynx. A negative pressure is exerted by movement of the buccal musculature in order to assist this movement towards the hypopharynx. The viscosity of food is important during this stage, especially for those with brain damage; slightly thicker pastes are easier to keep within the oral cavity as the bolus shape and adhesion is easier to maintain, but thicker foods require a greater pressure to be exerted by the tongue in order for movement to occur. It takes 1-1.5 seconds to complete this phase.

## Pharyngeal Phase

The pharyngeal swallow is triggered when the bolus reaches a point somewhere between the anterior faucial pillars and where the tongue base crosses the lower rim of the mandible. As the bolus progresses sensory receptors in the tongue and oropharynx are stimulated, allowing information about the quality of the bolus to be processed centrally. The pharyngeal phase requires closure of the velum and velopharyngeal port to prevent spillage into the nasal cavity, along with retraction of the tongue base, elevation and anterior motion of the larynx and closure of the vocal cords and epiglottis in the larynx to protect the airway. Breathing is suspended during the pharyngeal phase, again to assist with airway protection. The normally tonic upper oesophageal sphincter then relaxes and food is channelled via the pyriform fossae into the oesophagus.

## Oesophageal Phase

Oesophageal peristalsis carries the bolus through the cervical and thoracic oesophagus and into the stomach, whilst the lower oesophageal sphincter opens to allow smooth transit. Oesophageal transit usually takes 8-20 seconds and once initiated the peristalsis can propagate without higher control [3-5].

## Neural Control

As already discussed deglutition involves the synchronised activation of numerous muscles via the central nervous system. The amount of voluntary control that can be exerted over the swallow diminishes as it progresses through the different phases; the oral preparatory phase is a predominantly voluntary action whereas the oesophageal phase is mainly involuntary.

Swallowing is thought to be a reflex action generated by a central pattern generator within the upper medulla, composed of the nucleus ambiguous, tractus solitarius and reticular formation, which also have relays to and from the pons. There are two regions in the pons, one ventral which can stimulate swallowing and mastication and one dorsal region which relays sensory information to the thalamus and is involved in the initiation and organization of the swallow sequence [6, 7]. This central pattern generator in the medulla is able to integrate information both from descending efferent pathways from higher cortical and subcortical centres and from peripheral afferents in order to modulate the swallow according to the characteristics of the bolus [4, 8]. Mastication and deglutition are heavily dependent on afferent feedback so that loss of sensation either through lack of stimulation, anaesthesia or loss of receptors, can impair their function [9].

Sensory information from the oral cavity, pharynx and larynx is transmitted to the brainstem via the trigeminal, facial, glossopharyngeal and vagus nerves (cranial nerves V, VII, IX and X respectively). This sensory input, via the cranial nerve nuclei within the brainstem, synapses within the nucleus tractus solitarius at the medullo-pontine junction and is then relayed to the reticular formation, pons and higher centres. The extensive interconnection of these regions, including bilaterally, facilitates the coordination of swallowing.

Higher control of swallowing is multiregional with known areas of involvement in the caudal sensorimotor cortex, anterior cingulate, premotor cortex, frontal operculum, insular and temporal cortex, cerebellum, substantia nigra, ventral tegmentum, hypothalamus, amygdala and basal ganglia [10]. There is some evidence that these areas are involved in different stages of deglutition, as will be discussed later in the chapter. Initiation of voluntary swallowing requires the integrity of the cerebral cortex, the locus of swallowing muscle control within the primary motor cortex lies anterocaudal to the face area [11] and representation of oral muscles in the sensorimotor cortex tends to be symmetrical, whereas those of the pharynx and oesophagus are more asymmetrically represented [12].

Afferent information is channelled back through the nucleus tractus solitarius in brainstem to the nucleus ambiguus which innervates all of the intrinsic muscles and most of the soft palate musculature and initiates the pharyngeal motor pattern. The hypoglossal nucleus in the caudal medulla receives input from the nucleus solitarius and the trigeminal sensory nucleus as well as corticobulbar afferents from both hemispheres; it controls all of the motor supply to the tongue. The hypoglossal nerve is thought to be under bilateral control with the input from the hypoglossal nuclei being symmetrical, but supranuclear control of the nucleus itself more likely to be asymmetrical [13].

Motor output to the oropharyngeal musculature is via cranial nerves V, VII, IX, X, XII and the cervical spinal nerves C1-4 which innervate the infrahyoid muscles.

The upper oesophageal muscles are controlled centrally by the nucleus ambiguus motor neurons and some lower musculature by the dorsal vagal motor nucleus, but there is some transition in neural control more distally where striated muscle turns to smooth, the oesophageal musculature then acts more like the muscles of the small intestine which can function without higher control.

The control of respiration is also important during swallowing and interneurons in the brainstem which control breathing are inhibited by inputs which elicit deglutition [3, 5, 14].

### Normal Ageing Changes

Strokes tend to occur in the elderly and although age-related changes in deglutition usually cause only subclinical problems, any acute illness in this group may produce a temporary decompensation leading to clinical dysphagia [3, 15]. Symptoms may also be exacerbated by poor dentition, oropharyngeal muscle atrophy and oesophageal dysmotility [16]. It is also of note that many medications commonly prescribed in the elderly and stroke populations may also interfere with swallowing, including some antihypertensives and anticonvulsants which can cause xerostomia, antidepressants which are known to cause xerostomia and slowing of swallow coordination and centrally acting drugs such as benzodiazepines which may result in slowing and impaired coordination of swallowing [3].

## Functional Imaging of the Brain during Healthy Human Swallowing

### Functional Magnetic Resonance Imaging (fMRI)

Functional magnetic resonance imaging has been extensively used to investigate swallowing, but as with most of the other functional imaging modalities has not yet been commonly used to investigate dysphagia following stroke.

Blood oxygen level dependent images on 1.5T MR systems were acquired for most of the swallowing studies done so far, with 3T scanners occasionally used. Magnetic resonance has good spatial resolution, of at least 2 mm, but the temporal resolution of a few seconds does limit its use when studying deglutition. Newer fast magnetic resonance methods, using echo-planar imaging or diffusion imaging, are able to give much better temporal resolution of around 40-100ms.

Functional MRI was originally fraught with difficulties when used to assess brain signals associated with swallowing, because of large movement artefacts due to the swallow itself, especially in the inferior regions of the brain. Newer analysis techniques have allowed us to overcome these problems and obtain useful images [17]. Traditional block trial studies require repeated swallows within short spaces of time and this can induce inhibition of oesophageal peristalsis, which may then mask some of the cortical activity that may otherwise be seen. fMRI, unlike some of the other functional imaging modalities, may also be used with a single event-related approach where the cerebral activity is correlated with each specific task. Event-related studies have advantages over block trial designs, especially with swallowing, as they can provide better functional information and are less likely to produce artefacts due to motion.

The simplest studies using functional imaging have looked at the areas of increased cortical activation during voluntary swallowing of either saliva or water, prompted by cues. Other studies have used a number of different techniques to investigate swallowing more thoroughly and to try to isolate the various neural components controlling each phase of deglutition; for example using comparisons with tongue or hand movements and non-cued, involuntary swallowing.

Although multiple regions are activated during swallowing there appears to be some variability between subjects and between studies. During volitional swallowing the most consistent cortical activation is seen in the primary motor cortices and primary somatosensory cortices [2, 18-22]. The greatest area of fMRI activation in the primary motor cortex is over the mid-inferior lateral portion of the precentral gyrus which corresponds with what is already known from direct cortical stimulation to be a region representing the face, tongue and pharynx. This activation in the lateral precentral gyrus during swallowing tasks occurs dorso-caudally to the hand area [19].

Most studies have also shown increased BOLD signal in the majority of subjects during volitional swallowing in the anterior cingulate cortex (BA32, 33), anterior insular cortex (BA16), frontal operculum (BA44), anteromedial temporal cortex (BA21, 22), superior premotor cortex (BA6,8) and the precuneus. There is less consistently increased activation across subjects in the cerebellum, supplementary motor area, prefrontal cortex, posterior parietal cortex (BA5), middle and inferior frontal gyri, cuneus, parietal opercula, motor association areas, sensory-motor integration areas, posterior cingulate (BA23,31), basal ganglia, thalamus and internal capsule [2, 18-23]. When fMRI is used specifically to look at the cerebellum and basal ganglia during volitional saliva swallowing there is evidence of bilateral cerebellar activity more on the left, bilateral putamen, globus pallidus and substantia nigra activation [23].

Volitional swallowing will result in activation of areas involved not only in the organisation of a swallow itself, but also in the cue recognition and response and planning of the event. One method of differentiating these components is to study reflexive swallowing, which can be stimulated by injecting tiny amounts of water directly into the pharynx. Different swallowing tasks produce slightly different cortical maps, the areas most consistently and prominently activated in all tasks are the lateral precentral gyri, postcentral gyri, supplementary motor area and insular cortex [19, 24].Reflexive swallowing induces bilateral activation concentrated in the primary somatosensory and motor cortices (BA4,6) which is present in all subjects [23]. When automatic saliva swallowing is compared to volitional saliva swallowing there is more activation of the caudal anterior cingulate cortex during the reflexive swallow [24].

Using visually cued go/no-go swallowing tasks during fMRI shows marked activation in the pericentral gyri and anterior cingulate cortex during the go condition suggesting these areas are specifically involved in the act of swallowing whereas there is activation in the cuneus and precuneus during both go and no-go tasks supporting the view that these areas are more concerned with processing of cues [25].

By comparing volitional movement of individual muscles involved in the swallow, such as the tongue, with a full swallow sequence it begins to be possible to identify areas that may have more to do with the control of swallowing itself rather than motor planning areas. Tongue contraction alone produces bilateral signal increases within the sensorimotor cortex and operculum as well as some activation in the supplementary motor area, putamen, thalamus and cerebellum; there is also activation within the medulla corresponding to the regions known to contain the hypoglossal nuclei [26]. Tongue movement and swallowing both produce activation of left lateral pre- and post-central cortices, the anterior parietal cortex and the anterior cingulate cortex. Tongue movements in these areas show a greater overall activation than that seen with volitional swallowing, perhaps because of a larger volitional component to tongue movement tasks compared with swallowing where much of the processing may be within the brainstem. Movements of the tongue also produce more activation than swallowing in the right pericentral gyri, supplementary motor area, premotor cortex, right putamen and thalamus. Superimposed mapping of areas with increased activity suggests that only swallowing activates the most lateral extent of left pericentral and anterior parietal cortex, the rostral anterior cingulate cortex, precuneus, cuneus, middle frontal gyrus and right parietal operculum, although the main areas where activation is stronger in swallowing than tongue elevation are the precuneus and cuneus [2]. Cortical activation in volitional swallowing also shares many regions with jaw clenching , lip pursing and tongue rolling, activation during all of the above functions can be found in anterior cingulate cortex, motor and premotor cortices and occipital/parietal regions (BA7.19,31) [27]. There is little agreement between studies about the activation of the insula some having found it predominantly during swallowing tasks and others during both swallowing and tongue movement tasks [2, 23, 26].

Hand grasping and finger movement exercises have also been compared to swallowing tasks, they activate more superior and posterior parts of the motor and sensory cortices than swallowing [22]. The hand tasks also show much more strongly and consistently lateralised activation than that seen during swallowing [22].If subjects are asked to perform dry and bolus swallows and the resulting activation is compared to that seen during a finger movement task, there is preferential activation during the swallowing tasks of primary motor cortex, primary somatosensory cortex, the supplementary motor area, prefrontal cortex, superior temporal gyrus, insular cortex, transverse temporal gyrus, cingulate gyrus, association areas, sensory-motor integration areas, thalamus and internal capsule [18, 19].

Peripheral stimulation can also have a direct effect on cortical reorganization, following electrical stimulation of the pharynx bilateral increases in fMRI activation can be seen in the lateral sensorimotor cortex [28].

During volitional swallowing the activation is usually bilateral, but with some areas having hemispheric dominance, 63% of subjects show left hemisphere dominance, this may be why some studies in stroke patients have shown a preponderance of left hemispheric lesions causing dysphagia [29].

Most subjects show asymmetry of the postcentral gyrus activation(BA4) [2, 29]. There also appears to be strong lateralisation of increased activity in the mid lateral precentral gyrus and somatosensory cortices (BA1,2,3), supplementary motor area (BA6), prefrontal cortex (BA9,10), transverse temporal gyrus (BA42),insula, operculum, cingulate gyrus, internal capsule and premotor cortices[21, 22, 29]. This dominance of one hemisphere is more often left, but if it is dominant on the right then the lateralisation is stronger; the asymmetry of activation may also vary depending on the type of swallow performed [29]. In another study, of right handed subjects, all had significantly more activation in the right insular than left [24].

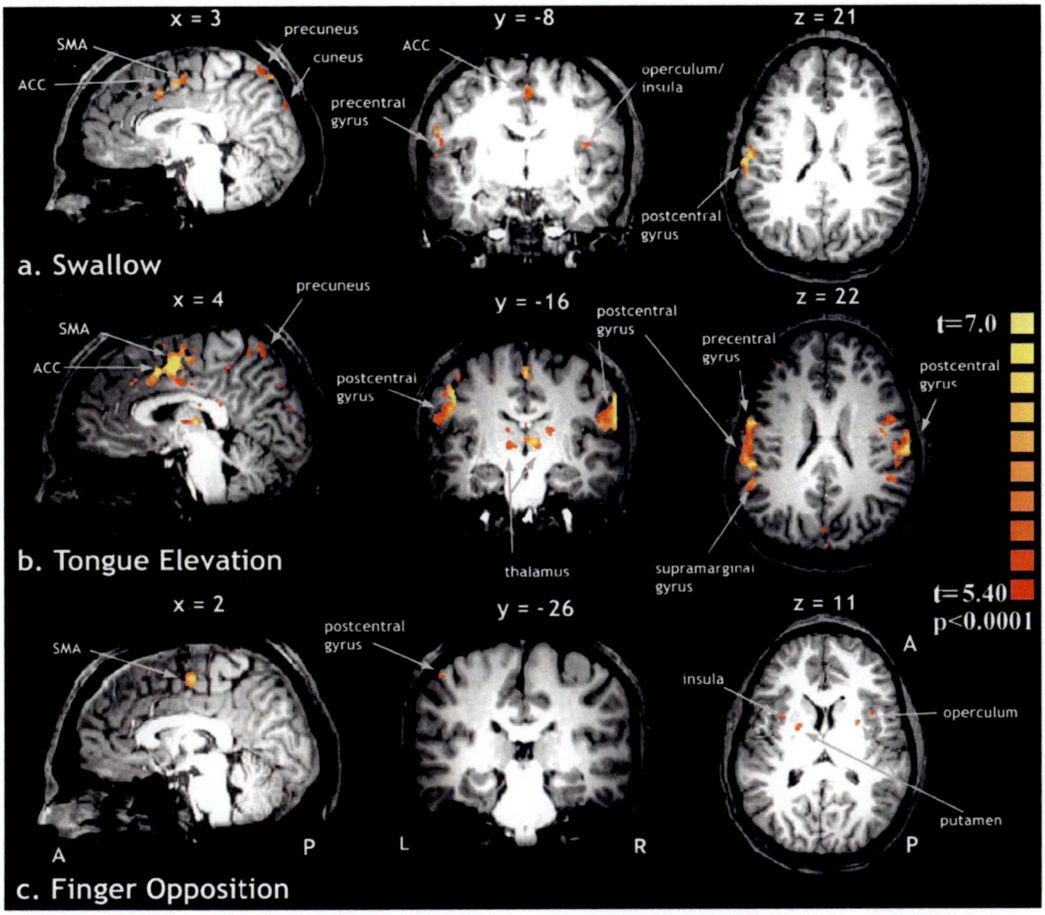


Figure 1. Voxelwise analysis of BOLD responses for a group of 14 subjects to (a) voluntary saliva swallow , (b) tongue elevation and (c) voluntary finger-thumb opposition. Regions of significant activation are displayed on sagittal (left), coronal (middle) and axial (right) brain slices. Talaiach-Tornoux plane coordinates are displayed above each image. Used with kind permission of R.E. Martin [2].

There have been few studies looking specifically at the pattern of activation within the brainstem, but some of the brainstem nuclei involved in swallowing have been localised using fMRI and the sites correlate with what has previously been observed from pathological and animal studies.

During dry swallowing activation within the nucleus ambiguous of the medulla can be seen and tongue movements activate a region of the medulla consistent with the location of the hypoglossal nucleus [30].

The cerebral regions that are most activated during dry swallowing in adults are similarly active in the brains of children. The main activation is seen in pre and post-central gyri (BA3,4), superior motor cortex (BA24), insula, inferior frontal cortex (BA44,45), Heschl gyrus(BA41,42), putamen, globus pallidus, superior temporal gyrus(BA38) and the nucleus ambiguous in the brainstem. Even in those children who have never eaten orally, where quite different patterns of activation or diminished signal may be expected, the areas of increased activity within the brain remain the same during dry swallows [31].

fMRI can also be used to investigate the functional connectivity of different areas of the brain. When used during volitional swallowing it has shown that the central organization appears to function in a number of different clusters – the sensorimotor and cingulate gyrus; the inferior frontal gyrus, S2, corpus callosum, basal ganglia and thalamus; the premotor cortex and posterior parietal cortex; the cerebellum; the insula cortex. They also appear to function in two parallel systems with connections to either the cerebellum or insula and connected through the sensorimotor-cingulate module [20].

The delay between swallowing and time of maximal BOLD signal in the motor cortex is approximately 6-8sec [31]. When event-related fMRI tasks are used to obtain improved temporal information the cingulate and premotor cortices can be seen to be activated earlier in the swallowing sequence than the sensorimotor cortex and other areas [21].

## Positron Emission Tomography (PET)

PET is currently being used along with the other functional imaging techniques to try and unravel the neural control mechanisms of swallowing. PET is limited as its temporal resolution is inferior to that of fMRI and only provides better spatial resolution when imaging subcortical regions. It also exposes the participants to ionizing radiation, making repeat studies undesirable.

Most work has been done in healthy subjects using $H_2{}^{15}O$ injection in order to estimate regional blood flow.

Voluntary swallowing of saliva produces strong bilateral increases in cortical blood flow particularly in the inferior precentral gyrus, extending into primary somatosensory cortex (BA43), the right insula and left cerebellum, there is also some activation in the putamen and thalamus, although less consistently [32]. Volitional water swallows produce a similar picture of increased blood flow in both caudolateral sensorimotor cortices (BA3, 4, 6) and the superiomedial cerebellum. There is also a less consistent activation in the temporopolar cortices (BA38), right anterior insula, right orbitofrontal cortex (BA11), left mesial premotor areas (BA6,24), dorsal brainstem and amygdale [1]. In both these types of swallowing there is bilateral, but often asymmetrical, increased cerebral blood flow within the sensorimotor cortex. In water swallowing most subjects were strongly lateralised, whereas in saliva swallows only 25% showed significant asymmetry; this dominance is unrelated to handedness and correlates well with data on the same subjects using transcranial magnetic stimulation to assess asymmetry of swallowing motor cortex [1, 32]. Swallowing of infused water causes an associated decrease of blood flow within the posterior parietal cortex, right anterior occipital cortex, left superior frontal cortex, right prefrontal cortex and superiomedial temporal cortex [1].

PET has also been used to try and localise the cerebral areas involved in particular components of deglutition. Oesophageal sensation elicits activation of the primary somatosensory cortex bilaterally, insular cortex, frontal/parietal operculum and to a lesser extent the right anterior insula and anterior cingulate cortex. This is associated with decreased activation of the right prefrontal cortex[33].

If the blood flow changes seen in swallowing are compared to those seen with tongue movement alone the peak activations in precentral cortex are still present, although approximately 1 cm away. Tongue movement also produces bilateral rather than predominantly right insula activation, again this is in a slightly different region of the insula than that seen with swallowing [32].

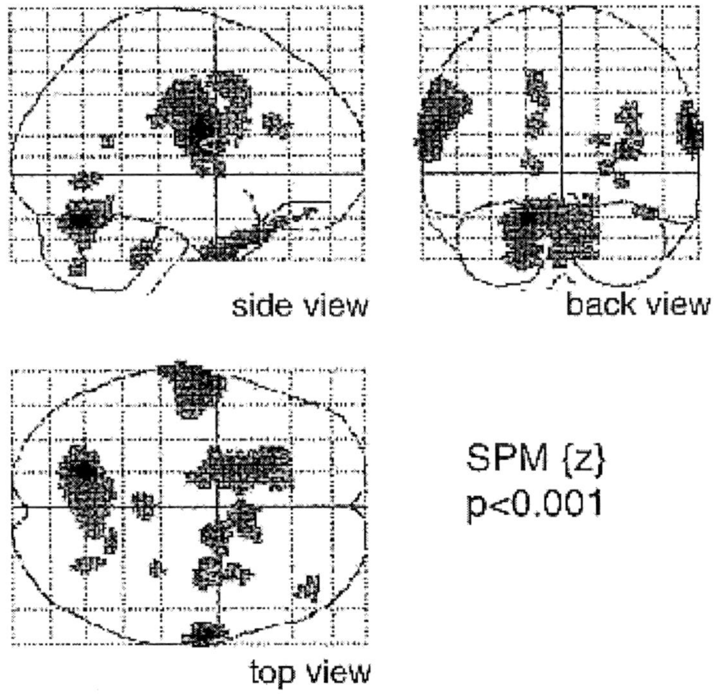


Figure 2. The group mean Statistical Parametric Mapping (SPM*z*) maps of the areas of increased regional cerebral blood flow (rCBF) associated with swallowing are shown as 3 orthogonal projections through sagittal (*side view*), coronal (*back view*), and transverse (*top view*) views of the brain. A threshold of *P* , 0.001 was applied. A number of areas are activated, including regions corresponding to sensorimotor cortex, bilaterally, right insula, left cerebellum, left mesial frontal cortex, temporopolar cortex, and dorsal brain stem. (Used with kind permission of S. Hamdy[1]).

FDG PET ($F^{18}$ labelled fluorodeoxyglucose) may be used as an alternative to water PET, it uses a glucose analogue to quantify regional glucose metabolism rather than blood flow and this gives a better spatial resolution. It also allows tasks to be performed outside the scanner as FDG-6-phosphate, the metabolic product of FDG, remains trapped within brain tissue for an extended period of time and this allows swallowing to be performed in the more physiological sitting position before being scanned supine.

When volitional swallowing is assessed using FDG PET there is evidence of increased glucose metabolism in left sensorimotor cortex (BA3,4,6), right prefrontal cortex (BA10), bilateral lateral postcentral gyri (BA43), right temporal cortex (BA39),cerebellum, thalamus, precuneus (BA31), anterior insula and bilateral occipital cortex (BA18,19). Decreased activity is seen in right premotor cortex, bilateral sensory and motor association cortices, left posterior insula and left cerebellum [34].

## Magnetoencephalography (MEG)

MEG is able to give very good temporal resolution (milliseconds) of brain activation as it detects the post-synaptic magnetic fields generated by active cortical neurons. Thus it is particularly useful when studying dynamic functions such as swallowing. The basic MEG instrument contains magnetic detection coils called a superconducting quantum interference device (SQUID) which is placed over the head and records magnetic field changes. The original equipment was unable to provide useful data on dynamic functions such as tongue movement or swallowing as they produced EMG signals and which masked any cortical activity [35], more advanced analysis techniques are now available and this allows investigation of MEG signals during motor tasks. MEG has more recently been used with synthetic aperture magnetometry analysis which provides much better resolution of the resulting images [36-38].

This high temporal resolution compared to other functional imaging techniques allows some analysis of the sequence in which central activation occurs during swallowing in addition to localization of active regions.

At 1000-1500ms before volitional water swallowing activation can be identified in the anterior cingulate gyrus (BA24,25,32,33) and supplementary motor areas of both hemispheres [39]. The insula and inferior frontal gyrus(BA44) are also particularly active prior to the onset of motor swallowing activity and at the same time there is also some simultaneous lesser activity in the posterior cingulate and middle frontal gyrus(premotor and motor areas BA8,9) [36, 40].

Activity starts within the insula and cingulate cortex and then progresses to the frontal gyri. The activation within the cingulate cortex is relatively short and mostly prior to the swallow and therefore thought to be involved in the initiation of voluntary swallowing and its cognitive processing. In comparison the activation of the frontal gyri and insula are longer lasting and continue into the motor phase of swallowing [40]. It should also be noted that the activation within the insula and cingulate cortex is specific to deglutition, when it is compared with MEG during finger movements there is no comparable activity in these areas [40]. During the execution of volitional water swallows frontal operculum are activated as well as the continued activation of left insula, sensorimotor cortices and integration areas [36].

The pericentral gyri and inferior parietal lobule show sustained decreases in power throughout water infusion, during tongue thrusting and at the initiation of swallowing, but this disappears immediately following the volitional phase of swallowing. During the swallow activity moves from the caudal pericentral cortex rostrally to the superior postcentral gyri and paracentral lobule [37].

The planning and processing of volitional swallowing has been studied by comparing it to reflexive swallowing, where tiny amounts of fluid are infused into the pharynx in order to directly stimulate a swallow. These swallows differ in that no cue is required and there is usually little or no oral phase to the swallow. The primary sensorimotor cortices (BA1,2,3) become bilaterally activated prior to the volitional movements of both swallowing and tongue movement, but there is no activation prior to reflexive swallowing [36]. Prior to volitional swallowing there is also some lesser activation of the sensorimotor integration areas (BA5, 7) and primary motor cortex (BA4). During the volitional swallowing and tongue movements bilateral mid-lateral sensorimotor cortices (BA 4,3,1,2) and sensorimotor integration areas are activated whereas during the reflexive swallowing movements there is more medial activation of the primary sensorimotor cortex [36].

The degree of lateralisation of activation within the primary sensorimotor cortex (BA1,2,3) seen with MEG appears to relate to the particular movement, it is most lateralised to the left during volitional water swallows, less strongly lateralised during reflexive swallowing and not lateralised during tongue movements [36]. The areas of activation within a region may also vary depending on the task performed; oral water infusion preferentially activates the caudolateral sensorimotor cortex whereas volitional swallowing and tongue movement activate the superior sensorimotor cortex. Sensory input from the tongue simultaneously activates caudolateral sensorimotor and primary gustatory cortex[37]. Interestingly, following electrical stimulation of the pharynx MEG activity can be seen in caudolateral sensorimotor cortex (BA4,1,2), suggesting that sensory inputs converge on the same higher centres that produce the motor output [38].

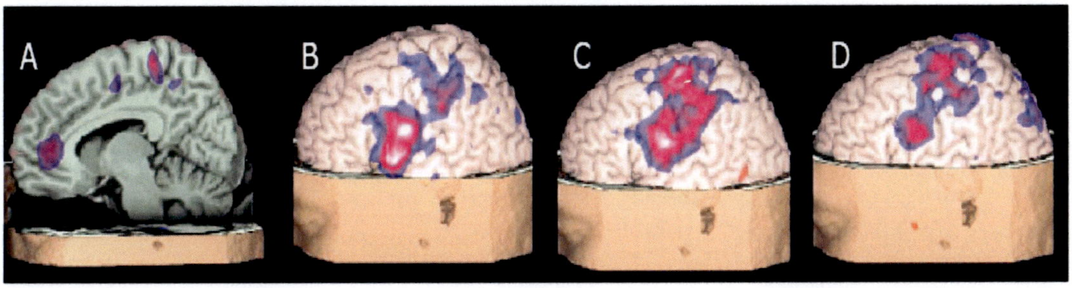


Figure 3. Group MEG data which ahs been spatially normalised and superimposed onto a template brain, showing activation during progression of the swallowing sequence (A) and (B) during water infusion into the mouth, (C) tongue movement, (D) swallowing. Reproduced with kind permission of Dr. A.R.Hobson.

## Transcranial Magnetic Stimulation (TMS)

Transcranial magnetic stimulation uses an electromagnetic field to generate electric currents in the neural tissue beneath the stimulator site; the site of stimulation is not as well localised as direct current electrodes placed on or in the brain tissue itself, but has the advantage of being non-invasive [41].

Using transcranial magnetic stimulation maps can be created of the cortical areas devoted to motor representation of swallowing by plotting the areas that elicit an EMG potential in the oropharyngeal muscles. Motor excitability, another marker of the strength of the cortical motor projection, can be measured by the size of the EMG responses resulting from stimulation of these areas.

It has been shown that magnetic stimulation over the motor and premotor cortex of either cerebral hemisphere is able to produce EMG responses in the pharyngeal and oesophageal muscles, suggesting that swallowing is bilaterally represented. In most people these pharyngeal responses are larger in one hemisphere than the other and this lateralization is unrelated to handedness [12]. This contrasts with the oral musculature, which is thought to be symmetrically represented [42].The site of cortical control of swallowing in humans was originally localised to an area antero-caudal to the face area of primary motor cortex [11] using direct electrical stimulation and this is confirmed by magnetic stimulation studies. The mapping is also able to show the arrangement of cortical projections to the different groups of swallowing muscles. Oesophageal, mylohyoid and pharyngeal muscles are all discretely represented within the motor cortex; mylohyoid being more anterolateral than the pharyngeal muscles and those more anterolateral than the oesophageal muscles [12].

If both hemispheres are stimulated almost simultaneously then the size of the pharyngeal response is larger and the latency shorter, than if either hemisphere is stimulated alone; this suggests that summation occurs, perhaps within the brainstem where input from both hemispheres could converge on shared interneurons [43].

## Summary of Functional Imaging in Healthy Swallowing

The use of functional imaging techniques during healthy swallowing has given us detailed information about the central control mechanisms involved in the swallowing process, but data does not always correlate between trials using the same imaging techniques or between different imaging modalities. This may be partly explained by the slightly different protocols used, different types of swallowing examined and relatively small numbers of subjects studied. Cortical areas that consistently show increased activation during normal swallowing include the primary motor and somatosensory cortices and anterior insula, but multiple other areas within the brain show increased or decreased activation during swallowing. Activity of some regions is strongly lateralised during swallowing, but not always to the same side and in some areas varies depending on which type of imaging is used, the reasons for these differences remain unclear.

# Dysphagia and Stroke

Dysphagia is very common following stroke, affecting hundreds of thousands of people each year and occurring in up to 70% of stroke patients on admission to hospital [44-53]. Most patients with swallowing difficulties make some spontaneous recovery although reported rates are very variable and depend on the definitions used. By 3 months 41% of stroke patients remain dysphagic when videofluoroscopy is used to assess swallowing [47], whereas other studies show 75%-90% of initially dysphagic patients are able to consume normal diet at this stage[46, 51, 52, 54]. At 6 months post-stroke 87-99% of patients have returned to a normal diet, but when investigated with videofluoroscopy half of them will still have some evidence of dysphagia [49, 55].

Dysphagia is important to recognise as it is an independent risk factor for mortality and morbidity and results in significant increases in these rates when compared to non-dysphagic stroke patients as well as predisposing to a range of complications [52, 56]. About 16% of people admitted to hospital with stroke are malnourished and any subsequent swallowing problems or feeding difficulties may exacerbate this. Aspiration of oral contents occurs in 22% of all stroke patients [51] and in 40-50% of dysphagic patients [57]. One third of these patients at risk of aspiration will go on to develop pneumonia [50]. Dysphagic stroke patients are also much more likely to have prolonged hospital stays [45] and chest infections [49].

# Lesional Studies - CT and MRI

Strokes are able to provide useful information in the study of swallowing due to the discrete nature of the lesions in a wide variety of locations. Much work has been done trying to correlate the site of the lesions with resulting deficits, in order to try and predict the type of difficulties in swallowing that patients may present with. Originally the only methods of determining the function of particular cerebral areas was by looking at animal studies, using direct cortical stimulation in humans for example during neurosurgical operations or awaiting pathological results following death. One of the first descriptions of stroke causing dysphagia was by Bastian in 1898 [58] when he described a man who 'before admission to hospital had fallen down without loss of consciousness and ......at first he had difficulty in deglutition and putting out his tongue, but these symptoms passed away in a few days' on necropsy he was found to have two limited lesions within the left hemisphere; but since that time there have been long held assumptions that swallowing has bilateral central control and that only bilateral cortical lesions or brainstem lesions were able to cause dysphagia. The advent of computerised tomography (CT) and magnetic resonance imaging (MRI) has allowed non-invasive study of stroke lesions and their relationship to dysphagia as well as allowing progress to be assessed during recovery. It is important to note however that many of the earlier studies relied on neurological examination rather than imaging findings to determine lesion location [44, 59, 60] and since then many studies have used only CT or a combination of CT and MR [54], despite the fact that MRI has been shown to be more sensitive in detecting smaller, more acute lesions [61-63]. It is therefore possible that patients originally diagnosed as having single lesions, may have also had further unidentified lesions bilaterally or at other sites within the same hemisphere.

There is great variability in the site and size of lesions that can cause swallowing problems. Most of the current data available regarding the localisation of human swallowing centres is from lesion studies following cerebral injury and these provide a very varied picture of the areas that are important in addition to the primary motor areas and brainstem, for example the thalamus and cerebellum [64], basal ganglia [57, 64], pyramidal tracts [65, 66], frontal operculum [67] and insula [68], all of which have been associated with swallowing problems when damaged.

In general, studies have failed to identify any single lesion site on MR analysis to account for aspiration and often lesions of a similar size and in identical locations may show differing results on swallowing assessments [64]. One of the more consistent findings is that the larger the lesion the more likely a patient is to develop swallowing problems [52, 69, 70] and those with brainstem [53] or posterior circulation strokes are more likely to aspirate [71] as are those with bilateral lesions [71]. It has also been shown that patients with haemorrhagic stroke are significantly more likely to have swallowing problems than those with ischaemic stroke, irrespective of lesion site, having an incidence of dysphagia of 49% compared with 32% [52].

Because of the variety of lesions within the central nervous system that can lead to abnormalities of swallowing and the number of different components of the swallow that can be affected the lesions will be discussed primarily by location.

## Cortex

Traditionally swallowing difficulties following stroke have been associated with brainstem damage or bilateral cortical lesions, but more recent studies have shown that dysphagia is also common in patients with unilateral hemispheric lesions [54, 66, 67].

The cerebral cortices, although probably the main contributor to volitional swallowing, are also associated with parts of the more automatic pharyngeal and oesophageal phases. Hemispheric lesions have been noted to delay the pharyngeal phase of swallowing [57, 67], increase pharyngeal transit time [72], impair coordination of movement [57, 65, 67] and reduce peristalsis [57].

Although some studies report a slightly greater proportion of left hemisphere strokes compared to right in dysphagic stroke patients there appears to be no significant correlation between which hemisphere is damaged and the chance of dysphagia [44, 55, 57]. There has been much debate about the role of each hemisphere and there are many inconsistencies between the studies trying to associate lesion site with particular swallowing abnormalities, some have associated oral phase problems with CT identified left hemispheric lesions and impairment of the pharyngeal phase to right hemispheric lesions [65-67, 73-75] whilst others have not confirmed these findings and found no correlation between site and swallowing characteristics, suggesting that control is more complex [53, 57, 64, 72, 75-77]. Even very similar lesions seen on MRI can produce a variety of swallowing abnormalities [64, 72]. Ischaemic lesions in the territory of the left middle cerebral artery have been shown to cause impaired oral stage, problems with labial, lingual and mandibular coordination, apraxia and a prolonged pharyngeal transit time; right hemispheric damage appears to significantly affect all aspects of deglutition including all the pharyngeal stage durations and increase aspiration, penetration and pharyngeal pooling [65, 66].

Aspiration has been shown to occur in both right and left hemispheric lesions, but is much more likely when the damage is bilateral or involves large vessel infarcts[48, 54, 64], some studies suggest that most middle cerebral artery territory stroke patients who aspirate have right hemisphere strokes [66]. Patients most at risk of aspiration are likely to have lesions of the periventricular white matter, isolated lesions of the periventricular white matter are uncommon in patients with no risk of aspiration [53].

When right handed patients with first ischaemic strokes identified on either MRI or CT were divided into groups of either anterior or posterior middle cerebral artery territory stroke and lesion volume was calculated a number of differences could be seen in specific videofluoroscopic measures. Anterior lesion subjects had significantly longer swallow durations of oral transit, stage transition, pharyngeal transit and duration to upper oesophageal sphincter opening as well as increased total swallow time, posterior lesion patients had only longer pharyngeal transit times of liquids, in general the anterior strokes were worse than posterior, but the anterior ones also tended to have a larger lesion volume [66]. Other studies of patients with hemispheric stroke identified on CT or MRI support these findings and show there is a greater incidence of anterior lesions in those with dysphagia [53].

Lesions verified on MRI to be within the frontal cortex are associated with a significant risk of prolonged dysphagia and slow recovery [69].

## Insular and Subcortical Areas

Strokes involving the insula cortex are relatively rare, but they are caused by infarction of the middle cerebral artery territory with the anterior insular predominantly supplied by the M3 division. In Ceredas study only 4 of 4800 strokes were limited to the insula and all of these were in the posterior insula; none of which developed dysphagia[78]. Other work does suggest that the insular cortex is involved in swallowing, it being the most common site of unilateral hemispheric stroke in patients with dysphagia, especially prolonged dysphagia [68, 69, 75]. In particular, lesions of the anterior insular identified on CT resulted in dysphagia, whereas those of the posterior insular were not associated with swallowing difficulties [68]. This would fit with known connections of the anterior insula to the motor and premotor cortices, gustatory and olfactory structures, thalamus and nucleus tractus solitarius, all of which are important in swallowing[68]. Of those stroke patients demonstrated to be at risk of aspiration 36% have lesions involving the insular cortex and 86% of those with insular lesions have dysphagia[53].

Strokes isolated to the subinsular region are also rare (0.4% of strokes); infarcts in this region have been defined on CT or MRI as a linear subinsular lesion extending parallel and subjacent to the insular cortex for at least one third of the anteroposterior extent of the insular. The subinsular component has to be continuous with the paraventricular component and the infarct should not primarily involve the insular cortex [79]. The subinsular infarcts tend to lie in a border zone between small insular penetrating arteries and branches of the lenticulostriate arteries [80]. Half of patients with subinsular lesions show evidence of dysphagia on initial admission following the stroke, but the rate of spontaneous recovery is good and most have resolution of symptoms by 1 month [79]. Wong et al studied deep cerebral infarcts extending from paraventricular white matter to the subinsular region, 5 of 8 (71%) patients had dysphagia in combination with other symptoms [80].

There is little information on swallowing difficulties following strokes involving the basal ganglia although it has been shown that the incidence of pneumonia in patients with basal ganglia infarction is more than twice that seen in hemispheric stroke patients and if bilateral involvement of the basal ganglia occurs then the incidence of pneumonia trebles [81]; this is shown to be independent of patient mobility and severity of stroke. Although there is no videofluoroscopic data available in this group the latency of oral bolus injection to swallowing time can be analysed by measuring submental EMG responses following injection. The swallowing latencies are longest in those demonstrated to have bilateral basal ganglia lesions on CT followed by those with unilateral basal ganglia lesions and then those with hemispheric lesions not involving the basal ganglia. The latencies are even more delayed when measured at 1am, thus it may be the case that pneumonia in basal ganglia infarcts is related to silent aspiration during the night [81].

## Brainstem

The brainstem is often difficult to image with CT because of artefact and the majority of infarcts can be missed when compared to MRI [82]. Brainstem strokes have long been associated with swallowing difficulties, 44-65% of patients have aspiration and 75-81% are dysphagic [53, 83, 84]. When investigated with videofluoroscopy an even greater proportion of these patients have mild abnormalities of deglutition that do not significantly affect their function [54, 85, 86]. A number of areas essential to swallowing are located in the dorsolateral medulla oblongata; including the nucleus tractus solitarius, nucleus ambiguous and the reticular formation. Medullary strokes may often also affect cranial nerves IX and X resulting in incoordination of the pharyngeal muscles.

Lesions in the pons and medulla have been associated with dysphagia, although no specific site has been identified as solely responsible those with bilateral, large, large-vessel lesions are more likely to aspirate [54]. Approximately 47% of patients with lesions isolated to the pons have dysphagia [85] and 55% of those with lesions in the medulla [85].

When dysphagic patients with brainstem strokes are evaluated using surface EMG of the perioral muscles, masseter and infrahyoid, they are found to have less coordination of activity than controls; videofluoroscopic data shows that they all have pharyngeal residue post swallow and laryngeal penetration [84]. Those with lesions involving the medulla have a poorer outcome in terms of recovery of oral feeding [83].

Pure medullary lesions are associated with clinically identified dysphagia in 55% and the majority of these patients will have pharyngeal residuum or confirmed aspiration on videofluoroscopy [45, 86]. The risk of aspiration is also related in some degree to the extent and laterality of lesions. Sites particularly associated with aspiration when damaged are in the middle, combined middle/lower or upper medulla. Even patients with extensive longitudinal lesion may not aspirate depending on their lateral extent, paramedian lesions may miss the more laterally situated nuclei, whereas those patients with inferodorsolateral and dorsolateral lesions have a much higher incidence of aspiration [86].

Lateral medullary stroke (Wallenberg syndrome) is due to occlusion of the vertebral artery, its posterior inferior cerebellar branch or their lateral medullary penetrating arteries. In those diagnosed with unilateral lateral medullary infarction on magnetic resonance imaging between 52 and 65% of patients will have dysphagia [61, 82, 87]. An interesting case report of dysphagia in lateral medullary syndrome that was closely followed up with videofluoroscopy revealed intact oral and oesophageal phases of swallowing, but a failure of laryngeal elevation and coordination of the pharyngeal musculature; on MRI the lesion was centred in the right dorsal medulla, rostral to the obex [88]. This is supported by a study using electrophysiological measures of dysphagia including laryngeal elevation times and length of the reflex pharyngeal phase which shows that patients with lateral medullary syndrome fare worse than those with hemispheric strokes. Lateral medullary lesions cause an increase in the length of laryngeal elevation, delay to elevation and length of pharyngeal swallow, in contrast they have less problems with the oral phase of swallowing than those with hemispheric strokes[89]. In Kim's study of 33 patients the lesions were divided into rostral, caudal and middle groups; all patients who had rostral lesions required nasogastric feeding for dysphagia and 75% of those with middle medullary lesions had dysphagia although this was generally less severe [61]. The only large study correlating pure lateral medullary infarcts on MRI with clinical outcomes involved 130 patients and again the classification used divided the lateral medulla into rostral, middle or caudal and dorsal. 83% of the group with lesions in the rostral medulla had dysphagia compared with 47% of those in the caudal group; those in the rostral group were also more likely to have severe dysphagia and 40% them required a nasogastric tube for feeding [87].

Medial medullary stroke is less common (0.3% of strokes) and usually involves tongue weakness and atrophy ipsilateral to the infarct as part of Dejerine's syndrome. When lesions are identified on MRI they are associated with rates of lingual palsy of 11-82% and loss of the gag reflex in just under half of patients; only 11-27% have dysphagia. It has been postulated that the cases with dysphagia may be due to extension of the lesions towards the lateral medulla with involvement of the nucleus ambiguus [90, 91].

## Cerebellum

There is little information about the precise swallowing difficulties found in patients with cerebellar stroke, but videofluoroscopy of one 54y old with haemorrhagic cerebellar stroke showed disruption of initiation of swallowing and impairment of the pharyngeal stage with resulting aspiration. During her recovery the oral function remained slow, but pharyngeal and laryngeal function improved over the course of 3 years [92]. Up to 40% of those with strokes in the cerebellum aspirate [85], but no specific lesion location within the cerebellum has been implicated as being particularly likely to cause dysphagia.

## Cerebral Lesions Affecting Specific Phases of Swallowing

Whilst most studies have examined the effect of lesion location on swallowing few have looked at the individual components of swallowing to try and identify the areas involved. One exception to this is tongue movement, difficulties with coordination of tongue movements during swallowing are found in 19% of stroke patients and approximately half of these will also have pharyngeal dysphagia. Other studies have found that 29% of all hemispheric stroke patients will have tongue deviation compared with 5% of controls and that this is always to the same side as the limb weakness [13]. It is interesting that tongue deviation is associated with dysphagia in only 43% of patients, although this may be an underestimation as assessment was only carried out using bedside tests of swallowing [13].

A number of studies in stroke patients have tried to establish lesion locations associated with lingual incoordination, but there is no clear consensus. Some have concluded that the oral phase of swallowing is predominantly a function of the left hemisphere [65, 66, 73], some the right side was more commonly affected (64%right versus 27% left) [76] whilst others found no difference between hemispheres [75, 76]. There are no strong associations with anatomical site identified on CT or MRI, although those stroke patients with subcortical involvement, particularly in the periventricular white matter, are more likely to have tongue deviation[76] and those with lacunar infarct on CT are less likely [13]. In those stroke patients with lingual discoodination the lesions are found in purely cortical areas in 10%, purely subcortical in 40% or in both sites in 50% [76].

Buccal hemineglect is associated with other neglect phenomena and is especially seen after right hemisphere lesions due to right middle cerebral artery territory strokes, causing left buccal neglect; causes dribbling, impaired swallowing, loss of saliva, choking, inability to initiate chewing when food is on the left side of the mouth or swallowing when food or saliva is on the left [93].

## Summary of Lesion Studies in Stroke Using CT and MRI

The idea that swallowing is a complex task requiring intact function of numerous muscles and neural networks is supported by the fact that a lesion in any one of a number of different areas within the brain is able to cause significant impairment of swallowing. Lesions causing dysphagia may be unilateral or bilateral and can be found in cortical, subcortical or brainstem sites. Although some studies have suggested associations between particular lesion sites and specific abnormalities of swallowing most show no consistent correlations; an exception is that patients with large, haemorrhagic or bilateral strokes are more likely to become dysphagic. Some of the earlier studies using CT to identify lesion location may have missed small or multiple lesions that could be detected by MRI, as scanning quality improves the information obtained from lesion studies may improve and allow prediction of the type of swallowing abnormality to be expected from damage to certain areas.

## TMS in stroke

Patients with unilateral hemispheric stroke identified by CT have been shown to have different pharyngeal EMG responses to transcranial magnetic stimulation depending on whether or not they have difficulty swallowing. Dysphagic stroke patients evoke a smaller response in the pharynx than non dysphagic patients when the unaffected hemisphere is stimulated. In contrast, stimulation of the affected hemispheres of both groups results in smaller responses than stimulation of the unaffected hemispheres, but the responses are similar in all patients irrespective of dysphagia. This suggests that dysphagia is more likely to occur after unilateral hemispheric stroke if it is the hemisphere with the larger cortical projection (i.e. dominant swallowing hemisphere) that contains the lesion [42].

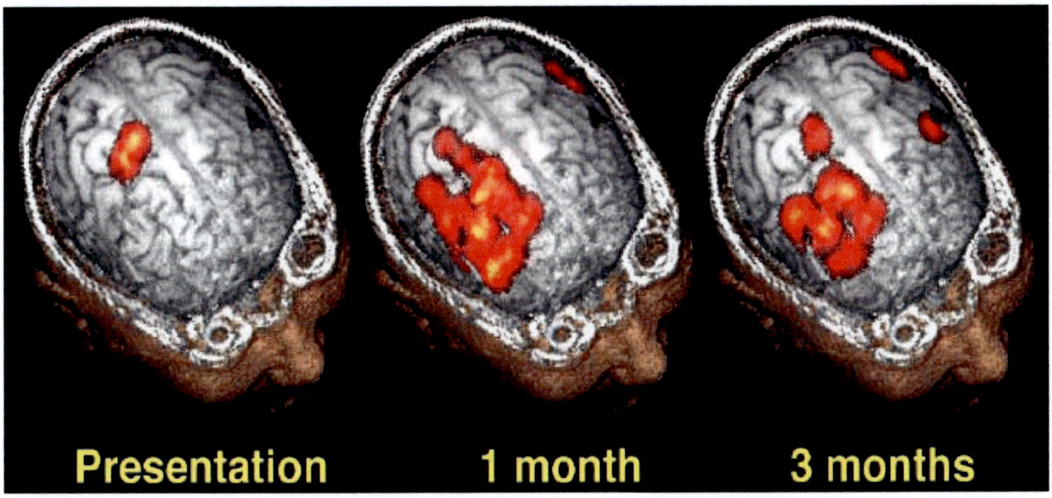


Figure 4. TMS topographic maps superimposed on MRI images showing the size of pharyngeal cortical representation during recovery of a dysphagic patient from stroke. The patient had a left hemisphere cortical stroke affecting the lower sensorimotor cortex and recovered functional swallowing by one month. The unaffected hemisphere is shown to have an increasing representation during recovery whereas that of the affected hemisphere exhibits little change. (used with kind permission from Hamdy, S. et al. [47]).

Transcranial magnetic stimulation has also demonstrated that, over time, there is a marked increase in size of the pharyngeal motor map in the undamaged hemispheres of stroke patients whose swallowing improves. This heightened response to stimulation of the cortex is seen only in the undamaged hemisphere and is not found on the affected side. It is of note that this increase in excitability precedes any functional resolution of dysphagia and therefore the findings are not merely due to the recovery of normal swallowing, but rather, suggest that the recovery of swallowing is dependent on this cortical reorganization. Patients who are not dysphagic or those showing no resolution of dysphagia do not exhibit any of these changes in excitability or increase in motor map size [47]. If the pharynx of stroke patients is stimulated electrically there is an greater increase in response to TMS stimulation seen in the unaffected hemisphere than in the undamaged hemisphere even though the peripheral stimulus will stimulate both cortices [28].

In stroke patients with supranuclear tongue palsy transcranial magnetic stimulation of the unaffected hemisphere produces normal ipsilateral responses whereas there is no response to stimulation of the damaged hemisphere.

In those that functionally recover, the response to stimulation of the affected hemisphere continues to be absent, suggesting that the tongue also relies on the unaffected hemisphere taking over function in order to recover following stroke [94]. This is in direct contrast to the recovery seen in limb muscles, where TMS studies show functional improvement is due to reorganization of cortex in the damaged hemisphere.

In summary, transcranial magnetic stimulation has been able to show that the representation of swallowing cortex is strongly lateralised in most people, that it is damage to the dominant hemisphere following stroke that usually causes dysphagia and that functional recovery relies on an increase in excitability of the undamaged hemisphere.

### fMRI in Stroke

The brains of patients with dysphagia up to 4 weeks following subcortical stroke have been imaged during swallowing using fMRI; there is much less activation within the pericentral cortex compared to controls and most stroke patients show asymmetry of activation with greater activity of the contralesional whole-brain as well as the post-central gyrus in the unaffected hemisphere[95].

## Swallowing Imaging Post Stroke

### Videofluoroscopy

Videofluoroscopy, also referred to as modified barium swallow, is an essential tool for investigating swallowing problems following stroke, less than half of patients who manifest aspiration on videofluoroscopy are diagnosed with abnormalities on bedside evaluation [96, 97]. Videofluoroscopy uses small volumes of barium as a contrast medium to study the anatomy and physiology of the swallowing process in addition to its temporal characteristics. It is able to provide detailed information on the oral preparatory, oral, pharyngeal and oesophageal stages of swallowing and structural information about the pharynx and oesophagus. It allows real time assessment as well as the ability to record data and play it back frame by frame at a later date and can assess the benefit of compensatory techniques such as positioning and changes in bolus viscosity in those patients with dysphagia[3, 98]. Small quantities of barium are given to minimise the risks of aspiration and these are mixed with food of varying consistencies in order to thoroughly evaluate the swallow. The patient must remain seated throughout the study in order to best mimic normal feeding posture, this may cause some difficulties in those who are frail or have significant other symptoms as a result of their stroke. The other disadvantages of videofluoroscopy are the radiation exposure, greater costs compared to endoscopy and a lack of concordance between reports with some studies showing only 76% agreement between reporting of aspiration, whether by radiologists or speech and language therapists [99-102].

Aspiration is defined as penetration of material past the true vocal cords, if this elicits no cough reflex or other signs of difficulty then this is defined as silent aspiration. Silent aspiration occurs in up to 40% of dysphagic patients who aspirate and it is often unnoticed in bedside examinations, therefore examination with videofluoroscopy becomes increasingly important [60].

Even in those patients without aspiration, who have functionally safe swallows, there are still readily identifiable abnormalities on videofluoroscopic examination. Dysphagic stroke patients most commonly exhibit a delayed swallow reflex, but more than half also have decreased control of the tongue and reduced pharyngeal peristalsis [57, 72] as well as reduced oral and tongue mobility, delayed swallow initiation and poor pharyngeal peristalsis [103].

As discussed earlier there is no great correlation between the site of the stroke lesion and the resulting abnormality of swallowing although some trends have been identified in some studies. The majority of stroke patients, whether with cortical, subcortical or brainstem lesions, may exhibit some abnormality on videofluoroscopy, most having a delayed swallow reflex [48, 57, 72, 103]. Hemispheric strokes have been associated with variety of swallowing deficits including hesitancy in triggering pharyngeal phase [3, 57, 67], incoordination of swallow related movements [57, 65, 67], increased pharyngeal transit time [72] and reduced pharyngeal peristalsis [57]. A study of patients with brainstem strokes showed oral phase abnormalities in 57%, delayed initiation in 91%, pharyngeal residue in 74%, aspiration in 65% and impaired relaxation of the upper oesophageal sphincter in 44% [54]. Patients with single small basal ganglion/ internal capsule infarcts diagnosed on CT have a low probability of significant clinical dysphagia when confirmed by videofluoroscopy, but although considered safe to eat the remaining non-dysphagic patients all show mild differences on videofluoroscopy compared to controls including increased oral transit time and reduced oropharyngeal swallow efficiency; with thicker boluses they also had longer pharyngeal transit times and pharyngeal delay times [104].

Those that aspirate are more likely to have oral slowness, prolonged pharyngeal transit times or pharyngeal residue post swallow [48, 105]. Delayed or absent swallowing reflex in VFS is the best independent predictor of subsequent chest infection, whilst delayed oral transit predicts failure to return to normal diet by 6 months [49].

Increase of the bolus volume may shorten the pharyngeal delays experienced by stroke patients whereas there is little change in the normal population [103]. It may be that increasing the volume increases the sensory feedback and so overcomes some of the delay.

Quantitative scales for stroke patients have been proposed as a guide to assessing the severity of dysphagia and to allow more objective evidence of recovery, they can be scored using a number of variables including bolus formation, residues, oral and pharyngeal transit times, laryngeal elevation and nasal penetration [106].

## Videoendoscopic Swallowing Study (VESS)

Videoendoscopic examination of swallowing uses a fibreoptic nasopharyngoscope to directly visualise the pharynx and larynx before and after swallowing; the swallow itself cannot be visualised due to contraction of the pharyngeal musculature and little of the oral stage can be visualized. It is able to give detailed information on the timing and movement of food through the hypopharynx, ability to clear the bolus, palatal movement and anatomy of pharyngeal and laryngeal structures [3, 107, 108]. In up to 33% of patients nasendoscopy may be limited by inadequate visualisation of the preswallow spillage and postswallow residue and there is only moderate reproducibility of findings during swallowing of solids [109]. In addition to the anatomical and physiological data obtained laryngopharngeal sensation may be assessed by delivering pulses of air to the mucosa, known as flexible endoscopic evaluation of swallowing with sensory testing (FEESST) [110]. Although most studies assessing oral and pharyngeal sensation have detected reduced sensation post stroke [111-113] there are cases where electrical stimulation was used and which then found sensory thresholds were reduced in most areas, contrary to expectation [109].

Aspiration may be determined by the presence of food residue postswallow. Because of the inability to visualise the actual swallow it is not possible to determine the exact cause of the swallowing disorder or aspiration although it may be inferred indirectly. Reports of the tolerability of the procedure vary, but it does have the advantage of being radiation free and it can be used at the bedside in poorly mobile or bedbound patients [3, 107, 108], the rates of pneumonia and pneumonia free interval are comparable whether videofluoroscopy or FEESST is used except in stroke patients where 4.8% of patients develop pneumonia following FEES compared to 29% of those who have videofluoroscopy [114].

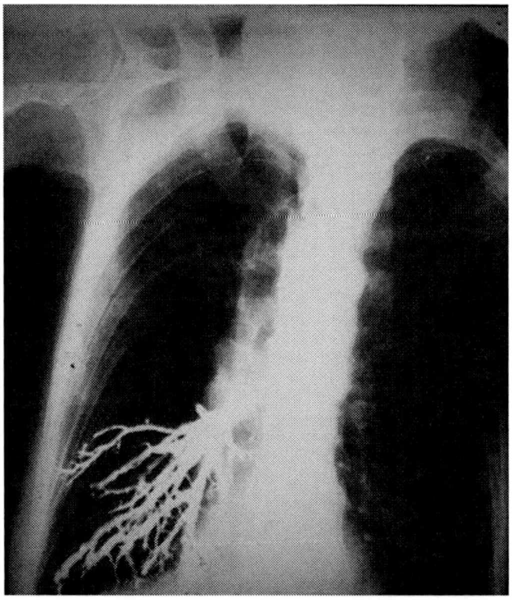

Figure 5. CXR showing barium within the bronchial tree following aspiration during a videofluoroscopy. (Barium white).

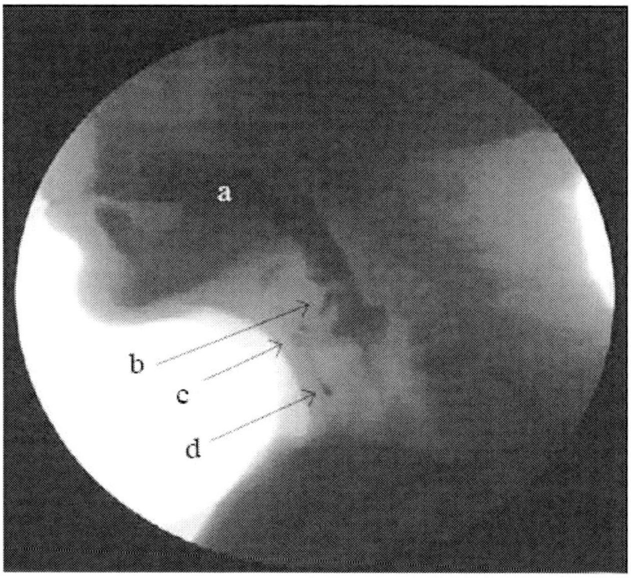


Figure 6. Videofluoroscopic image showing aspiration of barium. (a) Tail of bolus in oral cavity (b) Barium tracks under epiglottis due to incomplete laryngeal elevation (c) Barium on the vocal cords (d) Barium in the trachea. (Barium black).

When compared with control subjects half of stroke patients examined endoscopically have an impairment of voluntary pharyngeal motor activity and 14% have pooling of secretions in the pyriform fossae, they also have a a generally longer time to initiation of epiglottic tilt and prolonged total duration of swallow although few have post swallow laryngeal residue [109].

# Possibilities for the Future

## Functional Imaging in Stroke

As previously discussed PET, MEG and fMRI have all been used extensively as research tools to investigate the central control of healthy swallowing. They have the potential to provide detailed information in stroke patients about the immediate effects of the injury itself and the mechanisms of subsequent recovery.

## Ultrasound

When small ultrasound probe is placed submentally activity of the hyoid bone, oral cavity muscles, tongue movements, laryngeal motion and oral transit times may be assessed[115-117]. It is not useful for the pharyngeal phases of swallowing due to interference from other structures within the head and neck. Although it isn't commonly used in stroke patients at present it has been used to assess other neurological causes of dysphagia such as twelfth cranial nerve palsy [115] and progressive supranuclear palsy in which it is able to demonstrate significant delays in the duration of swallows[118]. It has the advantage of being non-invasive and well tolerated and may therefore find a complementary role to other swallowing imaging modalities in the future.

## High-Speed MRI

These techniques are now able to dynamically capture images of the swallowing process whilst avoiding the risks of radiation exposure and allowing better soft tissue imaging. At present their application is limited as the faster imaging sequences, which allow evaluation of the swallow, limit the spatial resolution of the soft tissues. Magnetic resonance imaging is able to visualise all of the anatomy of the soft tissues and has proved better than videofluorography at assessing the oral phase of swallowing, unfortunately the images of pharyngeal transit and laryngeal movement are less clear and at present most MR scanners will only allow supine assessment; the scanning speed of echo-planar or FLASH MRI is 0.2 – 0.33 sec/frame compared with videofluoroscopy which gives 30 frames/sec[119]. Turbo-FLASH sequences provide a reasonable combination of temporal and spatial resolution during swallowing assessment with magnetic resonance imaging [120-122]. Echo-planar MRI sequences also have a good temporal resolution, but so far have only been used to study tongue and vocal cord movement during swallowing [123-125]. Dynamic MRI with single shot fast spin echo has also been assessed in healthy volunteers and although it gives good anatomical data on laryngeal elevation, oropharyngeal diameter, tongue base and velum displacement the temporal parameters are not well seen as the scanning speeds are slower[126]. Multi-gradient-echo MRI with projection reconstruction has also been used to assess swallowing with good temporal resolution, but poor spatial resolution[127] and real-time True allows better quality soft tissue contrast, but less temporal resolution[128]. With continued improvements in scanners and analysis techniques high-speed MRI may become much more commonly used in clinical practice and rival videofluoroscopy as the gold-standard for investigation of dysphagia.

## Scintigraphy

This uses rapid sequential acquisition of images of a single bolus, labelled with technetium [99] sulfur-colloid, which is recorded by means of a gamma camera [3].

Although this hasn't been used specifically in stroke patients, it can be used to assess and quantitate bolus transit, oropharyngeal residue and aspiration, but is unable to visualise the anatomy and physiology of the mouth and pharynx directly [3, 129]. One advantage is that it is able to pick up delayed aspiration as subjects may be rescanned up to several hours later to see if there is any material in the airway or lungs [3]. It is therefore possible that Scintigraphy could be used as an adjunct to other investigations when assessing the safety of swallowing post stroke.

# Take Home Message

Swallowing is a complex action requiring the coordinated action of a large number of muscles and involving numerous cortical, subcortical and brainstem areas under both voluntary and involuntary control. Knowledge of the physiology and pathophysiology of swallowing is important as dysphagia following stroke is associated with a high risk of morbidity and mortality. Functional imaging techniques including functional magnetic resonance imaging, positron emission tomography, magnetoencephalography and transcranial magnetic stimulation are being increasingly used to investigate the physiology of normal swallowing and show multiple areas of activation, including the primary motor and sensory cortices, anterior cingulate cortex and insula.

CT and particularly MRI have become more widely used in the investigation of stroke in recent years and patients are having scans earlier in the days following the stroke; this is allowing better identification of even very small areas of infarction and therefore more detailed analysis of the effect of lesions in specific cerebral locations is possible. There is a high likelihood of recovery of swallowing function following stroke, the mechanisms of this recovery have been investigated with transcranial magnetic stimulation and appear to relate to the bilateral, albeit asymmetrical, control of swallowing and the ability of the brain to reorganise following injury. Hopefully with the increasing use of the other functional imaging techniques more studies will explore the effect of disease on swallowing and further insight will be gained into the pathogenesis and recovery of dysphagia following stroke.

Videofluoroscopy, although far from perfect, remains the gold standard investigation for assessment of swallowing post stroke, giving detailed information on swallowing physiology and aspiration risk. Endoscopic assessment of swallowing has also proved to be a valuable tool in the investigation of dysphagia and it is possible that other imaging modalities such as high speed MRI will also contribute in the future.

# References


[1] Hamdy, S., et al., Identification of the cerebral loci processing human swallowing with H2(15)O PET activation. *Journal of Neurophysiology*, 1999; 81: 1917-26.

[2] Martin RE. et al. Cerebral areas processing swallowing and tongue movement are overlapping but distinct: A functional magnetic resonance imaging study. *Journal of Neurophysiology,* 2004; 92: 2428-2443.

[3] Logemann JA , *Evaluation and treatment of swallowing disorders*. 2nd ed. 1998.

[4] Kennedy JG, Kent RD, Physiological substrates of normal deglutition. *Dysphagia*, 1988; 3: 24-37.

[5] Miller AJ. Deglutition. *Physiological Reviews*, 1982; 62:129-84.

[6] Car A, Jean A, Roman C. A pontine primary relay for ascending projections of the superior laryngeal nerve. *Experimental Brain Research*, 1975; 22:197-210.

[7] Kessler JP, Jean A. Identification of the medullary swallowing regions in the rat. *Experimental Brain Research*, 1985; 57: 256-63.

[8] Smithard DG. Dysphagia following stroke. *Reviews in Clinical Gerontology*, 1999; 9: 81-93.
[9] Schaerer P, Legault JV, Zander HA. Mastication under anesthesia. *Helvetica Odontologica Acta,* 1966; 10:130-4.
[10] Hockman CH, Bieger D, Weerasuriya A. Supranuclear pathways of swallowing. *Progress in Neurobiology,* 1979; 12: 15-32.
[11] Penfield W, Boldrey E. Somatic motor and sensory representation in the cerebral cortex of man as studied by electrical stimulation. *Brain*, 1937; 60:389-443.
[12] Hamdy S, et al., The cortical topography of human swallowing musculature in health and disease. *Nature Medicine*, 1996; 2:1217-1224.
[13] Umapathi T. et al., Tongue deviation in acute ischaemic stroke: a study of supranuclear twelfth cranial nerve palsy in 300 stroke patients. *Cerebrovascular Diseases* 2000; 10:462-5.
[14] Perlman AL. Neuroanatomy and neurophysiology: Implications for swallowing. *Topics in Stroke Rehabilitation*, 1996; 3:1-13.
[15] Bucholz DW; Bosma JF, Donner MW. Adaptation, compensation and decompensation of the pharyngeal swallow. *Gastrointestinal Radiology*, 1985; 10:235-239.
[16] Tack J, Vantrappen. The aging oesophagus. *Gut*, 1997; 41:422-424.
[17] Birn RM, et al. Magnetic field changes in the human brain due to swallowing or speaking. *Magnetic Resonance in Medicine*, 1998; 40:55-60.
[18] Martin RE, et al. Cerebral cortical representation of automatic and volitional swallowing in humans. *Journal of Neurophysiology*. 2001; 85:938-50.
[19] Mosier KDMDP, et al. Cortical representation of swallowing in normal adults: Functional implications. The functional neuroanatomy of voluntary swallowing. *Laryngoscope*, 1999; 109:1417-1423.
[20] Mosier K, Bereznaya I. Parallel cortical networks for volitional control of swallowing in humans. *Experimental Brain Research* 2001; 140:280-9.
[21] Hamdy S. et al. Cortical activation during human volitional swallowing: an event-related fMRI study. *American Journal of Physiology*, 1999. 277(1 Pt 1).
[22] Wakasa T, et al. Functional MRI study of cerebral cortical activation during volitional swallowing. *Oral Radiology*, 2002; 18:65-71.
[23] Kern, MK, et al. Cerebral cortical representation of reflexive and volitional swallowing in humans. *American Journal of Physiology Gastrointestinal and Liver Physiology*, 2001; 280: G354-G360.
[24] Martin R et al., Cerebral cortical representation of automatic and volitional swallowing in humans. *Journal of Neurophysiology.* 2001; 85:938-50.
[25] Toogood JA, et al. Discrete functional contributions of cerebral cortical foci in voluntary swallowing: a functional magnetic resonance imaging (fMRI) "Go, No-Go" study. *Experimental Brain Research*, 2005; 161:81-90.
[26] Corfield DR, et al. Cortical and subcortical control of tongue movement in humans: a functional neuroimaging study using fMRI. *J. Appl. Physiol.*, 1999; 86:1468-1477.
[27] Kern MK, Birn R, Jaradeh S. Swallow-related cerebral cortical activity maps are not specific to deglutition. *American Journal of Physiology Gastrointestinal and Liver Physiology,* 2001; 280:G531-538.

[28] Fraser C, et al., Driving plasticity in human adult motor cortex is associated with improved motor function after brain injury. *Neuron,* 2002; 34:831-40.
[29] Mosier KM, et al. Lateralization of cortical function in swallowing: A functional MR imaging study. *American Journal of Neuroradiology*, 1999; 20:1520-1526.
[30] Komisaruk B, et al. Functional localization of brainstem and cervical spinal cord nuclei in humans with fMRI. *American Journal of Neuroradiology*, 2002; 23:609-17.
[31] Hartnick CJMD, et al. Functional magnetic resonance imaging of the pediatric swallow: Imaging the cortex and the brainstem. *Laryngoscope*, 2001; 111: 1183-1191.
[32] Zald DH, Pardo JV. The functional neuroanatomy of voluntary swallowing. *Annals of Neurology*, 1999; 46:281-286.
[33] Aziz Q, et al. Identification of human brain loci processing esophageal sensation using positron emission tomography. *Gastroenterology*, 1997; 113: 50-59.
[34] Harris ML, et al. Mapping metabolic brain activation during human volitional swallowing; a positron emission tomography study using $^{18}$fluorodeoxyglucose. *Journal of cerebral blood flow and metabolism*, 2005. (In press March 2005).
[35] Loose R, Hamdy S, Enck P. Magnetoencephalographic response characteristics associated with tongue movement. *Dysphagia,* 2001; 16:183-185.
[36] Dziewas R, et al., Neuroimaging evidence for cortical involvement in the preparation and in the act of swallowing. *NeuroImage*, 2003; 20:135-144.
[37] Furlong PL, et al. Dissociating the spatio-temporal characteristics of cortical neuronal activity associated with human volitional swallowing in the healthy adult brain. *Neuroimage,* 2004; 22:1447-55.
[38] Gow D, et al. Characterising the central mechanisms of sensory modulation in human swallowing motor cortex. *Clinical Neurophysiology*, 2004. 115:2382-90.
[39] Abe S, et al. Magnetoencephalographic study of the starting point of voluntary swallowing. *Cranio*, 2003; 21:46-9.
[40] Watanabe Y, et al. Cortical regulation during the early stage of initiation of voluntary swallowing in humans. *Dysphagia*, 2004; 19:100-108.
[41] Barker AT, Jalinous R, Freeston IL. Non-invasive magnetic stimulation of human motor cortex. *Lancet*, 1985:1106-7.
[42] Hamdy S, et al. Explaining oropharyngeal dysphagia after unilateral hemispheric stroke. *Lancet,* 1997; 350: 686-692.
[43] Hamdy S, et al. Sensorimotor modulation of human cortical swallowing pathways. *Journal of Physiology*, 1998; 506: 857-66.
[44] Gordon C, Hewer RL, Wade DT. Dysphagia in acute stroke. *British Medical Journal Clinical Research Ed*, 1987; 295: 411-4.
[45] Teasell R, et al. The incidence, management, and complications of dysphagia in patients with medullary strokes admitted to a rehabilitation unit. *Dysphagia*, 2002; 17: 115-120.
[46] Finestone HM, et al. Tracking clinical improvement of swallowing disorders after stroke. *Journal of Stroke and Cerebrovascular Diseases*, 2002; 11:23-27.
[47] Hamdy S, et al. Recovery of swallowing after dysphagic stroke relates to functional reorganization in the intact motor cortex. *Gastroenterology,* 1998; 115:1104-12.

[48] Horner J, et al. Aspiration following stroke: clinical correlates and outcome. *Neurology*, 1998; 38:1359-1362.
[49] Mann GB, et al. Swallowing function after stroke: Prognosis and prognostic factors at 6 months. *Stroke* 1999; 30: 744-748.
[50] Kedlaya D, Brandstater ME. Swallowing, nutrition, and hydration during acute stroke care. *Topics in Stroke Rehabilitation*, 2002; 9:23-38.
[51] Smithard DG, et al. The natural history of dysphagia following a stroke. *Dysphagia*, 1997; 12:188-193.
[52] Paciaroni M, et al. Dysphagia following stroke. *European Neurology*, 2004; 51:162-167.
[53] Daniels SK, Foundas AL. Lesion localization in acute stroke patients with risk of aspiration. *Journal of Neuroimaging,* 1999; 9: 91-98.
[54] Horner J, et al. Dysphagia following brain-stem stroke. Clinical correlates and outcome. *Archives of Neurology*, 1991; 48:1170-3.
[55] Barer DH. The natural history and functional consequences of dysphagia after hemispheric stroke. *Journal of Neurology, Neurosurgery and Psychiatry,* 1989; 52: 236-41.
[56] Smithard DG, et al. Complications and outcome after acute stroke: Does dysphagia matter? *Stroke,* 1996; 27: 1200-1204.
[57] Veis SL, Logemann JA. Swallowing disorders in persons with cerebrovascular accident. *Archives of Physical Medicine and Rehabilitation*, 1985; 66:372-5.
[58] Bastian HC. A treatise on aphasia and other speech defects. London. Lewis., 1898: 87.
[59] Barer DH. Lower cranial nerve motor function in unilateral vascular lesions of the cerebral hemisphere. *British Medical Journal*, 1984. 289:1622.
[60] Horner J, Massey EW. Silent aspiration following stroke. *Neurology,* 1988; 38: 317-9.
[61] Kim JS, et al. Spectrum of lateral medullary syndrome. Correlation between clinical findings and magnetic resonance imaging in 33 subjects. *Stroke,* 1994; 25:1405-10.
[62] Kidwell CS, et al. Comparison of MRI and CT for detection of acute intracerebral hemorrhage. *Journal of the American Medical Association*, 1823;292:1823-1830.
[63] Kertez A, et al. The sensitivity and specificity of MRI in stroke. *Neurology,* 1987;37:1580-1585.
[64] Alberts MJ, et al. Aspiration after stroke: lesion analysis by brain MRI. *Dysphagia*, 1992; 7: 170-3.
[65] Robbins J, Levin RL. Swallowing after unilateral stroke of the cerebral cortex: preliminary experience. *Dysphagia*, 1988; 3: 11-7.
[66] Robbins J, et al. Swallowing after unilateral stroke of the cerebral cortex. *Archives of Physical Medicine and Rehabilitation*, 1993; 74:1295-300.
[67] Meadows JC. Dysphagia in unilateral cerebral lesions. *Journal of Neurology, Neurosurgery and Psychiatry*, 1973;36: 853-60.
[68] Daniels SK, Foundas AL. The role of the insular cortex in dysphagia. *Dysphagia,* 1997. 12:146-156.
[69] Broadley S, et al. Predictors of prolonged dysphagia following acute stroke. *Journal of Clinical Neuroscience*, 2003. 10:300-305.

[70] Sharma JC, et al. Prognostic value of CT scan features in acute ischaemic stroke and relationship with clinical stroke syndromes. *International Journal of Clinical Practice,* 2000; 54:514-8.

[71] Horner J, Massey EW, Brazer SR. Aspiration in bilateral stroke patients. *Neurology,* 1990. 40:1686-8.

[72] Johnson ER, et al. Dysphagia following stroke: quantitative evaluation of pharyngeal transit times. *Archives of Physical Medicine and Rehabilitation,* 1992; 73:419-23.

[73] Irie H, Lu CC. Dynamic evaluation of swallowing in patients with cerebrovascular accident. *Clin Imaging*, 1995. 19: 240-3.

[74] Martin RE, Sessle BJ. The role of the cerebral cortex in swallowing. *Dysphagia*, 1993; 8:195-202.

[75] Daniels SK, Foundas AL, Iglesia GC. Lesion site in unilateral stroke patients with dysphagia. *Journal of Stroke and Cerebrovascular Diseases*, 1996; 6:30-34.

[76] Daniels SK, Brailey K, Foundas AL. Lingual discoordination and dysphagia following acute stroke: Analyses of lesion localization. *Dysphagia*, 1999;14: 85-92.

[77] Chen MY, et al. Oropharynx in patients with cerebrovascular diseasc: evaluation with videofluoroscopy. *Radiology,* 1990; 176:641-3.

[78] Cereda CM, et al. Strokes restricted to the insular cortex. *Neurology*, 2002;59:1950-1955.

[79] Kumral EMD, Ozdemirkran TMD, Alper YMD. Strokes in the subinsular territory: Clinical, topographical, and etiological patterns. *Neurology,* 2004. 63: 2429-2432.

[80] Wong EHMBC, Pullicino PMMDP, Benedict RP. Deep cerebral infarcts extending to the subinsular region. *Stroke*, 2001; 32: 2272-2277.

[81] Nakagawa T, et al. High incidence of pneumonia in elderly patients with basal ganglia infarction. *Archives of Internal Medicine*, 1997. 157: 321-324.

[82] Sacco RL, et al. Wallenberg's lateral medullary syndrome. Clinical-magnetic resonance imaging correlations. *Archives of Neurology*, 1993. 50: 609-14.

[83] Meng NHMD, Wang TGMD, Lien INMD. Dysphagia in patients with brainstem stroke: Incidence and outcome. *American Journal of Physical Medicine and Rehabilitation*, 2000; 79:170-175.

[84] Crary MA, Baldwin BO. Surface electromyographic characteristics of swallowing in dysphagia secondary to brainstem stroke. *Dysphagia,* 1997; 12:180-187.

[85] Teasell R, et al. Clinical characteristics of patients with brainstem strokes admitted to a rehabilitation unit. *Archives of Physical Medicine and Rehabilitation*, 2002;83:1013-1016.

[86] Kim H, et al. Aspiration subsequent to a pure medullary infarction: Lesion sites, clinical variables, and outcome. *Archives of Neurology*, 2000; 57: 478-483.

[87] Kim J. Pure lateral medullary infarction: clinical-radiological correlation of 130 acute, consecutive patients. *Brain* 2003;1864-72.

[88] Martino R, et al. Dysphagia in a patient with lateral medullary syndrome: insight into the central control of swallowing. *Gastroenterology* 2001; 12:420-6.

[89] Aydogdu IMD, et al. Dysphagia in lateral medullary infarction (Wallenberg's Syndrome): An acute disconnection syndrome in premotor neurons related to swallowing activity?. *Stroke* 2001; 32:2081-2087.

[90] Kumral E, et al. Spectrum of medial medullary infarction: Clinical and magnetic resonance imaging findings. *Journal of Neurology*, 2002; 249:85-93.
[91] Kim JS, Kim H, Chung CS, Medial medullary syndrome:report of 18 new patients and a review of the literature. *Stroke*, 1995; 25:1405-1410.
[92] Perie S, et al. Swallowing difficulties for cerebellar stroke may recover beyond three years. *American Journal of Otolaryngology Head and Neck Medicine and Surgery*, 1999. 20:314-317.
[93] Andre JM, et al. Buccal hemineglect. *Arch Neurol*, 2000:1734-41.
[94] Muellbacher W, Artner C, Mamoli B. The role of the intact hemisphere in recovery of midline muscles after recent monohemispheric stroke. *Journal of Neurology*, 1999; 246:250-256.
[95] Martin RE, et al. Neural mechanisms of swallowing impairment in hemispheric stroke: a functional magnetic resonance imaging (FMRI) study. *Dysphagia* 2005. In press.,
[96] Splaingard MI, et al. Aspiration in rehabilitation patients:videofluoroscopy vs bedside clinical assessment. *Archives of Physical Medicine and Rehabilitatio*n, 1988; 69:637-40.
[97] Kidd D, et al. Aspiration in acute stroke: a clinical study with videofluoroscopy. *Quarterly Journal of Medicine*., 1993; 86: 825-9.
[98] Freson M, Stokmans R. The radiologic investigation of dysphagia. *Acta oto-rhino-laryngologica belg*., 1994; 48:127-137.
[99] Mann G, Hankey GJ, Cameron D. Swallowing disorders following acute stroke: prevalence and diagnostic accuracy. *Cerebrovascular Diseases*. 2000; 10:380-6.
[100] Stoeckli SJ, et al. Interrater reliability of videofluoroscopic swallow evaluation. *Dysphagia,* 2003; 18:53-7.
[101] McCullough GH, et al. Inter- and intrajudge reliability for videofluoroscopic swallowing evaluation measures. *Dysphagia*, 2001; 16:110-118.
[102] Smithard DG, et al. Can bedside assessment reliably exclude aspiration following acute stroke? *Age and Ageing*, 1998; 27:99-106.
[103] Lazarus CL, et al. Effects of bolus volume, viscosity, and repeated swallows in nonstroke subjects and stroke patients. *Archives of Physical Medicine and Rehabilitation*, 1993; 74:1066-70.
[104] Logemann JA, et al. Oropharyngeal swallowing after stroke in the left basal ganglion / internal capsule. *Dysphagia*, 1993; 8:230-234.
[105] Johnson ER, McKenzie SW, Sievers A. Aspiration pneumonia in stroke. *Archives of Physical Medicine and Rehabilitation*, 1993; 74: 973-976.
[106] Han TR, Paik NJ, Park JW. Quantifying swallowing function after stroke: A functional dysphagia scale based on videofluoroscopic studies. *Archives of Physical Medicine and Rehabilitation,* 2001; 82: 677-682.
[107] Bastian RW. The videoendoscopic swallowing study: an alternative and partner to the videofluoroscopic swallowing study. *Dysphagia*, 1993; 8:359-67.
[108] Aviv JE, et al. The safety of flexible endoscopic evaluation of swallowing with sensory testing (FEESST): An analysis of 500 consecutive evaluations. *Dysphagia*, 2000; 15: 39-44.

[109] Sellars C, et al. Swallowing abnormalities after acute stroke: A case control study. *Dysphagia*, 1999; 14:212-218.

[110] Aviv JE, et al. Air pulse quantification of supraglottic and pharyngeal sensation: A new technique. *Annals of Otology, Rhinology and Laryngology*, 1993; 102:777-780.

[111] Aviv JEMD, et al. Laryngopharyngeal sensory testing with modified barium swallow as predictors of aspiration pneumonia after stroke. *Laryngoscope*, 1997; 107:1254-1260.

[112] Aviv JE, et al. Supraglottic and pharyngeal sensory abnormalities in stroke patients with dysphagia. *Annals of Otology, Rhinology and Laryngology*, 1996; 105: 92-97.

[113] Sacco RL, et al. Silent laryngopharyngeal sensory deficits after stroke. *Annals of Otology, Rhinology and Laryngology*, 1997; 106: 87-93.

[114] Aviv JEMD, Prospective, Randomized outcome study of endoscopy versus modified barium swallow in patients with dysphagia. *Laryngoscope*, 2000;110:563-574.

[115] Shawker TH, et al. Real-time ultrasound visualization of tongue movement during swallowing. *Journal of Clinical Ultrasound,* 1983; 11:485-90.

[116] Shawker TH, Sonies BC, Stone M. Soft tissue anatomy of the tongue and floor of the mouth: An ultrasound demonstration. *Brain and Language,* 1984; 21: 335-350.

[117] Shawker TH, et al. Ultrasound analysis of tongue, hyoid, and larynx activity during swallowing. *Investigative Radiology*, 1984; 19: 82-86.

[118] Litvan I, Sastry N, Sonies BC. Characterizing swallowing abnormalities in progressive supranuclear palsy. *Neurology*, 1997; 48: 1654-62.

[119] Honda Y. Kinetic MRI using high-speed sequence to evaluate swallowing - Comparison with videofluorography. *Oral Radiology*, 2003; 19: 14-21.

[120] Anagnostara A, et al. Evaluation of the anatomical and functional properties of deglutition with various kinetic high-speed MRI sequences. *Journal of Magnetic Resonance Imaging,* 2001; 14:194-199.

[121] Suto Y, Kamba M, Kato T. Dynamic analysis of the pharynx during swallowing using Turbo-FLASH magnetic resonance imaging combined with an oral positive contrast agent: A preliminary study. *British Journal of Radiology*, 1995; 68: 1099-1102.

[122] Foucart JM, et al. Kinetic magnetic resonance imaging analysis of swallowing: A new approach to pharyngeal function. *Surgical and Radiologic Anatomy*, 1998; 20:53-55.

[123] Flaherty RF, et al. Dynamic magnetic resonance imaging of vocal cord closure during deglutition. *Gastroenterology,* 1995; 109: 843-849.

[124] Gilbert RJ, et al. Echo-planar magnetic resonance imaging of deglutitive vocal fold closure: Normal and pathologic patterns of displacement. *Laryngoscope*, 1996; 106:568-572.

[125] Gilbert RJ, et al. Patterns of lingual tissue deformation associated with bolus containment and propulsion during deglutition as determined by echo-planar MRI. *Journal of Magnetic Resonance Imaging,* 1998; 8: 554-560.

[126] Hartl D, et al., Morphologic parameters of normal swallowing events using single-shot fast spin echo dynamic MRI. *Dysphagia*. 2003; 18:255-62.

[127] Rasche V, Holz D, Proksa R. MR fluoroscopy using projection reconstruction multi-gradient-echo (prMGE) MRI. *Magnetic Resonance in Medicine*, 1999; 42:324-334.

[128] Barkhausen J, et al. Visualization of swallowing using real-time TrueFISP MR fluoroscopy. *European Radiology*, 2002; 12:129-33.
[129] Galli J, et al. Postoperative dysphagia versus neurogenic dysphagia: scintigraphic assessment. *Annals of Otology, Rhinology and Laryngology*, 2003; 112: 20-8.

In: State-of-the-Art Imaging in Stroke, Volume 2
Editor: Bernhard Schaller, pp. 195-244
ISBN 978-1-60021-499-8


*Chapter VII*

# Differences in Imaging Arterial Infarction or Venous Infarction of the Brain

***S. E. J. Connor and H. Mehta***
King's College Hospital, London, UK

## Introduction

A primary goal in both venous and arterial ischaemia is to recognise diagnostic imaging features and exclude other conditions. Arterial infarction is usually diagnosed by directly visualising the typical imaging characteristics and distribution of the parenchymal changes. Vascular imaging in arterial infarction may be advocated as a secondary goal in order to increase diagnostic specificity and to refine the selection of patients for thrombolysis [130]. Venous ischemia or infarction is less stereotypical in its parenchymal imaging appearances but is more consistently associated with ongoing vascular occlusion so the emphasis is on vascular imaging of the causative CVT.

Cerebral venous sinus thrombosis (CVT) generally occurs in young or middle aged adults and accounts for 1-2% of strokes in these patients [26]. Although it is reported to be an uncommon condition, the diverse clinical presentation has made CVT a difficult and often delayed diagnosis,and the prevalence is likely to be underestimated [8,22]. Latent thrombus of the cerebral veins and dural sinuses has been shown to be present in 9.5% of cases in one autopsy series [188]. There are serious clinical consequences with more recent studies demonstrating a 5-15% mortality rate [6, 29, 39, 52, 59] and significant morbidity in survivors. However an increased awareness and developments in non-invasive imaging techniques have led to earlier and more frequent detection than was previously possible. This is important as earlier treatment may prevent serious neurological sequelae [22, 28].

## Clinical Presentation and Predisposing Factors

CVT presents with a diverse range of symptoms and signs so it should be considered in almost any cerebral syndrome [51]. However, there are certain clinical features, which provide clues to the presence of CVT. Although the onset may be acute [52], the symptoms typically evolve over days or weeks since growth of thrombus is usually slow, and venous collateralization may be extensive [8,201]. The severity of symptoms depends on the vessels involved and the chronicity of development. A headache is a key presenting feature, and since this may be associated with papilloedema, the clinical presentation may be confused with benign intracranial hypertension [BIH]. In fact, onventional angiography or magnetic resonance venography [MRV] has revealed CVT in 25% of patients with a previous clinical diagnosis of BIH. Another differential diagnosis that should be considered with this clinical presentation is dural arteriovenous fistula, particularly if the patient is male and not obese [185]. Focal deficits and seizures resulting from venous oedema or infarction may be variably present [8, 29, 39]. Visual disturbances consist of diplopia, increased central scotoma and other visual field defects. An uncommon but classical presentation is of bilateral alternating deficits and hemiparesis predominating in the legs due to superior sagittal sinus [SSS] thrombosis and parasagittal venous infarction [154]. Hemianopia and dysphasia may result from occlusion of the posterior SSS or transverse sinus and associated cortical veins. Thrombosis of the deep venous system has a variable clinical presentation ranging from neuropsychological symptoms [204] to impairment of consciousness. A sixth nerve palsy is usually secondary to intracranial hypertension, however, cranial nerve palsies may also result from thrombus extension to the transverse or sigmoid sinus [III-VIII], petrosal sinus [V] and jugular vein [IX-XI] [110,187].

Although a predisposing factor is identified in up to 80% of patients [198] and almost all children with CVT, its absence should not deter the radiologist from the diagnosis. The commonest aetiologies are pregnancy and puerperium [135], oral contraceptive use, dehydration, adjacent infection [e.g. mastoiditis or sinusitis], compressive tumour, trauma, blood dyscrasias and systemic disease [e.g. carcinoma, collagen vascular disease or endocrine disease] [39, 96, 154, 155, 198]. In those patients without known risk factors at presentation, inherited and acquired coagulation disorders such as protein C and S deficiency, antithrombin III deficiency or factor V Leiden mutation [30,126,200] must be excluded. Prothombotic disorders are reported in 33-96% of children and 15-21% of adults with CVT [54,175,216]. Neonates are particularly susceptible to CVT due to the maternal hypercoaguable states associated with the perinatal period, injury to the dural sinuses during delivery, higher haematocrits, slow venous blood flow and a decrease in the normal levels of protective clotting factors [175]. In addition, acute illness and dehydration are frequently precipitating factors for CVT in neonates whilst chronic disease, infection or coagulopathy are the commonest underlying conditions in children [55,134,198].

# Embryology, Anatomy and Anatomical Variants

An appreciation of the complex anatomy of the intracranial venous system is essential in order to understand the imaging appearances of the dural venous sinuses and cerebral veins as well as the consequences of venous occlusion. The embryological development will briefly be reviewed followed by consideration of the venous anatomy and significant anatomical variants. An emphasis will be placed on the anatomy of the major dural sinuses which are routinely visualized with MRV and CTV, however smaller dural sinuses, superficial and deep supratentorial and infratentorial veins will also be discussed, since they are increasingly visualised with contemporary imaging techniques [105,124,206] and their configuration and anastamoses influence the parenchymal effects of venous occlusion. In addition there are a number of anatomical variations which may mimic venous pathology and which are relevant to the later discussion of pitfalls in interpretation of imaging studies.

## Embryology

All stages of venous system development lag considerably behind development of the arterial system. The early venous system consists of a network of primitive collecting veins that drain into a superficial venous network on the surface of the neural tube. The primitive venous network is superficial to the primitive arterial network.

Basic early arterial flow is centrifugal whilst venous flow is centripetal. However growth of the cerebral hemispheres changes this pattern of blood flow. Deep medullary veins develop along the lines of the peripheral embryonic migration of gray cells, from the subependymal region of the cerebral ventricles outwards toward the superficial cerebral cortex. So whilst arterial flow remains centrifugal, venous flow becomes mixed as superficial cerebral tissues have centrifugal venous drainage, and deep cerebral tissues have centripetal venous drainage. The final development of the dural venous sinuses takes place following birth [88,115].

## Anatomy

### *A) Dural Sinuses*

The cranial dural venous sinuses are endothelial-lined channels located between the outer periosteal and inner meningeal layers of dura. They do not possess valves and their walls are devoid of musculature so drainage is passive. Most dural sinuses are complex trabeculated structures that have numerous crossing bands, chords and bridges [12].There are a plexus of adjacent venous channels which act as collateral pathways for drainage in the event of venous sinus occlusion. These include lateral lacunae, dural cavernous spaces and meningeal tributaries [147,171].

Dural sinuses collect blood from the superficial and deep cerebral veins, meninges and calvarium. The dural sinuses flow into the internal jugular veins however they also communicate with the extracranial venous system via a network of emissary veins that pass directly through the cranial vault and basilar foramina. These pathways may provide an important potential route for collateral venous drainage in cerebral venous occlusion [11]. The dural sinuses also link with the meningeal and diploic veins.

The major dural venous sinuses comprise of the superior and inferior sagittal sinuses, the cavernous and intercavernous sinuses, the superior and inferior petrosal sinuses, the occipital, straight, transverse and sigmoid sinuses.

The superior sagittal sinus [SSS] originates near the crista galli and arcs posteriorly in the midline along the attached border of the falx, progressively increasing in caliber as it collects the superficial cerebral veins. It demonstrates a clear triangular shape in crosssection. It terminates by joining with the straight sinus to form the torcular Herophili at the internal occipital protruberance [147,171].

The inferior sagittal sinus is a smaller channel which courses posteriorly in the free edge of the falx cerebri. It lies above the anterior aspect of the body of the corpus callosum and receives tributaries from the falx, corpus callosum, cingulum and medial cerebral hemispheres. The sinus terminates by joining the vein of Galen to form the straight sinus [147,171].

The straight sinus runs posteroinferiorly within the confluence of the falx and tentorium cerebelli to the torcular where it is usually continuous with the left transverse sinus. It is a single midline tentorial channel in 85% but in the remaining 15% segments can be doubled or tripled [147,171].

The torcular Herophili is formed by the confluence of the superior sagittal sinus, straight sinus and transverse sinuses. The confluence is often asymmetric and shows numerous variations since it is ontogenetically derived from a plexiform structure. It has been described as demonstrating a common pool, plexiform, ipsilateral or unilateral configuration [25, 47].

The occipital sinus is a small variable sinus, which starts at the posterior margin of the foramen magnum and passes superiorly to the torcular. The sinus communicates with the internal jugular vein, vertebral venous plexus and clival venous plexus via multiple small channels [31,171]. In about 2% of cases the occipital sinus forms a major draining channel for the SS or SSS and it is detected in approximately 10% of MR venogram [MRV] or CT venogram [CTV] studies [15,82].

The transverse sinuses curve anterolaterally from the internal occipital protruberance to the posterior border of the petrous temporal bone where they receive the superior petrosal sinuses and turn downward to form the sigmoid sinuses. The transverse sinus may receive inflow from the anastomotic cortical vein of Labbe together with veins from the inferolateral temporal lobe, occipital lobe and cerebellum. Prominent transverse sinuses will groove the adjacent occipital bone. The transverse sinuses communicate with extracranial veins via mastoid emissary veins [47]. In 75% of cases the right transverse sinus is larger than the left [215]. In 5-20% of anatomic specimens a narrowed or atreitic segment is identified in at least one of the transverse sinuses [15, 95, 215]

The sigmoid sinuses are the anteroinferior continuation of the transverse sinuses beyond the tentorial margin, lieing in the sigmoid sulcus of the temporal bone, and terminating as the internal jugular vein at the jugular fossa. There are numerous anastomoses between sigmoid sinuses and the vertebral plexuses, suboccipital muscular and scalp veins, and condylar emissary veins. Although the jugular veins have been thought to be the predominant draining pathway, recent findings have demonstrated this situation to apply only in the supine position, with redirection of flow to the vertebral plexus when in the upright position [197].

The marginal sinus is occasionally seen to be located within the dural leaves at the margins of the atlanto-occipital ligament. It connects the basal venous sinuses with the verebral veins inferiorly [14].

The superior petrosal sinus extends from the cavernous sinus to the sigmoid sinus. It runs along the attachment of the tentorium cerebelli to the dorsal ridge of the petrous temporal bones.

The inferior petrosal sinus lies in a groove between the petrous apices and clivus extending posterolaterally along the petro-occipital fissure. They demonstrate marked anatomic variation in size and anastomoses but also in their relationship with cranial nerves entering the jugular foramen and with the jugular foramen itself [70]. The sinus terminates by draining into the jugular bulb. There are numerous anastomotic channels between the sinuses, basilar venous plexus, vertebral venous plexus, pterygoid venous plexus and epidural veins. Absence of an anastomosis between the inferior petrosal sinus and internal jugular vein occurs in only 1% of cases [70,138].

The sphenoparietal sinus is the continuation of the middle meningeal veins [166]. The sphenoparietal sinus enters the cavernous sinus, or more rarely extends directly to the pterygoid venous plexus, the inferior petrosal or transverse sinus. The notion that it also drains the superficial middle cerebral vein has recently been challenged [166].

The cavernous sinuses lie on either side of the sphenoid body. The cavernous sinus extends from the superior orbital fissure anteriorly to the petrous apex posteriorly. Cavernous sinus tributaries and interconnections are complex and variable. Each cavernous sinus communicates with its counterpart on the opposite side via intercavernous sinus to surround the sella turcica. Posteriorly the sinuses empty into the superior and inferior petrosal sinuses through which they drain into the transverse sinus and jugular bulb respectively. The cavernous sinuses also communicate with a network of veins within the clival venous plexus which extends from the basiocciput to the foramen magnum and which communicates with the vertebral venous plexuses.

### *B) Superficial Supratentorial Venous System*

There are numerous veins extending over the surface of the brain which drain the cortex and the subcortical white matter. The superficial middle cerebral vein, superior anastamotic vein and the inferior anastamotic vein are the most consistently identified and any of these major superficial drainage rotes may dominate. The superficial middle cerebral vein runs along the sylvian fissure, curves around the temporal pole and enters the sinus of the lesser wing of sphenoid which then drains to the cavernous or paracavernous sinuses [166]. It anastomoses with the deep cerebral venous system and with other superficial veins and dural sinuses. It communicates with facial veins and pterygoid venous plexus through the foramen ovale. The superior anastamotic vein (of Trolard) extends from the posterior sylvian fissure and drains into the superior sagittal sinus [SSS] over the mid hemispheric convexity, along with 10-12 other superficial cortical veins [13]. The inferior anastamotic vein (of Labbe), also referred to as the occipito-temporal vein, courses over the temporal lobe along the occipito-temporal sulcus and enters the transverse sinus or, more frequently, the adjacent lateral tentorial sinus [137]. This vein is demonstrated on one or both sides in 75% of dissections [172]. Variable connections exist between these major routes of drainage which influences the ability to divert venous blood flow in the event of venous occlusion. The existence of venous anastamoses traversing the centrum semiovale between the superficial and deep venous systems remains controversial [11,115].

### *C) Deep Supratentorial Venous System*

The deep venous system drains the deep cerebral white matter, choroid plexus, cortical areas of the limbic lobe, diencephalon, together with the rostral brainstem and cerebellum [12,145]. This territory may be defined as that served by the vein of Galen or alternatively as that exhibiting centripetal venous drainage [12,171]. The capacity for collateral drainage is poor relative to the superficial veins. The internal cerebral veins are paired structures which are seen near the midline within the roof of the third ventricle. They receive venous blood from the septal, anterior caudate, ventricular choroidal and terminal subependymal veins at the level of the foramen of Monro. Anatomical variation is frequent at this site and there are probably separate tributaries from the deep grey matter and occipital horn which enter the internal cerebral veins more posteriorly [193]. The basal vein of Rosenthal arises in the sylvian fissure where it is formed by the confluence of veins draining the insula, cerebral peduncle and temporal lobe and it then extends posteriorly around the cerebral peduncle. There are potential communications with the vein of Galen, the sphenoparietal sinus, superior petrosal sinus, cavernous sinus, pterygoid plexus and infratentorial veins [11]. Although the basal veins flow into the vein of Galen in about 90% of cases [180], this anastamosis is frequently hypoplastic and so alternative rotes of drainage anteriorly and inferiorly may be dominant. The vein of Galen is an unpaired midline structure which extends from under the splenium of the corpus callosum and joins the inferior sagittal sinus to form the straight sinus [147,171].

### *D) Veins of the Posterior Fossa*

The infratentorial veins can be classified into four groups: superficial, deep, brainstem and bridging veins [132]. Superficial veins are divided in the neurosurgical literature according to whether they drain the tentorial surface (superior hemispheric and superior vermian veins), the suboccipital surface (inferior hemispheric and inferior vermian veins) and the petrosal surface (anterior hemispheric veins). The most consistently demonstrated superficial veins on angiographic studies are the precentral cerebellar and superior cerebellar veins in the midline and draining into the vein of Galen [81]. The deep veins course in the fissures between the cerebellum and brainstem and on the three cerebellar peduncles. The veins of the brainstem are named according to whether they drain the midbrain, pons or medulla, and they may be orientated transversely or longitudinally. The anterior pontomesencephalic vein is well documented in the angiographic literature [81] and may be particularly prominent on imaging studies [186].These superficial, deep and brainstem veins terminate as bridging veins which collect into three major systems: the galenic system to the vein of Galen, the petrosal system to the petrosal sinus and the tentorial system to the sinuses bordering the tentorium cerebelli [115, 132, 147].

## Normal Anatomical Variations

The appearance of the intracranial venous system is more asymmetrical and variable than its arterial counterpart. Although the SSS typically begins anteriorly at the level of the foramen caecum, its anterior segment may be hypoplastic or atreitic to the level of the coronal suture. When this configuration is apparent, the SSS may form from the union of a large superior anastamotic vein and a major superficial cortical vein. In contradistinction to an acutely occluded anterior SSS, this hypoplastic portion will appear small on imaging studies that directly visualize the sinus. The distal SSS may also be fenestrated or high splitting [147].

It is a frequent pattern for the SSS bifurcation at the torcula to be asymmetric and for the SSS to terminate as a dominant transverse sinus, most frequently on the right [82]. The contralateral transverse sinus may be hypoplastic or supplied by the deep venous system. Absence or hypoplasia of part or the entire transverse sinus is common and is frequently manifest on imaging studies [7, 15, 27, 82]. When the transverse sinus is absent, there may still be a well formed sigmoid sinus which drains the superior or inferior petrosal sinuses. The occipital bone is less likely to demonstrate an adjacent vascular groove adjacent to a hypoplastic transverse sinus. Segmental areas of hypoplasia and stenoses may be present [7, 15, 27, 62], however these are rarely seen in the dominant transverse sinus or bilaterally [7, 15, 78, 82]. It has recently been shown that there is a strong association between bilateral transverse sinus stenosis and benign intracranial hypertension [BIH] [78, 82]. Farb et al found substantial bilateral transverse sinus stenoses in 27/29 patients with BIH but in only 4/59 controls [62]. Unilateral aplasia of the sigmoid sinus and internal jugular vein may also be present with the dominant drainage occurring through emissary veins to the vertebral venous plexus [80]. Age related changes in venous sinus anatomy may be relevant in early life. The occipital sinus is more frequent in neonates and young infants [163] and primitive venous channels sometimes have the ability to recanalise [102].

Arachnoid granulations are normal anatomical structures which represent enlarged arachnoid villi. They invaginate into the dural sinus and may grow sufficiently to occlude and enlarge the sinus [5, 42, 71, 79, 119]. They have been demonstrated as filling defects in 24% of contrast enhanced CT scans and 13% of MRI studies [119] being most frequently identified in the transverse sinus and in the vicinity of draining veinS. They may cause diagnostic confusion with CVT on CTV and MRV studies; however they are distinguished by a round, clearly defined morphology, together with normal proximal and distal flow and luminal contrast opacification. They are hyperintense on T2-w and hypointense on T1-w MRI sequences and do not undergo contrast enhancement. They be quite prominent and should not be mistaken for thrombi on imaging. Ectopic polypoid nodules of fat, hamartomas, septations and air may also cause intrasinus filling defects on imaging studies [48,79]. This is particularly evident in the cavernous sinuses where normal filling defects may be distinguished from thrombus by their small size [usually <7 mm], low CT attenuation, and longitudinal, oval or rounded configuration [3, 170].

Intracranial developmental venous anomalies represent a congenital variation in the deep cerebral venous drainage, likely due to underdevelopment of the superficial or deep cerebral veins [35,165].They have a typical appearance on cross sectional imaging and conventional angiography, with a "candelabra" appearance of the proximal intramedullary veins.

## Differences between the Intracranial Venous and Arterial Systems

Vascular anatomy, blood flow and pathology of the intracranial venous system differs to that of the arterial system in a number of respects and this influences the design and success of imaging techniques. Venous flow is slower and multidirectional with a narrower velocity profile. There is a greater normal variance in venous anatomy and calibre with frequent normal intravascular filling defects. Isolated occlusions of small cortical veins are far less frequent than isolated occlusion of small arteries and the calibre of the vessels being imaged is generally larger. In addition, CVT only requires imaging of the intracranial venous system, whereas vascular imaging for arterial infarction requires imaging of both intracranial and extracranial vessels and assessment for a wider range of occlusive aetiologies such as dissection. Although venous ischemia may occasionally occur secondary to compressive tumour, haematoma or brain swelling, venous sinus occlusion will generally be present in the setting of venous ischaemia. In contradistinction, demonstrable intracranial arterial stenoocclusive disease will only be found in a minority of cases of arterial infarction [215]. Finally, the small veins are anatomically juxtaposed to the arterial system and may interfere with interpretation, whereas the arteries are remote from and can easily be separated from the dural sinus and major superficial veins.

### Imaging of the Cerebral Venous System

A number of imaging techniques are now available to study the intracranial venous system and these have also been applied to imaging intracranial arteries [93,169,176]. In general, most centres will have a preference for a CT and CT venography [CTV] based or an MRI and MRV based approach to diagnosis. There is only minor contribution from other paraclinical investigations [106]. In the following sections, the techniques will be discussed according to whether they are principally used to image the venous lumen, detect venous blood flow or directly image the venous thrombus (table 1). Technical aspects will be described and the imaging features of CVT and pitfalls in interpretation will be discussed. Advantages and disadvantages relative to other imaging approaches (table 2) will be outlined and more recent comparative clinical studies will be reviewed.

### Imaging of the venous lumen

The presence of venous thrombus can be implied if filling defects are demonstrated when the venous system is opacified with contrast agent.

**Table 1. Imaging modalities used for the investigation of CVT**

| | |
|---|---|
| Imaging of the venous lumen | Contrast enhanced CT |
| | CT venography |
| | Contrast enhanced SE and GRE T1-w sequences |
| | Dynamic contrast enhanced MRV |
| Imaging of the venous lumen and venous blood flow | Conventional angiography (with rotational angiography) |
| Imaging of venous blood flow | 3D PC MRV |
| | 2D TOF MRV |
| | Ultrasound (with power Doppler and echo contrast agents) |
| | Time resolved MRA |
| Imaging of the thrombus within the venous lumen and venous blood flow | MRI |
| Imaging of the thrombus within the venous lumen | CT |

**Table 2. Advantages and disadvantages of imaging modalities in the investigation of CVT**

| Imaging modality | Advantages | Disadvantages |
|---|---|---|
| Standard thick section CT (pre and post contrast) | Easily available and useful in excluding other pathology,<br>Demonstrates acute haemorrhage well | Oedematous parenchymal changes may be less well demonstrated,<br>Normal intrasinus filling defects more difficult to distinguish than with higher resolution techniques,<br>"pseudodelta signs" and causes of relative increased density of the venous sinus must be excluded,<br>Partial volume effects interfere with assessment,<br>Presence of signs are very dependent on age of CVT |
| CT venography | Can immediately follow CT which is usually the first investigation performed,<br>Applicable when contraindications to MRI,<br>Contrast "floods" venous system so no arterfacts due to unopacified inflowing blood,<br>Rapid so no motion artifacts and of particular benefit in unstable or young patients | Complex post processing which is operator and software dependent,<br>Radiation exposure and iodinated contrast medium required,<br>Chronic thrombus may not be detected due to enhancement |

**Table 2. (Continued)**

| Imaging modality | Advantages | Disadvantages |
|---|---|---|
| CE GRE MRI/MRV | Rapid sequence, Some parenchymal information, No vascular dephasing or saturation effects, Better demonstration of smaller venous structures than other MRV techniques (collateral flow better demonstrated) | Chronic thrombus may enhance and hence not be detected, Requires careful timing relative to the contrast bolus, Meningeal enhancement may obscure superficial veins |
| 2D TOF MRV | | Subacute thrombus leads to T1 shortening and may mimic flow, In plane saturation effects more significant than with PC MRV |
| 3D PC MRV | Sensitive to flow in all directions | Longer acquisition times, Superior contrast to noise of the venous blood flow makes it impossible to visualise structure of the sinus and distinguish hypoplasia from occlusion, Intravoxel dephasing problematic in areas of complex and turbulent flow |
| MRI | Parenchymal changes also well demonstrated | Multiple sequences used and time consuming, Overlapping signals returned by thrombus and normal venous sinus flow |
| Conventional angiography | Excellent spatial and temporal resolution, Demonstrates flow and luminal filling, Collateral flow and isolated cortical vein thrombosis demonstrated | Time consuming and invasive, Limited number of projectional images are usually available so partial CVT may not be detected, Filling defects due to unopacified inflowing blood may mimic CVT |
| Ultrasound | Easily available, Cheap and mobile with "bedside application" | Little clinical data available, Very operator dependent, Predominantly depends on indirect signs |

This can be achieved with the use of conventional contrast enhanced CT, CT venography (CTV), contrast enhanced MRV (CE MRV) or MRI (CE MRI) and conventional angiography.

### *A) Contrast Enhanced CT*

In the 1980s prior to the advent of helical CT, axial CT with thick collimation [5 or 10 mm sections] was routinely used to detect signs of CVT [32, 33, 117, 154]. When appearances were considered doubtful, it was suggested that thinner sections and higher doses of contrast agent should be employed [72] however the number of sections which could be obtained during peak venous enhancement was limited with this technology. Wider window settings and orthogonal views with multiplanar reformats have also been used to help detect CVT [8, 30].

The best described radiological sign of CVT on contrast enhanced CT is the empty delta sign [117,202]. It consists of a triangular area of enhancement or high attenuation with a relatively low attenuating centre on multiple contiguous slices obtained in the region of the superior sagittal sinus. No single explanation for the pathophysiology of this has been universally accepted. Possible aetiologies proposed include recanalisation of thrombus within the sinus, organization of clot, blood brain barrier breakdown and dilatation of collateral peridural and dural venous channels. The most likely explanation however, appears to be that proposed by Virapongse et al [202]. They suggested that enhancement of the rich dural venous collateral circulation, which consisted of lateral lacunae, dural cavernous spaces and meningeal venous tributaries, was responsible. Other indirect diagnostic clues to dural sinus thrombosis on contrast enhanced CT, which are less sensitive and specific, include strong tentorial or falcine enhancement [85] and dilated transcerebral veins [10]. These do not usually appear in the initial stages of CVT.

There are a number of difficulties in using this sign with thick section conventional contrast enhanced axial CT. The sign may be absent in the acute stage [in the first 5 days] when thrombus is of high attenuation or in the chronic stage [greater than 2 months] when the channel recanalises with thrombus [174] and the organized thrombus may be converted to vascularised connective tissue [57]. The empty delta sign is only relevant if the affected venous sinus is perpendicular to the scan plane. Hence it is only applied to the posterior third of the SSS [117,154]. In addition, partial volume averaging with the thicker sections has been felt to obscure the recognition of smaller venous sinuses such as the Galenic venous system. Consequently the sign was only described in 10-35% of cases with thick sections in earlier series [8, 30]. It should be noted that multislice CT with submillimetric collimation allows the empty delta sign to be visualized throughout the dural venous sinuses with much greater diagnostic accuracy. Even segments of thrombus parallel to the section plane will be detected using thin section axial images [143]. The frequency of the sign does vary with the site of thrombosis, timing of CT scanning and technical parameters used. Careful analysis of precontrast images should be routine since a "pseudodelta sign" can be seen on non-enhanced CT in patients with hyperattenuating acute subarachnoid haemorrhage, subdural empyema or posterior parafalcine interhemispheric haematoma around the sinus. In all of these cases intravenous contrast should opacify the sinus obliterating the pseudodelta. Sinus septations, arachnoid granulations and skull artifact are also reported to have led to false positive diagnoses of CVT [42, 202]

## CT Venography

Following the introduction of helical CT technology Casey et al [40] described the use of contrast enhanced CT with three-dimensional reconstructions to evaluate the cerebral venous system and termed it CT venography [CTV]. CTV overcomes many of the disadvantages of conventional CT by avoiding partial volume averaging and obtaining peak venous enhancement. Casey et al evaluated 33 patients with a 1mm collimated helical scan with a pitch of 2 scanning from vertex to skull base. Ninety millilitres, of non-ionic contrast was given intravenously by pump injector at 3ml/sec, following a 40 second pre-scan delay. A graded subtraction method was used to remove bone without deleting vascular structures and post processing by the radiologist took approximately 15 minutes. Casey and other authors [40,170] have suggested scanning from cranial to caudal in order to maximize the opacification of the venous system. Recently helical CTV has been refined by the development of multislice CTV which allows imaging of the entire brain within 30 seconds of peak vascular enhancement [128].

The use of maximum intensity projection [MIP] algorithms provides superior contrast between the high density intravascular enhancement and the brain, because it does not sum up the background across the projected volume but rather selects the maximum intensity voxel in the projected ray [9]. Bone elimination is required prior to the processing of the projectional images [40, 84, 128, 199]. Majoie et al have described the use of matched mask bone elimination [MMBE] in two patients as a technique for the automatic removal of bone pixels from CT angiography data sets. The technique was first described in CTA of the circle of Willis [199] and involves an unenhanced spiral CT scan prior to the contrast enhanced CTV examination. The principle of the MMBE method is that bone voxels are identified in the unenhanced data set and that the corresponding voxels in the CTA data set are given an arbitrarily low value [199]. A key step in the method is motion compensation between the two scans which is achieved by a fully automated 3D registration of the unenhanced CT scan with the contrast enhanced scan. After registration a threshold is applied to identify bone pixels, with a recommended level of 200 Houndsfield units. This technique is a better alternative than subtracting an enhanced scan from an unenhanced scan [84] as subtraction adds noise to the CTA images [199] and requires that the patient stays completely still which is often difficult to achieve. The graded subtraction technique described by Casey is a masking technique for removal of bone from the CT images. There is no precontrast scan and an initial mask is generated by thresholding followed by widening of the mask by multiple dilation steps. The technique is operator dependent and is best performed by an experienced radiologist with a detailed knowledge of the cerebrovascular anatomy to avoid elimination of dural sinuses and cortical veins during the procedure [40]. In contrast the MMBE procedure is fully automatic, operator independent and therefore reproducible. The simultaneous enhancement of the arteries does not generally interfere with evaluation however they may easily be subtracted out prior to producing MIP images since they are distant to the venous sinuses. MIP images are useful in providing a rapid overview of the venous system with a limitless number of projections and targeted MIP images may be produced for further accuracy. However muliplanar reformatted [MPR] images should be routinely reviewed since they have been shown to be the more sensitive post processing technique [206]. Wetzel et al found that MPR images were superior to MIP images with sensitivities of 95% and 80% respectively in depicting venous structures [206]. Whilst parenchymal evaluation may be obtained from the CTV data by summation of sets of several sections, optimal lesions evaluation requires plain CT and formal contrast imaging with a longer prescan delay.

CTV has the advantage that it can immediately follow an unenhanced CT, which is usually the first investigation requested, thus decreasing time to diagnosis and commencement of therapy. The technique is fast and less prone to motion artifact than MRV and therefore more suitable for acutely unwell patients. It can also be used in those patients with contraindications to MRI. The advantages of CTV over conventional venography are that it is less invasive, cheaper and quicker. There is complete "flooding" of the venous system so there is no potential confusion of unopacified blood with filling defects, and a single injection provides a limitless number of projectional views. The ability to view the bony appearances from the CTV data is also helpful. It may allow differentiation of a hypoplastic transverse sinus, where there is unlikely to be a vascular bony groove in the occipital bone, from an occluded venous sinus, where a groove may be present. A small jugular foramen on CT may also provide a diagnostic clue that the sigmoid sinus and internal jugular vein is hypoplastic rather than occluded.

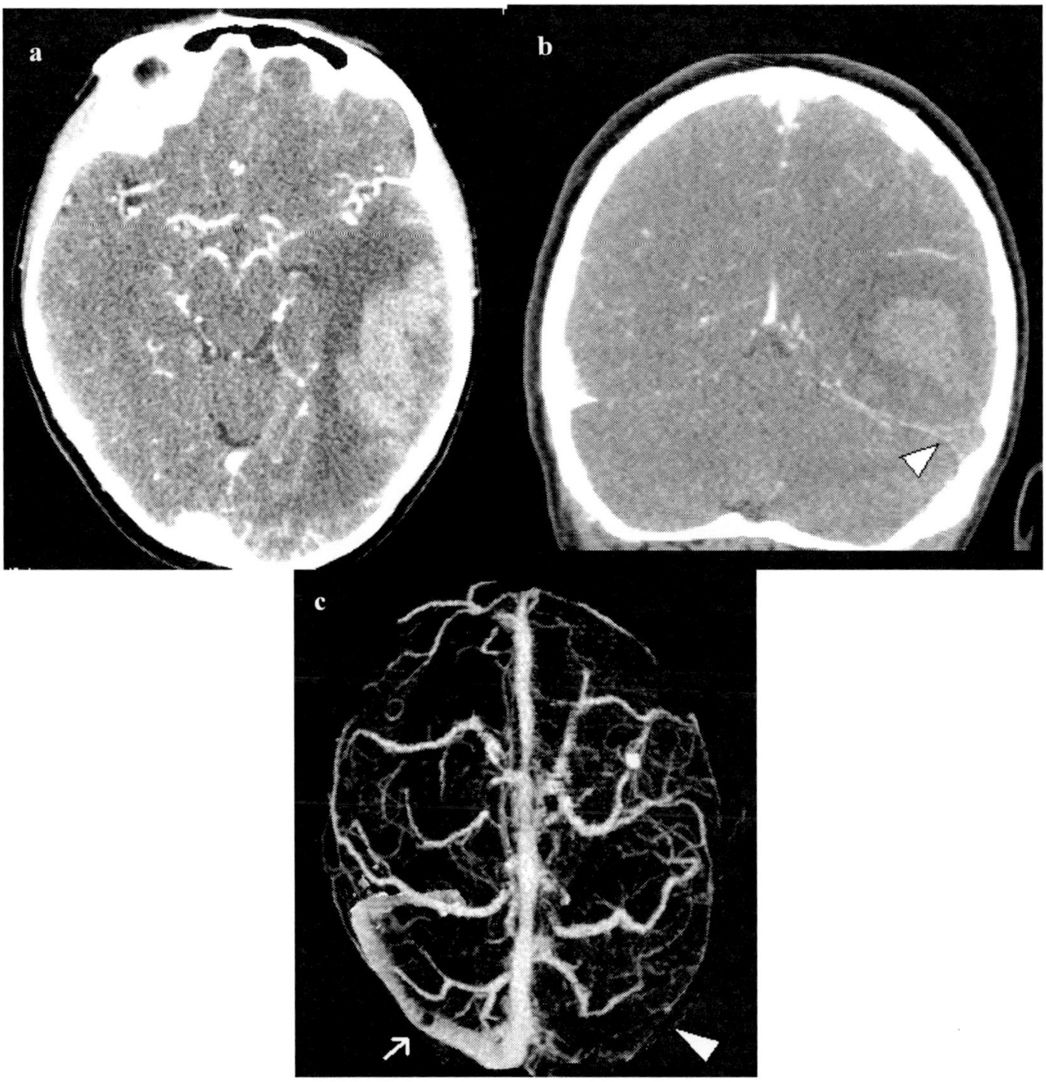


Figure 1. CT Venogram demonstrating left transverse sinus thrombosis and temporal lobe haemorrhage a) axial source image b) MPR coronal image and c) axial projection of a MIP . There is an acute haematoma with surrounding oedema in the left temporal lobe. The left transverse sinus is expanded by thrombus and demonstrates a "delta sign" (arrowhead in b). The sinus is not visualized on the MIP (arrowhead in c). Note the well defined, rounded arachnoid granulation in the contralateral transverse sinus (arrow in c).

CVT is demonstrated on CTV by the presence of a filling defect within the venous sinus on source or multiplanar reformatted images and segmental absence of enhancement on MIP images (figure 1) [44].

There are similar potential pitfalls with CTV as with contrast enhanced CT since it is using similar principles. CTV overcomes problems due to partial volume averaging, and whilst there remains the potential for misinterpretation of normal intrasinus filling defects and variations in venous anatomy, the improved detail and volumetric analysis makes this less likely. The possibility of contrast enhancing chronic thrombus merging with the intravascular enhancement should remain a consideration in the appropriate setting. Since the wall of the thrombosed sinus may enhance, as has been illustrated by the empty delta sign, there is a danger that there will be obscuring of the low attenuation voxels of intraluminal thrombus on MIP images. In both these settings, variable windowing of the MPRs may prove helpful. CTV does require complex post processing work. There are inherent limitations of the MIP algorithm which may lead to loss of the lower attenuation areas and thus poorer depiction of smaller vessels or vessel narrowing [9]. There requires proper selection of threshold values and since there is some overlap of density values and close proximity of the dural sinuses to the adjacent bone there is potential for removal of venous opacification following bone elimination. It is therefore always important to review source images and MPRs at the site of abnormalities highlighted on MIPs.

There are other potential disadvantages of CTV relative to other techniques. CTV lacks the detailed information regarding contrast media flow dynamics that is available with conventional angiography. Using a CT and CTV based approach to imaging CVT will be less sensitive to associated parenchymal changes than the combination of MRI and MRV. However the features are no less specific and it could be argued that the additional detection of parenchymal abnormality has little impact on patient management. Some investigators have reported that CTV is limited in its ability to depict thrombosis of the sigmoid sinus and jugular bulb [123]. The radiation dose with multislice CT is an important consideration. Wetzel et al reported an effective dose of 2.22mSv for CTV at a pitch of 2.5 compared with 2.48mSv for the contiguous unenhanced CT scan [206]. Radiation dose is of particular concern in the paediatric age group due to increased organ sensitivity, longer life time risk for cancer and lack of adjustment of CT parameters relative to the size of the patient [175]. Also a rapid injection rate is not feasible in the paediatric population however one group has shown that CTV may be effectively performed in children by using a hand injection [4].

Several studies have evaluated the utility of CTV in visualizing the cerebral venous system and in detecting CVT as compared with MRV and conventional angiography. In their original paper demonstrating the diagnostic utility of CTV, Casey et al [40] noted that the major dural venous sinuses, internal cerebral veins and vein of Galen were present in all cases and the inferior sagittal sinus, basal veins and cavernous sinuses were visualized in 90% of cases. An average of 4.4 cortical veins were demonstrated which compares favourably with MRV [113]. The few CTVs that were compared with MRV revealed greater small vessel anatomy and had fewer artifacts. They noted that slow flow subependymal veins and collateral venous drainage in dural sinus thromboses were better visualized with CTV than MRV. Ozsvath and Casey [149] reported a study comparing CTV with MRV in 24 patients of which 17 were investigated for suspected dural sinus thrombosis. They found that

CTV was at least equivalent to MRV in the diagnosis of dural sinus thrombosis with all MRV diagnoses being visible on CTV. In addition CTV was superior to MRV in the identification of smaller cerebral veins and dural sinuses. Wetzel et al [206] prospectively compared CTV with conventional angiography in 25 patients with three observers evaluating CTV and comparing them with intraarterial DSA which was the reference standard. They found that CTV was a reliable method to depict cerebral venous structures. CTV MPR images were superior to DSA images in showing the cavernous sinus, the inferior sagittal sinus and the basal vein of Rosenthal.

### *A) Contrast Enhanced MRI and MRV*

Standard post contrast spin echo T1-w images may be used to demonstrate filling defects due to thrombus [52]. Post gadolinium three dimensional [3D] low flip angle gradient echo [GRE] sequences have also been evaluated for their depiction of the cerebral venous system and CVT [123,170, 207]. These produce heavily T1-w contrast with relatively high signal to noise ratio, post processing capabilities, thin contiguous images and flow related enhancement [90]. This method also has the benefit of simultaneous depiction of the brain parenchyma. Flow is depicted by time-of-flight [TOF] effects and the T1 shortening effects of gadolinium [210]. Studies in a phantom [123] have illustrated that the signal intensity was no longer dependent on flow rate when the blood concentration of gadolinium reached approximately 1.0 mmol/l [123]. Long lasting injections of higher than normal doses of gadolinium resulted in improved signal to noise in the venous sinuses [123]. The signal was not affected by the angle between the direction of flow and the scan slab plane. Some investigators have aimed to refine the technique by subtracting an unenhanced data set from the enhanced data set [207].

Whilst MRV studies have until recently been aimed at detecting the flow within the venous sinus by depending on the in flow of unsaturated spins or velocity induced phase shifts, recent developments in contrast enhanced MR angiography techniques have enabled direct imaging of the venous lumen [62,105,125,160,171,207] during the first pass of an intravenously injected bolus of gadolinium [CE MRV]. A conventional gradient echo sequence is used with an intermediate flip angle to keep background tissue saturated. The bolus of gadolinium is timed to maintain a high intravascular concentration during the acquisition of low k-space frequency [62,105,125]. Post processing involves targeted MIPs following removal of the major arterial vessels. A novel auto triggered elliptic centric ordered [ATECO], three dimensional gadolinium enhanced MRV has been developed by one centre. This employs the initiation of a two dimensional single section bolus detection sequence at the level of the cavernous carotids, an intravenous power injection of contrast medium, a fully automated detection of the arrival of contrast medium and a triggering system for the angiographic sequence eight seconds later [62].

The presence of thrombus within the dural sinuses is demonstrated on spin echo or 3D GRE gadolinium enhanced T1-w MRI by a non enhanced central area of intermediate signal surrounded by an enhanced rim which is the MRI equivalent of the delta sign (figure 2). It may be more clearly visualized than with contrast enhanced CT due to the ability to acquire multiplanar images and because there is less artifact from the adjacent bone [57,183].There may also be intense enhancement of the tentorium, superficial and deep collateral channels

[8]. The intravenous enhancement sign [18, 60, 103] refers to abnormal contrast medium retention within the cerebral vessels and has been described in the setting of CVT although it is more frequently associated with arterial ischaemia.

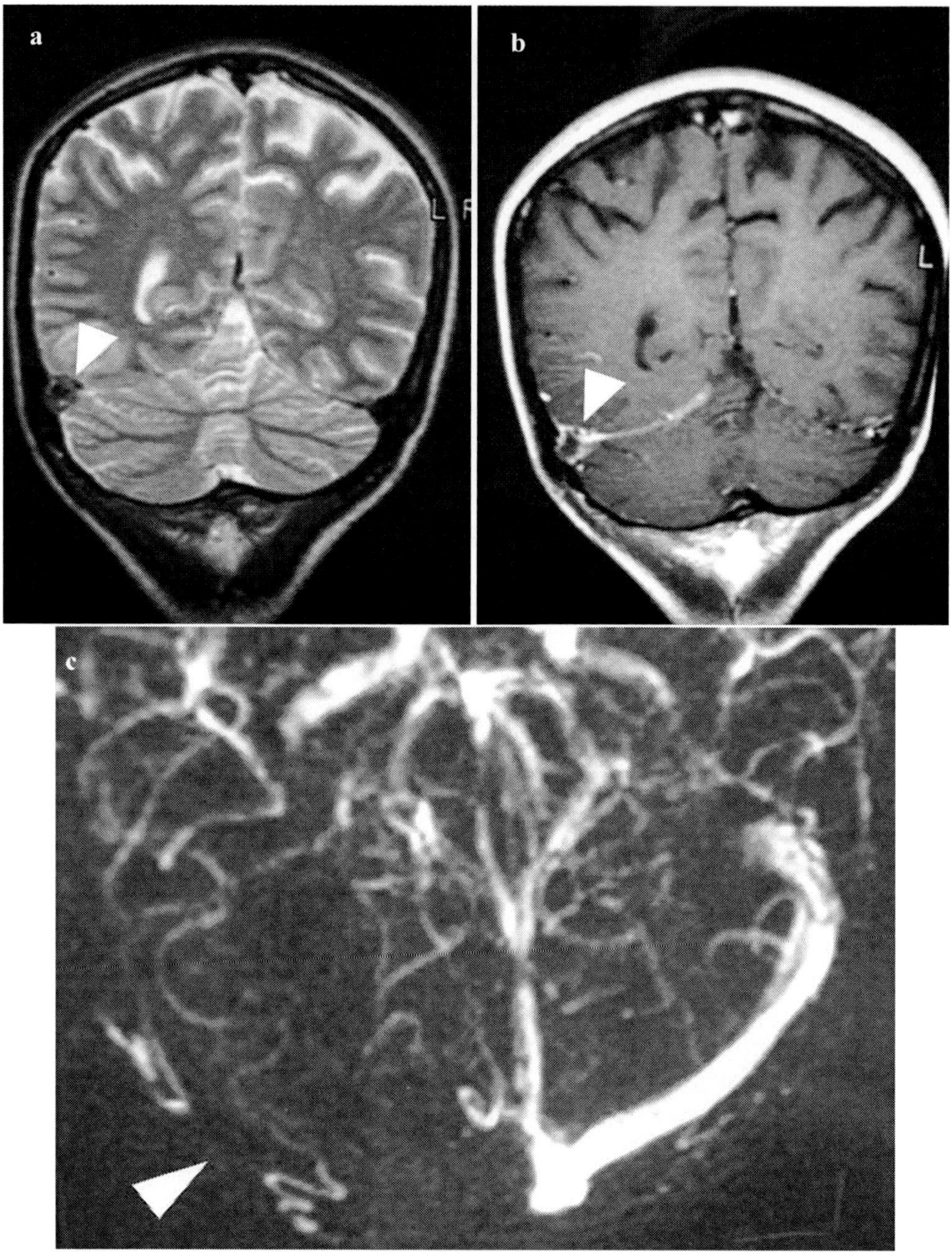


Figure 2. MRI , contrast enhanced MRI and MRV show acute right transverse sinus thrombosis. a) T2-w coronal image b) T1-w post gadolinium coronal image and c) 3D PC axial slab of the transverse sinuses. The acute thrombus (deoxyhaemoglobin) is seen as low T2 (arrowhead in a). There is an MRI equivalent of the "delta sign" (arrowhead in b) together with enhancement over the tentorium secondary to collateral flow and venous engorgement. The right transverse sinus is absent on the MRV study.

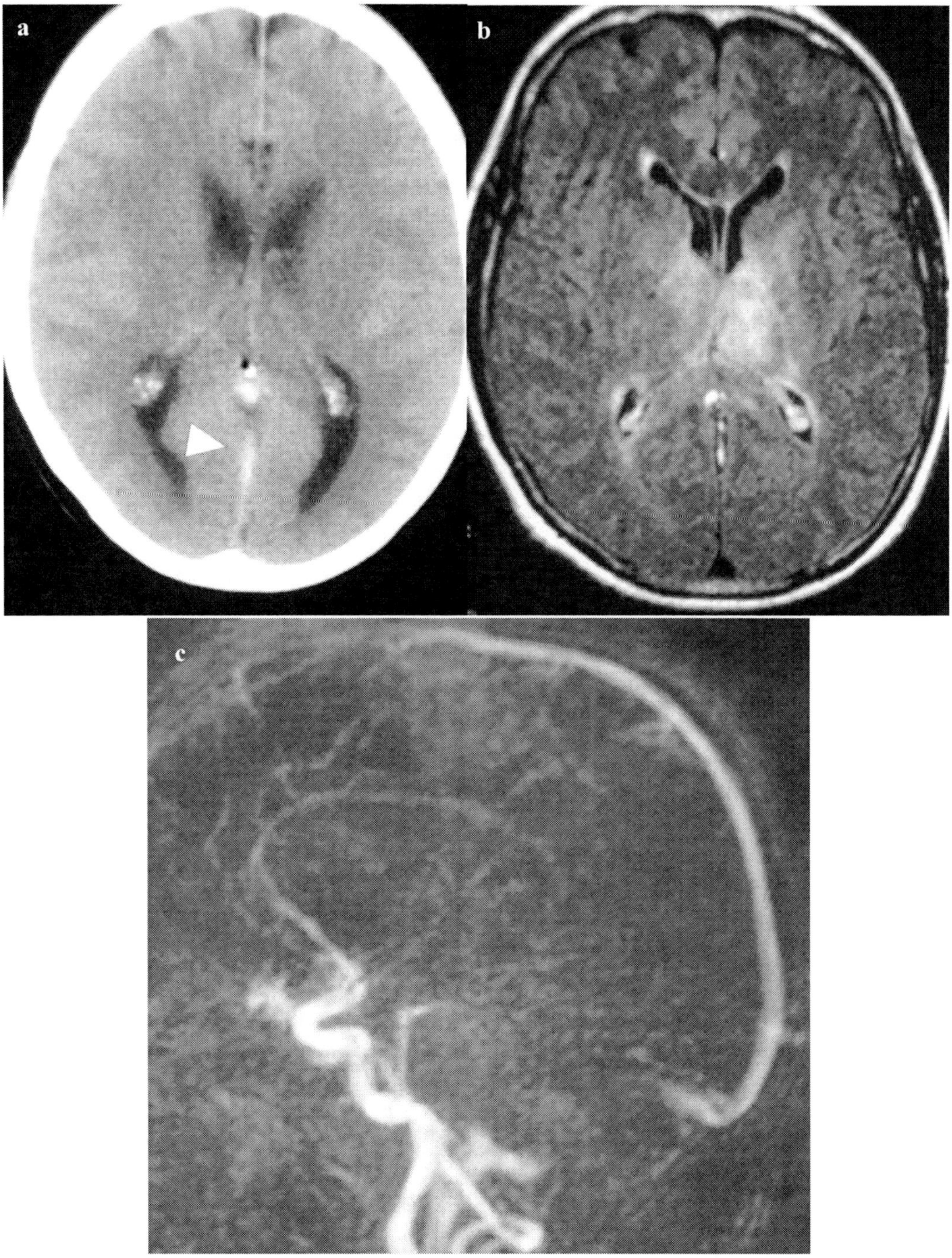


Figure 3. CT, MRI and MRV of deep venous sinus thrombosis. a) axial CT image b) axial FLAIR image and c) 3D PC sagittal slab. There is increased density of the straight sinus and vein of Galen on the CT image (arrowhead in a). The parenchymal changes involve the deep grey matter, capsular white matter and callosal splenium and is best shown on the FLAIR image (b). The MRV confirms absence of flow within the deep venous system.

CE 3D GRE MRI and CE MRV provide better demonstration of intraluminal filling defects [105,125] due to the marked T1 shortening of the venous blood resulting from the bolus passage of gadolinium. CVT is shown as filling defects on the projectional images with evidence of increased collateral drainage [125].

Spin echo and 3D GRE contrast enhanced MRI suffer from the same drawbacks as the other forms of luminal imaging, so it is poorly sensitive to cases of chronic enhancing thrombus and normal intrasinus filling defects lead to diagnostic confusion. On routine spin echo imaging, the administration of contrast medium often accentuates the overlap in signal intensities demonstrated by normal sinus and CVT [123]. CE MRA is unable to overcome the difficulties in detecting chronic thrombus since the uptake of contrast may be instant and undergoes a similar degree of T1 shortening to the lumen [90]. Normal anatomical structures and other intravascular pathology have also been reported to mimick sinus thrombosis [101]. A further disadvantage of CE MRV is that meningeal enhancement may obscure the superficial veins on MIPs and it must be ensured that the CE MRV acquisition is timed for peak passage of the contrast bolus to prevent misinterpretation resulting from inadequate vascular enhancement.

Recent clinical studies have evaluated CE 3D GRE techniques and dynamic CE MRV in terms of demonstrating normal cerebral venous structures and MRV. Liang et al [123] described the use of contrast enhanced magnetization prepared rapid acquisition gradient echo sequences [MP-RAGE] and compared it with 2D TOF MRA and digital subtraction angiography. Blinded receiver operating characteristic [ROC] analysis demonstrated that depiction of normal venous anatomy was better than 2D TOF MRA and comparable to or even superior to DSA. Another group [207] applied a contrast enhanced, interpolated 3D GRE sequence [VIBE] to imaging the cerebral venous system and compared it with 2D TOF MRV. The VIBE technique was superior to TOF MRV in visualizing the cerebral veins and using a subtraction technique further aided small vein conspicuity.

Early assessment of dynamic CE MRV has been similarly positive. Kirchof et al [105] studied 20 patients comparing contrast enhanced 3D radiofrequency spoiled FLASH [fast low angle shot] MRV with TOF and PC MRV. They found that the quality of visualization of the cortical veins and their first order branches was best with 3D FLASH MRA, followed by TOF and then PC MRV. The Trolard and Labbe veins were visualized equally well with FLASH and TOF sequences. PC MRV was inferior to FLASH and TOF MRV for septal, internal cerebral, and Rosenthal basal vein visualization. The thalamostriate, Vein of Galen, superior sagittal and transverse sinuses were seen equally well on all sequences. Lovblad et al [125] compared 3D contrast enhanced MRV with TOF MRV imaging in 32 normal and 10 CVT. The technique reliably detected all cases of CVT and demonstrated more detailed information by showing partially obstructed sinuses and by showing better the presence of cortical collateral venous drainage. The CE MRV technique provided more extensive small vein detail and provided a better demonstration of intraluminal defects, despite a slightly lower resolution. Finally, Farb et al studied patients with the ATECO technique and found it to be superior to TOF MRV in visualising venous structures [61].

*B) Conventional Angiography*

The venous phase of the conventional angiogram has traditionally been perceived to be the gold standard for demonstrating the cerebral venous system. It is possible to assess both luminal filling and flow dynamics and provides good demonstration of collateral flow. It superseded direct sinus venography which was a technique with a high risk of complications such as air embolism [68, 157, 158]. The venous anatomy is optimally demonstrated by greater volumes of contrast medium, and oblique positioning. Cross compression is useful to avoid mixing phenomena of opacified and unopacified blood which may be confused with CVT. The development of reliable non invasive methods for the demonstration of the venous system has made conventional angiography generally obsolete unless it is performed at the time of radiological intervention.

The essential finding of CVT on conventional angiography is a lack of contrast filling in the dural sinuses or cortical veins. Venous emptying is seen to be delayed and limited to collateral routes with resulting arterial stasis [158]. Dilated tortuous collateral veins develop following the onset of chronic venous hypertension which is referred to as a "pseudophlebitic pattern" [208]. Some authors report that it may still be necessary to rely on conventional angiography to diagnose rare cases of isolated cortical vein thrombosis without venous sinus occlusion when non invasive investigations are inconclusive [56,69]. It should be appreciated that non demonstration of portions of the venous system such as the cavernous sinus is frequent on a technically adequate angiogram [146].

A conventional angiogram is often considered as the standard of reference however the status of conventional angiography as a gold standard has been challenged by the development of high resolution multiplanar imaging of the vessel lumen [123]. It is now appreciated that partial recanalisation of the sinus can result in a normal projectional image and the number of preselected projections is usually limited. More recently, 3D rotational venography has been used to produce volume rendered images and a 3D data set which has the potential to overcome these disadvantages [142]. Conventional angiography is time consuming, invasive, expensive and has a 1.2% risk of stroke [1].

## Luminal Imaging in Intracranial Arterial Imaging

CE MRA and CT angiography have been successfully applied to assessment of the extracranial arterial circulation. There is theoretical advantage in employing such methods to the intracranial arteries for enhancing the visibility of small vessels, however this has proved less successful due to the close juxtaposition and overlap with small veins which interferes with visualization [68,176].

### A) Imaging of Venous Blood Flow

Whilst CVT may be detected by demonstration of filling defects following enhancement of the venous lumen, it may also be implied by the interruption of blood flow within the venous system. This principle has been widely applied in the clinical setting with the use of two dimensional time-of-flight [2D TOF] and three dimensional phase contrast [3D PC] techniques which are sensitive to slow flow. The choice of MRV technique may be machine limited. The loss of venous signal void on spin echo MRI is also an indicator of flow disturbance, however this replaced by directly visualized thrombus which will be discussed later in this chapter. Developments in ultrasound techniques have also allowed investigators to explore its utility in the diagnosis of venous sinus flow disturbance.

### *a) In flow MRV studies*

TOF MRV is based on the principle of flow related enhancement by demonstrating differences between the magnetization of inflowing spins and those of stationary tissues [83,100]. Stationary tissue is exposed to repeated radiofrequency pulses and thus becomes saturated, returning dark or intermediate signal, whereas inflowing blood in a plane perpendicular to that of the acquisition retains higher magnetization strength and hence returns higher signal. 2D TOF is performed by acquiring 1-2 mm thick sections through the entire intracranial venous system. A presaturation pulse is placed inferiorly in order to suppress arterial signal. A scan plane is chosen perpendicular to the direction of flow in order to avoid in plane saturation effects. Transverse sequences demonstrate poor visibility of the transverse sinuses and sagittal sequences reduce the visibility of the SSS [124]. A protocol acquiring images in three orientations would be too time consuming. Hence the coronal plane is most frequently used [124,133], although an oblique acquisition both reduces in plane saturation and allows head coverage with fewer sections [122].Spin saturation is also prevented by not making the repetition time too short [124] and using a low flip angle. Spin phase dipersion may be limited by decreasing the voxel size and shortening the echo times. Magnetisation transfer saturation is used to decrease the signal intensity of the background tissue. 3D TOF techniques are thought inferior in relation to the assessment of the cerebral venous system. Although 3D TOF benefits from increased spatial resolution and decreased intravoxel phase dispersion [122], there is more susceptibility to spin saturation because the effects are more likely in a selected volume compared with a single section and this is problematic with the slow venous flow [50,124,151]. 2D TOF MRV is sensitive to the order of 3-4 cm/s [133].

PC MRV uses velocity induced phase shifts to depict blood flow [83,192]. Flowing spins which move through the magnetic field will undergo phase shifts which depend on the velocity of flow, amplitude of the bipolar gradients and the time between the gradient lobes. PC MRV employs a gradient echo sequence with bipolar gradients along one or more axes and a velocity encoding [VENC] variable that adjusts the bipolar gradient to produce a phase shift of $180^0$ [105,124,192]. Low velocity encoding gradients of 20-30 cm/s should be collected, however these may be lowered to increase flow sensitivity if vessel patency cannot be confirmed. A reference data set without flow encoding is acquired simultaneously with data sets in which transverse, coronal and sagittal bipolar gradients are applied. Thus the imaging is sensitive to flow in all directions, which is useful in relation to the complex geometry of the intracranial venous system, and the imaging plane does not influence the visibility of the intracranial venous system [124]. 3D PC MRV acquisition times are generally longer than those of TOF MRV so they are more prone to motion artifact and this may be particularly relevant in the acutely unwell patient. MIPs of a sagittal slab covering the course of the SSS and straight sinus together with an axial slab incorporating the transverse and sigmoid sinuses may be employed for a complete evaluation of the venous sinuses. A single oblique 130 mm parasagittal slab has also been employed [2]. 2D PC MRV is generally unsuitable for applications in the venous circulation since there is marked intravascular signal loss due to intravoxel dephasing with the larger voxel size [124].

One further group has evaluated the clinical applicability of time resolved CE MRA to the demonstration of CVT. A 2D thick slice contrast enhanced subtraction MRA technique with subsecond temporal resolution was employed [159].

Using in flow MRV sequences, venous flow gives rise to high signal intensity and the absence of flow is indicated by reduced signal intensity in sinuses that do not appear hypoplastic or aplastic on individual source images/partitions. Thus CVT may be represented by a filling defect within or an amputation of the venous structure (figure 2, figure 4). Indirect signs of CVT such as increased signal in collateral veins may be recognized [203].

Artifacts may lead to both false positive and false negative interpretations for CVT on TOF MRV. Reduced signal intensity on TOF MRV can occur despite the integrity of flow, due to phenomena such as spin saturation and intravoxel phase dispersion [151]. Spin saturation results from spins which have not recovered from the previous radiofrequency pulse usually due to in plane flow of the venous blood. These effects have been described by some authors in the sphenoparietal and transverse sinuses [124] and by others in the posterior SSS [122] when using coronal acquisitions. Saturation effects are more pronounced in patients less than 25 months old [163]. Intravoxel spin phase dispersion occurs because of the wide spectrum of flow velocities within a voxel, the higher orders of motion, and the inhomogeneity of the magnetic field. Non uniform flow may be responsible for persistent phase dispersion and a resulting flow gap. This has been most frequently described in the transverse and sigmoid sinuses [15] and is probably secondary to of relative narrowing which should not be misconstrued as representing CVT. Artefactual signal drop out may also occur secondary to the inferior saturation band which is frequently used to saturate arterial flow. The more usual scenario is for the spins from cephalad flowing blood within the anterior SSS to become saturated; however there have been cases of arteriovenous shunting through a fistula to result in presaturated blood within the transverse sinus [92,154]. A persistent problem with TOF MRV for the detection of thrombus is the unsuppressed increased signal returned by subacute [methaemoglobin] intraluminal thrombus [154,212]. Other substances which shorten the T1-w values such as fat or gadolinium may also mimic flow on MIP images. Careful windowing of the source images or preferably review of T1-w images should overcome this pitfall.

PC techniques are not degraded by in plane saturation effects or the presence of stationary paramagnetic material such as subacute thrombus. They are however prone to artifactual signal drop out from intravoxel dephasing secondary to gradient imperfections and eddy currents [192] which are particularly prevalent in the sigmoid sinuses and jugular bulbs. Also, PC MRV only has the capability for a limited range of velocities and the optimal VENC is generally difficult to predict.

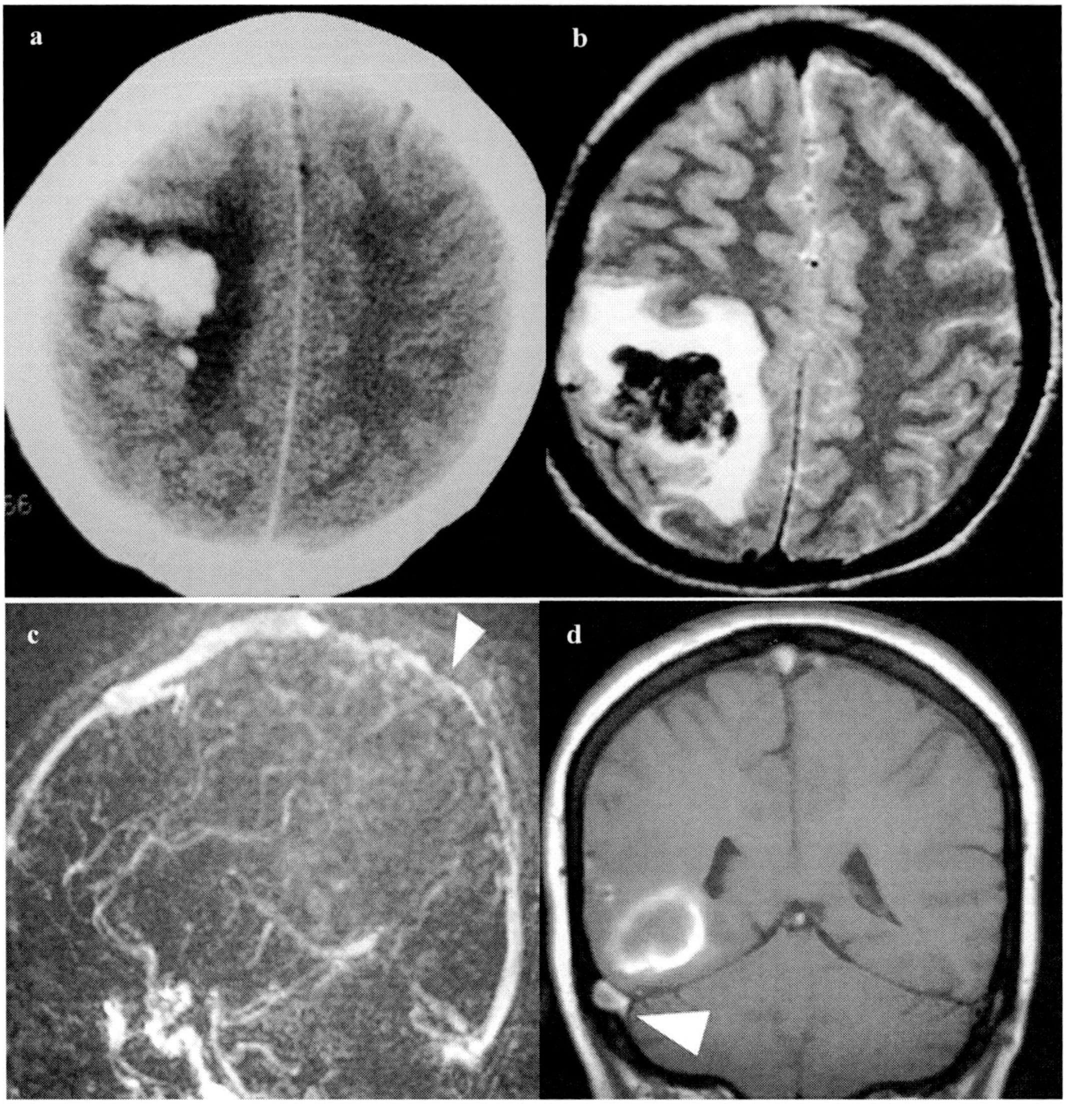


Figure 4. CT, MRI and MRV of haematomas secondary to CVT. a)axial CT image b) T2-w axial image, c) 3D PC sagittal slab in a patient with a right parietal haematoma secondary to posterior SSS thrombosis. The acute haemorrhage is of high CT density and low T2-w signal secondary to deoxyhaemoglobin. The MRI shows reduction of flow (arrowhead in c) within the posterior SSS. d) coronal T1-w image in a different patient demonstrates temporal haematoma secondary to right transverse sinus thrombosis. In this subacute haematoma there is evidence of increased T1-w signal representing methaemoglobin at the periphery which is mirrored by the evolution of the blood degradation products within the right transverse sinus thrombosis (arrowhead in d).

In particular, where there are developmental asymmetries in the transverse sinuses, there may be a wide range of velocities, leading to aliasing and signal drop out. PC techniques demonstrate such high contrast that it is difficult to visualize the anatomy of the sinus itself. Whereas the acutely thrombosed venous sinus [170] may be seen as an expanded structure on CTV, CE MRV, MRI or source images from a TOF MRV, the hypoplastic segment of transverse may be difficult to differentiate from an occluded sinus using PC MRV alone.

The breathing state has recently been highlighted as a pitfall in the interpretation of MRV flow studies [109,136]. Mehta et al [136] reported that deep inspiratory breath holding and deep expiratory breath holding resulted in a decrease in sinus blood flow and more recently Kudo et al [109] found that the breath holding manoeuvre affected the signal intensity of the sigmoid sinuses on MR venograms in about two thirds of subjects both increasing or decreasing signal intensity in different individuals. It was concluded that defects in venous sinuses on phase contrast imaging may be reversed by breath holding and that this maneoeuvre may be employed to reduce false positive interpretations in patients suspected of having CVT. Since drainage is principally passive, a reduction in systemic blood pressure may also result in stasis or flow reversal.

It is important to correlate the MRV MIPs with individual source images and with the spin echo MRI images in order to avoid misinterpretations. For instance, collateral veins can sometimes be seen as a collection of ancillary veins adjacent to an occluded venous sinus which will also simulate intact sinus flow on MIP images. In addition, the use of MIPs algorithms introduces additional potential artifacts, with distortion due to background variation and loss of lower intensity features. Finally, it should be remembered that differing MR parameters significantly influence the depiction of flow and normative data should be obtained for each scanner [148,184].

TOF and PC MRV have been compared with each other and with other modalities, including CTV, CE MRV, MRI and conventional angiography, for their ability to demonstrate the venous system and CVT. The flow related MRV techniques do not perform as well as luminal imaging [CE MRV and CTV] in terms of visualising cortical and other small veins [61,105,113,125,149,207]. An average of 4.3 cortical veins are reported to be visualized draining into each side of the SSS on TOF MRA [133]. Although they adequately demonstrate the dural sinus and major veins, there are relative reductions in caliber relative to luminal imaging at sites of turbulence such as the torcula and they are less often seen in completion relative to the contrast enhanced techniques. The most recent reports of TOF and PC MRV in the detection of CVT [113,125,149] indicate wide variations in sensitivity, however 2/3 of the studies demonstrated detection of all cases of CVT. In terms of comparing TOF and PC techniques, Liauw et al [124] confirmed the superiority of 2D TOF MRV and 3D PC MRV over 3D TOF MRV and 2D PC MRV in visualising 28 different intracranial venous structures.

### *b) Doppler Ultrasound*

Transcranial Doppler sonography [TCD] has been an established method for the evaluation of the arterial cerebral circulation for more than a decade. Until recently its use for the assessment of the intracranial veins was limited because of the considerable anatomic and hemodynamic variabilities of the venous system. More recently due to technical advances it is now possible for real time visualization of the cerebral venous system with information on blood flow dynamics. Conventional transcranial Doppler ultrasound using 2 MHz transducers have been used via a posterior temporal window, to evaluate flow within the deep venous system in the setting of SSS thrombosis in order to detect increased velocities resulting from collateral flow [37,196]. Other investigators have aimed to sonographically assess the SSS [21] and transverse sinus [161] directly. An adequate acoustic window to the venous system is more readily available in neonates [191]. Both power Doppler [191] and the use of echo contrast agents provide better diagnostic information concerning blood flow [161,179,191]. These techniques are primarily investigational however there may be a role in the monitoring of collateral venous flow and one study has shown echo contrast enhanced transcranial Doppler to reliably exclude transverse sinus thrombosis [161]. There has been normative data collected on normal deep veins [37,161,179].

Doppler ultrasound indicators of CVT are disturbed venous haemodynamics and absence of flow in venous sinus segments. Increased peak systolic velocities, end diastolic velocities and mean blood flow velocities in the collateral deep veins have been documented in the setting of SSS thrombosis [37,196] as has a pathological side difference of flow velocities in the paired deep cerebral veins and a flow reversal in the basal veins [179]. Segmental occlusion of the major dural sinuses may occasionally be detected [21,161].

The sonographic assessment of the venous sinuses remains in its infancy, however investigators recognise significant pitfalls. Firstly, there is difficulty in distinguishing CVT from congenitally hypoplastic sinuses since sonographic visualisation of the thrombus is impossible and there may be difficulty in distinguishing sinus blood flow from adjacent pathology such as a dural fistula [161]. It has not been possible to interrogate the anterior and mid portions of the SSS directly and it is difficult to obtain an adequate insonation angle to view the entire transverse sinus [161]. Its application is therefore limited by its dependence on indirect signs such as increased velocity in collateral veins.

# Flow Imaging in Intracranial Arterial Imaging

Imaging of the intracranial arteries presents differing challenges to that of the venous system. The arteries are generally smaller and thus benefit from the superior resolution of 3D techniques. They have a wider velocity profile, sharper bends and demonstrate rapid flow with focal acceleration and deceleration leading to greater phase dispersion which is less well tolerated by PC techniques. However spin saturation is less problematic due to the rapid flow. Hence, unlike the venous system, arterial system is best demonstrated with 3D TOF techniques.

Insonation of the basal cerebral arteries is easier to achieve than is the case with the venous sinuses, so it is possible to directly visualize the vascular pathology in the majority of patients, rather than depending on indirect signs [91].

## Imaging of Thrombus within the Venous Lumen

Perhaps the most direct imaging evidence of CVT is provided by direct visualization of the thrombus within the venous lumen. Imaging features of thrombus may be identified on both CT and MRI.

### A) Computed Tomography

Plain intracranial CT is readily available and since patients with CVT, frequently present with non specific neurological findings, it is likely to be the initial investigation performed in order to exclude differential diagnoses. It has a short scanning time and is readily able to detect acute haemorrhage. Although conventional thick section CT has been thought to be of limited diagnostic accuracy, it is important to recognize the imaging features of CVT in order to direct appropriate confirmatory imaging. In fact, with multislice helical CT techniques, there is high resolution capability in the z axis with isotropic voxels and high quality multiplanar reformats which demonstrate these findings with greater diagnostic accuracy.

Acute thrombus within the dural sinus or cortical veins may be seen as areas of high attenuation (figure 3). This is owing to the high protein concentration of haemoglobin and retraction of the clot. The dense triangle sign is used to describe the appearance within the cross section of the posterior SSS and torcula and the cord sign refers to the elongated increased density of a thrombosed cortical vein [32, 33, 72, 117, 156, 184]. It may be useful to measure the Houndsfield units in order to differentiate thrombus [60-80 Houndsfield units] from flowing blood in questionable cases. Selective venous hyperattenuation rather than generalized vascular hyperdensity is necessary in order to attribute the features to CVT.

The dense triangle sign was reported to be present in 20-55% of cases in older studies of thick section CT [184,202]. In these cases, the detection of the dense triangle sign is hindered by partial volume effects if the sinus was not perpendicular to the imaging plane [154,184] and therefore it was usually only detected in the posterior SSS. Thin collimation multislice CT frequently demonstrates these signs although the sensitivity is not well defined since the conspicuity will change with the age of the thrombus. It should be remembered that hyperattenuation of the venous structures may be secondary to polycythaemia [77] and they may also appear of relative high density in children or patients with cerebral oedema [107,154,202] due to the relative low density of the adjacent brain. The dense triangle sign is occasionally mimicked by a thick dural wall [202]. Confirmatory imaging studies should be suggested if there is any plain CT suspicion of CVT either due to these signs of luminal thrombus or the presence of suggestive parenchymal changes.

### B) Magnetic Resonance Imaging

Spin echo MRI is both able to detect flowing venous blood and to directly visualize intraluminal thrombus. At least two orthogonal imaging planes should be used in order to distinguish slow flow, in which the signal changes with orientation of data acquisition, from thrombus, there is constant abnormal signal returned [89,182]. A combination of axial and coronal sections permits an exploration which is perpendicular to most of the venous sinuses. High resolution "black blood" imaging is possible and provides an effective means of detecting small veins [159]. T2-w images with a sufficiently long echo time [40-60 ms] [56] should be employed and gradient moment nulling turned off to further ensure that hypointense signal is returned by the flowing blood. In addition T2*-w sequences maybe useful in detecting thrombus within the cortical veins [36].

Spin echo MRI can provide diagnostic criteria for CVT by demonstrating the replacement of flow voids with the signal of intraluminal thrombus [182, 214].

The MR signal intensity of venous thrombus is affected by both the degree of residual flow and the age of the thrombus [56, 127, 182]. A thorough knowledge of the evolving signal change of thrombus is required to avoid diagnostic confusion and to date thrombus. The MRI signal of thrombus changes with the time according to the biochemical status of the haemoglobin (table 3). In the acute stage of venous thrombosis [up to 5 days], the haemoglobin moiety is deoxyhaemoglobin and this is of intermediate T1-w and low T2-w signal (figure 2, figure 5). In the subacute phase [between 5 and 30 days] [56], there is conversion of the moiety to methaemoglobin such that the thrombus is seen as both T1-w and T2-w hyperintensity. The conversion to methaemoglobin first occurs at the periphery, and as with an intracerebral haematoma, subsequently progresses centrally. Some authors have also documented another phase of thrombotic occlusion in which there is isointense T1-w and hyperintense T2-w signal returned [56]. In the later stages, the signal returned by the venous sinus is increasingly dependent on the degree of recanalisation. Abnormal signal may persist for months or years [56,131]. A similar time course for signal changes has been described in isolated cortical vein thrombosis [53]. In the case of septic dural sinus thrombosis there may be inflammatory debris within the venous sinus which alters the typical signal characteristics of thrombus [75].

There are several pitfalls in relying on MR images alone. In view of this, the MRI appearances should be correlated with a corresponding MRV study. In the assessment of acute intraluminal thrombus there is potential for confusion of hypointense T2-w signal due to deoxyhaemoglobin with that of the normal venous sinus flow void. Variable windowing of the MR images helps to avoid this problem. Variable signal change within slow flowing blood of the venous sinus may confuse the interpretation. The observer must become expert in interpreting the signal obtained with their particular scanner and scanning parameters [56,184].

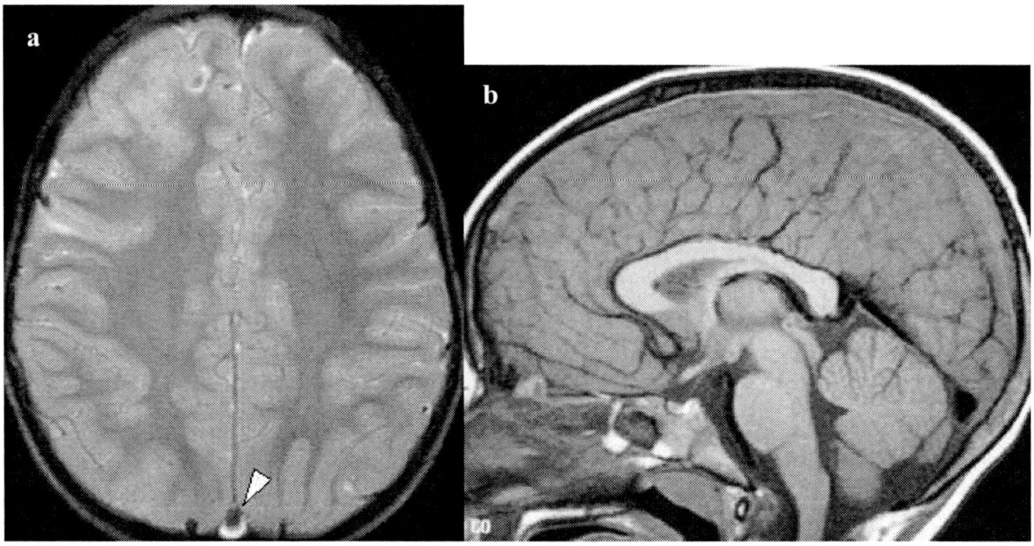


Figure 5. Continued on next page.

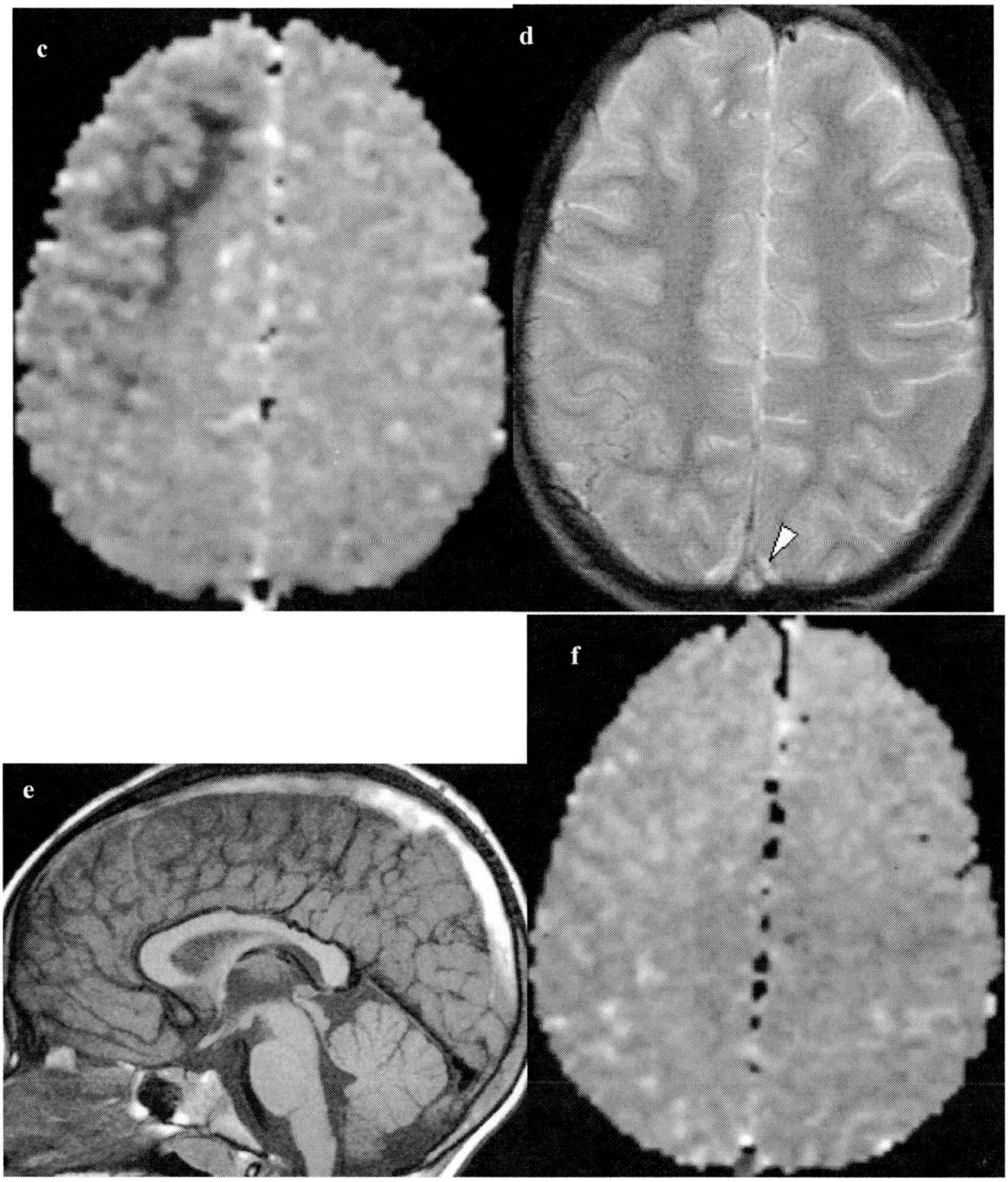


Figure 5. MRI with ADC maps in SSS thrombosis and reversible restricted diffusion. a)axial T2-w image b) T1-w sagittal image c) axial ADC map at clinical presentation and d) T2-w image e) T1-w sagittal image f) axial ADC map 12 days later. At presentation there is evidence of acute SSS thrombosis (intermediate T1-w signal and low T2-w signal (arrowhead in a) is seen in the SSS) with low signal seen on the ADC map representing restricted diffusion. 12 days later the SSS thrombus has evolved (increased T1-w signal and increased T2-w signal (arrowhead in d)). There is no evidence of residual parenchymal damage and the ADC changes have reversed.

**Table 3. MRI signal of the thrombosed venous sinus [56, 113, 127, 182]**

| | Normal sinus (with acquisition plane perpendicular to the venous sinus) | Acute thrombus (up to 5 days) | Subacute thrombus (5-30 days) | Late appearances (>30 days) |
|---|---|---|---|---|
| T1-weighting | Variable (low to high) | Intermediate | High | Variable, depending on recanalisation |
| T2-weighting | Signal void | Low | High | Variable, depending on recanalisation |

Flow related or paradoxical enhancement with blood flow perpendicular to the plane of acquisition and even echo rephasing of the blood flow with blood flow parallel to the plane of acquisition may both increase the intravascular signal and thus mimic the appearance of intraluminal methaemoglobin [56, 113, 203]. Increased T2-w high signal is noted within relatively hypoplastic transverse sinuses. Vascular signal induced by vessel pulsation and complex flow is frequently seen at the sigmoid sinus and jugular bulb. There are other indicators of vascular patency when increased intraluminal signal is returned. Higher signal on flow compensated sequences [49], loss of signal after the application of a presaturation band, propagation of flow artifact in the phase encoding direction, variation of signal with orthogonal scan planes and enhancement with gadolinium, may all be used to reflect the presence of venous blood flow and thus the absence of thrombus.

There are several studies comparing MRI with other modalities in its ability to detect CVT. Lafitte at al [113] used a 0.5 Tesla MR system to study 20 patients with CVT documented by conventional angiography. T1-w sagittal images and T2-w axial images were performed and a small number of the patients also underwent coronal T1-w imaging and gadolinium enhancement. The mean time from onset of symptoms was 7 days. MRI alone provided the diagnosis in 90 % [18/20] patients and CVT was evident on MRV in the remaining 2/20 patients. Dormont et al [56] studied 53 patients with CVT, of whom 43/53 had undergone confirmatory angiography, on either a 0.5, 1T or 1.5 T systems. A combination of T2-w, T1-w gradient echo and T2-w images in differing planes were employed. The sensitivity of MRI for CVT was reported as 91% with most of the false negative results being due to isolated cortical vein thromboses [56].

## Imaging of Intracranial Arterial Thrombus

Intracranial thrombotic occlusion is less frequently present in the setting of arterial ischaemia than is the case with venous ischaemia. It is also less easy to visualize due to the small vessel calibre. Hence assessment of arterial thrombus with CT in the form of the "hyperdense middle cerebral artery sign" or "the sylvian fissure dot sign" is relatively specific but poorly sensitive [19].

## Imaging of Parenchymal Change

The pathophysiology of parencymal changes secondary to CVT remains controversial however a spectrum of changes are recognized, including localized or generalized brain swelling, venous oedema, venous infarction and haemorrhage [39,43,56,153,203,213]. The parenchyma may however be normal [214]. MRI is more sensitive than CT to the detection and characterisation of the parenchymal abnormalities and they are reported in 40-70% of patients with CVT [39, 56, 203].

### *a) Oedema*

Oedema is seen as a diffuse low attenuation lesion on CT and increased T2-w or FLAIR signal on MRI. The parenchymal signal change is typically subcortical [98] but it may involve the overlying cortex [43]. Changes may be subtle in the early stages however severe parenchymal damage has been associated with gadolinium enhancement and a tumour like appearance [120,154]. The oedema observed with CVT corresponds to vasogenic oedema, cytotoxic oedema or both. Cytotoxic oedema occurs after energy failure of the cell with depolarization of the cell membrane [loss of Na+/K+ pump activity] and influx of ions and water into the cell, which quickly leads to irreversibly damaged brain tissue. In contrast vasogenic oedema develops with disruption of the blood-brain barrier [capillary tight junctions] and is not primarily associated with cellular damage [168]. Traditional models hold that the increased retrograde venous pressure results in breakdown of the blood brain barrier with leakage of fluid which results in vasogenic oedema [67,195]. Yuh et al [214] argued that the oedema was principally interstitial in origin. He postulated that venous obstruction disturbed the normal physiologic shift of bulk interstitial fluid from the capillary bed towards the ventricle. Initially when venous drainage was blocked the compliant venous system dilated and a slight increase in transudate was handled by drainage into the ventricle without significant oedema developing. However as venous pressure and transudate volume increased, the transependymal drainage route became saturated. In addition CSF absorption was decreased because of increased venous pressure. This resulted in interstitial oedema and mild hydrocephalus. These were felt to be reversible changes if venous drainage was restored and venous pressure reduced and they did not necessarily result in infarction. They noted that abnormal T2-weighted signal change and brain swelling and that T2 signal change could persist up to two years.

Tsai et al [190] carried out a retrospective review of 29 patients with angiographically proven acute dural sinus thrombosis, of which 11 had venous sinus pressure measurements. They correlated parenchymal brain changes, venous sinus pressure measurements and outcome in these patients. They were able to identify five distinct stages of brain parenchymal changes: stage 1, no parenchymal change, stage 2, swelling with mass effect but no signal change, stage 3, signal change with mild oedema, stage 4, severe oedema with or without haemorrhage, stage 5, massive oedema with or without haemorrhage. They noted that dural sinus pressures seemed to increase in 10-15mm Hg increments per stage and that this correlated with brain parenchymal changes on imaging studies. It was recognized that when the venous occlusion was successfully treated with thrombolytics, the abnormal signal, and clinical symptoms may rapidly resolve. They therefore also postulated that the parenchymal changes probably reflected interstitial oedema rather than the cytotoxic oedema, although there were noted to be irreversible changes with the higher stages.

However an alternative origin to the oedematous changes has been proposed, wherein increased retrograde venous pressure and decreased cerebral blood flow [94] and decreased cerebral perfusion pressure [164] result in tissue damage. There is data from dynamic contrast enhanced perfusion imaging in patients with CVT which shows changes in perfusion.. Keller at al documented a patient with deep venous cerebral thrombosis in whom there was increased cerebral blood flow and prolongation of the time to peak in an area of T2-w hyperintensity [99]. Manzione et al [129] demonstrated widespread prolongation in mean transit time in another patient with CVT. No reduction in cerebral blood flow has yet been confirmed in CVT patients, however animal studies have revealed that the reduction in cerebral blood flow associated with CVT is sufficient to cause cytotoxic oedema and tissue infarction [112,195]. In fact Ungersbock [195] in a rat model of CVT noted that experimentally induced superior sagittal sinus thrombosis only caused parenchymal damage in concurrence with reduced blood flow values. Certainly irreversible parenchymal changes resulting from CVT are well recognized and occur in approximately 50% of cases and portends to a poor outcome [43, 190].

Conventional MRI is unable to distinguish vasogenic from cytotoxic oedema, however diffusion imaging has recently provided further insight into the relative contributions of vasogenic and cytotoxic oedema to the initial parenchymal changes of CVT [45, 58, 65, 99, 129, 140, 167, 205, 211]. Diffusion imaging is based on the random motion of diffusion of water molecules [116] and it provides apparent diffusion coefficients [ADCs] [168,173]. Experimental results in ischaemia suggest that decreased ADC values reflect cytotoxic oedema and that increased ADC values correspond to vasogenic oedema [86, 111].

Some studies have shown that the parenchymal lesions demonstrate predominantly decreased ADC values [45, 5, 211] as a result of vasogenic oedema. Yoshikawa et al [211] retrospectively reviewed 16 patients with CVT whom had undergone diffusion imaging. Abnormal foci of T2-w signal were present in 10/16 patients and ADC values were assessed in these regions. ADC was predominantly increased in 9/10 patients of which three patients showed heterogeneous changes and ADC was normal in 1 patient. Other investigators have demonstrated increased or heterogeneous ADC values within these lesions [58, 65, 129, 140, 205]. Ducreux et al [58] carried out a retrospective review of nine patients with CVT and diffusion weighted imaging 3 hours to 4 days post onset of acute neurological deficit to determine the initial diffusion weighted abnormalities in these patients and found that ADC values were both increased and decreased. Forbes et al [65] assessed diffusion weighted imaging in 12 patients with acute CVT confirmed by MR venography. They found that restricted water diffusion suggesting cytotoxic oedema was found in the majority of subjects with acute CVT. Mullins et al [140] evaluated diffusion weighted images and ADC maps for increased, decreased or unchanged signal intensity MR images in 13 patients with CVT complicated by intraparenchymal abnormality on T2-w images. They discovered three lesion types: lesions with elevated ADC that resolved [vasogenic oedema]; lesions with decreased ADC that persisted [cytotoxic oedema] in patients without seizure activity; and lesions with decreased ADC that resolved [cytotoxic oedema] in patients with seizure activity.

The progress of these ADC values has also been studied. Those areas of increased ADC presumed to represent vasogenic oedema have been consistently shown to be reversible [58, 99, 140]. These are likely to represent areas of impaired but viable tissue which is shown to be free of sequelae on follow up MRI [58]. These regions may demonstrate increased regional cerebral blood volume on perfusion weighted MRI indicating extensive venous congestion without any perfusion deficit [99]. A decrease in ADC value has been previously assumed to represent a more severe pathology predisposing to subsequent infarction and haemorrhage [140,211].However reversal of these initially low ADC values and resolution of these parenchymal lesions has now been demonstrated in a number of CVT patients [129,140,167]. In experimental studies with animal models, lesions which showed partial normalistion of signal intensity changes with diffusion weighted imaging following thrombolysis, were demonstrated to show histopathological improvement [164]. Mullins et al [140] identified a group of patients with seizure activity who demonstrated resolution of cytotoxic oedema. The patients imaging findings were located appropriately for the venous thrombosis, seizure activity and symptoms. It was postulated that the decreased ADC in these patients may have resulted from seizure activity. One author [129] has suggested that quantitative assessment of ADC may be helpful in predicting the permanent neurological damage. He found that the area of less severe reduction in ADC never developed a corresponding area of anatomical abnormality and appeared to reverse completely after thrombolysis. Others have speculated that normalization of low ADC values may be due to increasing vasogenic oedema [60], however this does not explain the associated resolution of T2-w and FLAIR hyperintensity and excellent clinical recovery in these cases [140,167].

In interpreting these studies, it is important to consider two parameters which may hinder ADC measurement: the exact time point for brain damage and haemorrhagic transformation. The exact time of CVT in humans is often unknown as the course of disease in humans can proceed over days and weeks in a multistep process. Secondly ADC values may be calculated incorrectly in areas of haemorrhage due to signal loss induced by blood products on strongly susceptibility weighted MR sequences such as echo planar diffusion weighted imaging.

### *b) Haemorrhage*

Haemorrhage associated with CVT is seen as increased attenuation on CT. CT is currently the modality of choice in imaging acute intracranial haemorrhage although the diagnostic accuracy on contemporary CT scanners has not been investigated. It is dependent on time after onset, concentration of haemoglobin and size of haemorrhage. Haemorrhage is seen as low T2-w or low T2*-w imaging on MRI in the early stages and some studies have suggested the detection of acute haemorrhage rivals that of CT (figure 4) [150]. At later time points in haematoma evolution with the development of increased T1-w signal methaemoglobin, MRI is more specific and sensitive than CT (figure 4) [144].Micro haemorrhages are more reliably seen on gradient T2 weighted sequences than on CT.

Between 27-40% of symptomatic patients show CT evidence of haemorrhage [23, 58, 190, 214]. There may be a large subcortical haematoma or more typically small petechial haemorrhages. Yuh et al postulated that intraparenchymal haemorrhage results when venous pressure exceeds the integrity of the vascular wall [214]. Cortical vein thrombosis and dural sinus thrombosis have both been reported to present with subarachnoid haemorrhage

[41,181]. Deep vein thrombosis should always be considered as a cause of intraventricular haemorrhage in the neonate [162].

### c) Hydrocephalus

Communicating hydrocephalus secondary to elevated pressure in the dural sinuses is well recognized [24]. Bering and Salibi produced hydrocephalus in 74% of dogs by occluding cephalic venous drainage. They postulate that not only is CSF absorption reduced by elevated dural pressures, but that there is increased CSF production secondary to increased pulsation of the choroid plexus As described previously, Yuh et al attributred hydrocephalus to saturation of the transependymal drainage route and decreased cerebrospinal fluid absorption due to the raised venous pressure [214].

### d) Location of Parenchymal Changes and the Importance of Collateral Circulation

Due to the variability of venous drainage anatomy and collateral flow, the distribution of oedema or haemorrhage is not stereotypical. Despite this, unilateral or bilateral parenchymal change near the midline frontal, parietal or occipital regions should raise the possibility of SSS thrombosis (figure 4, figure 5), and changes in the posterior temporal lobe may result from thrombosis of the transverse sinus and associated vein of Labbe (figure 1, figure 2) [154, 203]. Bilateral or unilateral periventricular, striatal, thalamic or superior cerebellar abnormalities may occur secondary to deep vein CVT (figure 3) [114].

Tsai et al [190] noted that, whilst parenchymal changes were usually in close proximity to the occluded venous sinus, they were also found remote to the sinus. One patient presented with basal ganglia oedema secondary to superior sagittal sinus thrombosis and thrombosis of the deep cerebral veins, and another patient presented with supratentorial changes secondary to a posterior fossa dural sinus thrombosis [190]. This correlated with the findings of Bergui et al [23] who discovered that no significant correlation existed between the extent and site of thrombosis in dural sinuses and the extent and location of brain lesions in the 26 patients they studied. They postulate that this may be because the most relevant disturbances that arise from thrombosis are of 'critical veins', which were not well shown on neuroradiological investigations [such as cortical, bridging and medullary veins]. Bergui et al did demonstrate a correlation between the site of thrombosis and brain lesions when there was involvement of cortical or medullary veins. This is well recognized in experimental animal models [164, 167, 195] where thrombosis of the superior sagittal sinus is well tolerated, while infarcts develop if thrombosis involves the cortical veins. Similarly in neurosurgical practice it is recognized that occlusion of a single bridging vein may lead to a haemorrhagic infarct, whilst sinus occlusion of the ventral half of the superior sagittal sinus or transverse sinus may be well tolerated as collateral circulation compensates. The cortical veins and bridging veins are vital for the provision of collateral flow. It is possible to speculate that CVT evolves gradually with major symptoms occurring only if the thrombus expands from the sinus into bridging and cortical veins and occluding collateral venous outflow pathways. Slow SSS occlusion with better developed collateral veins in an experimental study with dogs was associated with less brain oedema, both radiologically and histopathologically, compared with more rapid SSS occlusion [194].

# Differences between Venous and Arterial Ischaemia and Infarction

Apart from the exclusion of stroke mimicks, imaging protocols in arterial infarction are aimed at early detection of the parenchymal changes including haemorrhage, and the determination of tissue viability. In the setting of venous ischaemia, it is the positive evidence of CVT rather than parenchymal changes which primarily influences management. There are also a number of key differences between parenchymal change due to CVT and that due to arterial ischaemia in terms of distribution, radiological appearance, pathogenesis and subsequent course (table 4).

CT appearances of parenchymal CVT changes have been noted to demonstrate more marked low density with earlier and more generalized brain swelling. Haemorrhage is more frequent in CVT infarction and is noted to spread from the centre to the periphery, whereas it is usually noted at the margins of an arterial infarct [16, 98]. Parenchymal changes of CVT will clearly not correspond to an arterial territory and are more often subcortical than cortical in distribution [98]. Multiple or bilateral haemorrhagic changes may result from arterial infarction or primary intracerebral haemorrhage, however it is more suggestive of CVT [16, 18]. CVT associated haematoma is reported to demonstrate an earlier onset of associated low density relative to primary intracerebral haemorrhage [16].Although the cerebellar hemispheres and brain stem may be damaged secondary to deep CVT, the combination of thalamic and posterior fossa changes is more suggestive of basilar artery thrombosis [114].

**Table 4. Imaging features of venous relative to arterial ischaemic parenchymal changes**

| |
|---|
| Variable location and not conforming to an arterial territory |
| Haemorrhage is more frequent |
| Subcortical rather than cortical location |
| More frequently multiple and bilateral |
| More associated brain swelling |
| May be associated ventriculomegaly |
| Evidence of free diffusion in early parenchymal changes |
| Areas of restricted diffusion are of lesser magnitude and are more frequently completely reversible |

Yuh et al carried out a retrospective review of 25 patients with venous sinus thrombosis to assess differences from patterns of arterial ischaemia on MRI. They observed three overall MR patterns: mass effect without T2 signal change, mass effect with abnormal T2 signal change and/or ventricular dilatation and intraparenchymal haematoma with surrounding oedema [214]. In venous occlusive disease there was recorded to be an absence of abnormal arterial or parenchymal enhancement, persistent brain swelling that was greater than the associated signal abnormality, abnormal venous enhancement, periventricular effusion with associated ventriculomegaly and a greater incidence of haematomas than seen with arterial infarction [46, 60, 213]. They postulated that these differences from arterial ischaemia reflect a different underlying pathophysiology, often with preservation of the integrity of the blood-brain barrier explaining the lack of vasogenic oedema and parenchymal enhancement in many cases.

The pathophysiology of haemorrhage in CVT is due to increased venous and capillary pressure whereas in arterial disease bleeding occurs during reperfusion of tissue damaged by ischaemia [201]. This explains why heparin treatment is effective in venous ischaemia, even in the context of haemorrhage as it shifts the equilibrium away from the prothrombotic state and is able to save large areas of brain tissue that are only reversibly damaged. Heparin therefore improves venous outflow, thereby reducing the risk of parenchymal haemorrhage, in contrast with arterial thrombotic disease where it can increase the risk [201].There is therefore less emphasis on the detection of minor haemorrhage in CVT imaging protocols relative to those used for imaging arterial infarcts where major symptomatic haemorrhage may be precipitated by therapies.

The initial ADC changes in acute venous ischaemia, together with their temporal evolution and significance, differ from those of arterial ischemia. In the setting of arterial stroke cytotoxic oedema typically predominates due to energy failure and loss of sodium/potassium pump activity so the finding of restricted diffusion has proved a useful diagnostic approach [177]. However in both clinical and animal studies, there is more evidence of free diffusion resulting from vasogenic oedema in early CVT [66, 99, 164, 211]. These appearances are less specific so diffusion imaging of less diagnostic utility in venous ischaemia and infarction.

When areas of low ADC are present, their prognostic significance appears different to those due to arterial ischemia. Diffusion abnormality that appears during acute arterial insufficiency is virtually always associated with permanent parenchymal injury [129]. In animal models of arterial infarction, the extent of ADC reduction is usually although not always predictive of subsequent tissue damage [76,139]. Whereas it is rare for diffusion abnormalities to reverse in clinical studies of arterial ischaemia [108], the CVT lesions with restricted diffusion are amenable to complete recovery if successfully treated (figure 5).

It is postulated that these differences are due to discrepancies in pathogenesis. The initial event in venous ischaemia is the increase in venous pressure which leads to disruption of the blood brain barrier and vasogenivc oedema. These lesions are completely reversible if there is successful recanalisation of the CVT [99]. Unlike arterial stroke, the relief of this venous obstruction may result in clinical benefit even if it is delayed. If there is continued venous occlusion, hypoperfusion develops [123]. In severe blood flow reduction in arterial thrombosis, the tissue is rapidly and irreversibly damaged, resulting in ischaemic cell necrosis. Cerebral blood flow of 6 ml or less per 100g per minute has been shown on xenon CT studies of human arterial stroke to lead to irreversibly infarcted tissue [97]. In contradistinction to arterial ischaemia, it is unlikely that the cerebral blood flow is reduced to this degree, particularly if some collateral drainage is possible [58, 66]. In these flow conditions the swollen cells may result in areas of restricted diffusion but are not irreversibly damaged and therefore have the potential for recovery. The hypothesis that the viable tissue is more likely to recover following successful recanalistion has not been tested in clinical studies.

The magnitude of ADC reduction appears to be greater in arterial infarction, where ADC is usually reduced by 50% or more, than with venous parenchymal injury. Some authors have suggested that areas of venous ischaemia with more severe restriction of diffusion may correspond to more marked hypoperfusion and irreversible parenchymal damage [129].

There has been noted to be a difference in the temporal evolution of ADC values in venous ischaemia relative to arterial infarction. Whilst there is a trend for the ADC in increase, as with arterial infarction, these changes are found to be more rapid. In a clinical study, Forbes et al [65] showed ADC values to normalise by approximately day 4 compared to day 7 in arterial infarcts [34] and ADC values returned to normal in 48 hours in one animal study [164]. This is likely to represent a combination of resolving cytotoxic oedema and the earlier development of vasogenic oedema in CVT. Analysis of the temporal evolution in clinical studies has been hindered by difficulties in defining the onset of venous ischaemia.

Finally, the perfusion pattern in venous ischemia differs from that of an arterial origin [99]. A characteristic feature is reported to be increased cerebral blood volume with delay in the bolus passage, resulting from venous congestion. According to the theories of secondary hypoperfusion, it is expected there would be subsequent development of decreased cerebral blood flow however this is not yet documented in clinical studies.

## Impact of Imaging on Therapeutic Options

Since CVT is uncommon and clinical presentation and outcome is so variable, current therapeutic management of patients is individual to each case [22].The role of heparin treatment has been investigated with two randomized trials and one meta-analysis [8, 28, 52, 59]. The first randomized, blinded, placebo controlled trial concluded that intravenous heparin was an effective treatment and that associated intracranial haemorrhage was not a contraindication [59]. This trial was criticised due to an unvalidated outcome assessment and a significant delay from onset of symptoms to treatment. A second randomized placebo controlled trial investigated therapy with low molecular weight heparin and only demonstrated a significant statistical improvement with relative to controls when low molecular weight heparin was followed by oral anticoagulation [52]. A meta-analysis of these two trials demonstrated a 14.3% mortality reduction but no overall statistically significant improvement in outcome [52]. Only cohort studies have been conducted in children with CVT and it may not be possible to extrapolate the data from research in adults.

Endovascular treatment has also been employed in the setting of rapidly progressive CVT and clinical deterioration despite adequate anticoagulation (figure 6). Direct infusion of thrombolytic agent and mechanical disruption using guidewires, rheolytic thrombectomy catheters and balloon angioplasty have all been reported [17, 22, 38, 104,118]. Utilisation of endovascular techniques in CVT is based on observations in uncontrolled case series [22, 38] and there has been no randomized controlled trial.

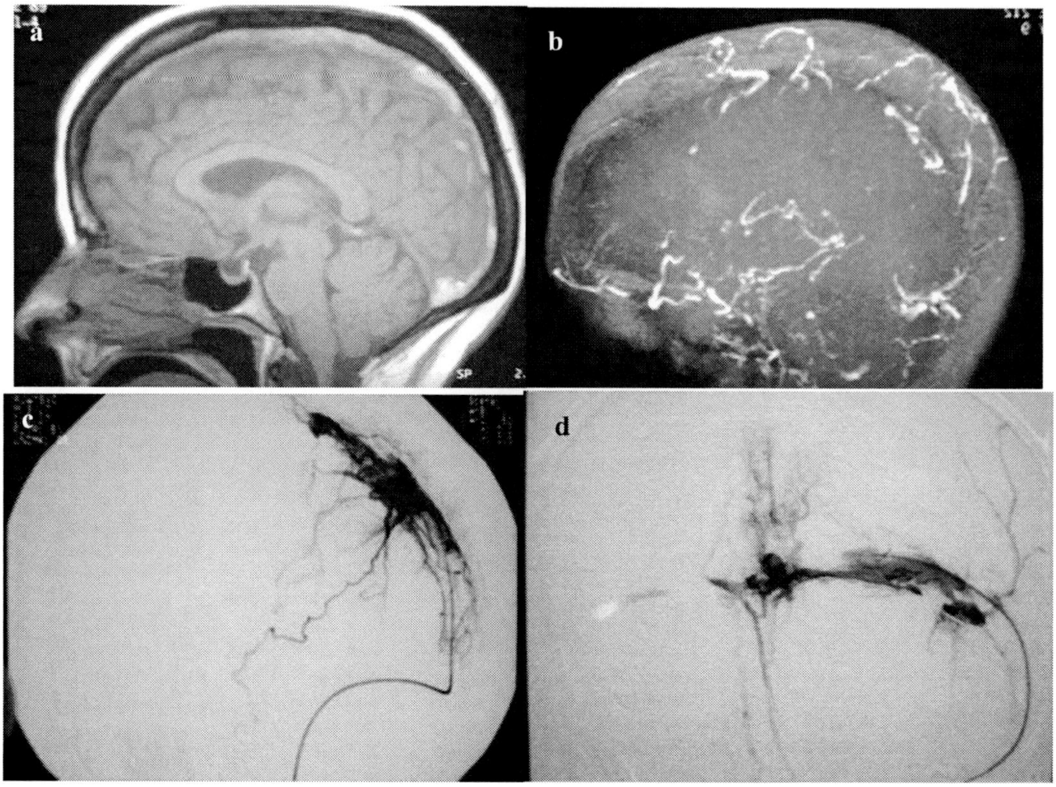


Figure 6. MRI, MRV of SSS with endovascular intervention. a) T1-w image b) 2D TOF MRV MIP confirm SSS thrombosis. There was clinical deterioration despite adequate anticoagulation c) lateral projection with microcatheter injection of SSS d) frontal projection with microcatheter injection of the transverse sinus. Partial recanalisation has been achieved however there remain thrombotic filling defects.

It should be remembered that investigations for and treatment for the underlying cause of CVT will be imperative so rehydration, antibiotics and surgical treatment of septic foci may be relevant. Therapy is also aimed at maintaining blood pressure, correcting metabolic abnormalities and treating seizures. If there is diffuse cerebral swelling and persistent intracranial hypertension, acetazolamide, serial CSF drainage and lumboperitoneal shunting may be employed.

There are now studies of long term outcome in CVT [63,64]. A number of multivariate predictors of death an dependence have been identified in a prospective, multicente study [63]: age >37 years, male sex, mental status disorder, coma, haemorrhage on admission CT scan, deep venous system involvement, and concomitant central nervous system infection or cancer. It is postulated that the high risk patients may benefit from more aggressive therapeutic intervention. Risk stratification would also allow randomization to appropriate therapeutic trials. Most current imaging strategies would identify haemorrhage and thrombotic involvement of the deep venous system, which appear to be the most important prognostic imaging criteria.

Other authors have identified other imaging features which may influence management and prognosis. Haemorrhages that are enlarging or involve the temporal lobe have been used by some as criteria to avoid anticoagulation [209] by one centre. Since the potential for parenchymal damage increases with involvement of the subependymal, bridging and cortical veins [66], some investigators have aimed to ensure visualisation of these veins in order to help predict the course of CVT [105]. However, since there are not well established imaging dependent therapeutic protocols, the emphasis should be on identification of CVT rather than the subtleties of thrombus extent and parenchymal effects.

MR perfusion weighted imaging and diffusion weighted imaging may be used to define early management and provide prognostic information in arterial infarction and some authors have proposed that these techniques could be used to help select patients with CVT who are suitable for more invasive therapy [129,211]. Manzione et al [129] presented a case of a patient with acute sagittal and lateral sinus thrombosis whose symptoms progressed despite heparin administration, and in whom diffusion and perfusion weighted MR imaging revealed abnormalities considerably beyond those revealed by conventional MR imaging. These functional deficits regressed following thrombolysis and this was accompanied by clinical improvement. It was suggested that diffusion and perfusion imaging may be useful in the triage between conservative [heparin only] and aggressive management [thrombolysis] of patients with CVT. Both the extent and the severity of diffusion abnormality may be important. However it is recognized that reduced ADC may not reflect a more severe pathological condition or predict sequelae on follow up imaging, so caution is needed in basing therapeutic decisions on the results of diffusion imaging. There is far less experience in these techniques as applied to venous insufficiency compared with arterial insufficiency, and the basis for the abnormalities remains poorly understood.

There is currently no consensus concerning the duration of oral anticoagulation treatment following initial intravenous heparin [152]. Although it may be assumed that recanalisation should indicate whether oral anticoagulation may be discontinued, there has been no study confirming this relationship between recanalisation and clinical outcome.

Both MRI and MRV have been used for follow up imaging in patients with CVT in order to tailor continued oral anticoagulation. CE MRI and MRV techniques are not suitable for follow up since organization and therefore vascularisation of chronic thrombus results in enhancement which is difficult to distinguish from the normal sinus. Baumgartner [20] studied 33 consecutive patients with CVT who were diagnosed on MRI/MRV and then had follow up imaging at 4 months and 12 months. Patients were treated with intravenous heparin and subsequently warfarin for a minimum of four months. They observed good recanalisation rates correlated with improvement in clinical outcome. However recanalisation rates were unchanged between 4 and 12 months irrespective of oral anticoagulation. This suggests that the benefits of anticoagulation and repeat imaging are limited after four months. Stolz et al [178] prospectively studied recanalisation in 37 consecutive patients who were treated with intravenous heparin acutely and then oral anticoagulation for 12 months. Imaging follow up was with MRV and in a few cases CT or conventional angiography on discharge, and then at 6 and 12 months. They observed that a 60% recanalisation rate was observed on discharge [mean 22 days], which did not increase significantly thereafter. This early recanalisation had no influence on clinical outcome parameters. Their 12 month functional outcome was excellent in 89% of patients. They also concluded that frequent imaging follow-ups were not useful since they provide no useful information on patient outcome.

## Conclusion

There are significant differences in the aims of imaging in venous ischaemia and infarction compared to arterial infarction. In the setting of potential venous ischaemic parenchymal changes, the emphasis is on vascular imaging with demonstration of CVT. Magnetic resonance imaging [MRI] and computed tomography [CT] techniques are now the mainstay of imaging in the cerebral venous system. They may be employed in the setting of CVT to visualise the patency of the venous lumen, the integrity of venous blood flow, the presence of venous thrombus. Recent studies have supported the use of luminal imaging with CT venography or CE GRE MRI and MRV to provide the most detailed demonstration of the intracranial venous structures and maximise detection of CVT. The parenchymal effects of venous ischaemia also differ from arterial ischaemia in terms of imaging appearances, pathophysiology and prognostic significance. They have recently been investigated with diffusion imaging and this approach seems likely to provide useful information concerning the degree of irreversible injury, and guide therapeutic options in the future.

## References

[1] ACAS. Endarterectomy for asymptomatic carotid artery stenosis: Executive Committee for the Asymptomatic Carotid Atherosclerosis Study. *JAMA* 1995; 273: 1421-1428.

[2] Adams WM, Laitt RD, Beards SC, Kassner A, Jackson A. Use of single slice thick slab phase contrast angiography for diagnosis of dural venous sinus thrombosis. *Eur. Radiol.* 1999; 9: 1614-1619.

[3] Ahmadi J, Keane JR, Segall HD, Zee CS. CT observations pertinent to septic cavernous sinus thrombosis. *AJNR Am. J. Neuroradiol.* 1985; 6: 755-758.

[4] Alberico RA, Barnes P, Robertson RL, Burrows PE. Helical CT angiography: Dynamic cerebrovascular imaging in children. *AJNR Am. J. Neuroradiol.* 1999; 20:328-334.

[5] Alexander C, Mamourian, Towfighi J. MR of giant arachnoid granulation, a normal variant presenting as a mass within the dural venous sinus. *AJNR Am. J. Neuroradiol.* 1995; 16: 901-904.

[6] Allroggen H, Abbott RJ. Cerebral venous sinus thrombosis. *Postgrad Med.* J 2000; 76: 12-15.

[7] Alper F, Kantarci M, Dane S, Gumustekin K, Onbas O, Durur I. Importance of anatomical asymmetries of transverse sinuses: MR venographic study. *Cerebrovasc. Dis.* 2004; 18: 236-239.

[8] Ameri A, Bousser MG. Cerebral venous thrombosis. *Neurol. Clin.* 1992; 10: 87-111.

[9] Anderson CM, Saloner D, Tsuruda JS, Shappeero LG, Lee RE. Artifacts in maximum-intensity-projection display of MR angiograms. *AJR Am. J. Roentgenol.* 1990; 154:623-629.

[10] Anderson SC, Shah CP, Murtagh FR. Congested deep subcortical veins as a sign of dural venous thrombosis: MR and CT correlations. *J. Comput. Assist. Tomogr.* 1987; 11: 1059-1061.

[11] Andeweg J. The anatomy of collateral venous flow from the brain and its value in aetiological interpretation of intracranial pathology. *Neuroradiology* 1996;38: 621-628.

[12] Andeweg J. Consequences of the anatomy of deep venous outflow from the brain. *Neuroradiology* 1999; 41: 233-241.

[13] Andrews BT, Dujovny M, Mirchandani G, Ausman JI. Microsurgical anatomy of the venous drainage into the superior sagittal sinus. *Neurosurgery* 1989; 24: 514-520.

[14] Arnautovic KL, Al-Mefty O, Pait TG, Krisht AF, Husain MM. The suboccipital cavernous sinus. *J. Neurosurg.* 1997; 86: 252-262.

[15] Ayanzen RH, Bird CR, Keller PJ, McCully FJ, Theobald MR, Heiser JE. Cerebral MR venography: normal anatomy and potential diagnostic pitfalls. *AJNR Am. J. Neuroradiol.* 2000; 21: 74-78.

[16] Bakac G, Wardlaw JM. Problems in the diagnosis of intracranial venous infarction. *Neuroradiology* 1997; 39: 566-570.

[17] Baker MD, Opatowsky MJ, Wilson JA, Glazier SS, Morris PP. Rheolytic catheter and thrombolysis of dural venous sinus thrombosis: a case series. *Neurosurgery* 2001; 48: 487-493.

[18] Bakshi R, Kinkel WR, Bates VE, Mechtler LL, Kinkel PR. The cerebral intravascular enhancement sign is not specific: a contrast enhanced MRI study. *Neuroradiology* 1999; 41:80-85.

[19] Barber PA, Demchuk AM, Hill MD, Warwick Pexman JH, Hudon ME, Frayne R, Buchan AM. The probability of middle cerebral artery MRA flow signal abnormality with quantified CT ischaemic change: targets for future therapeutic studies. *Journal of Neurology, Neurosurgery and Psychiatry* 2004; 75: 1426-1430.

[20] Baumgartner RW, Studer A, Arnold M, Georgiadis D. Recanalisation of cerebral venous thrombosis. *J. Neurol. Neurosurg. Psychiatry* 2003;74: 459-461.

[21] Becker G, Bogdahn U, Gehlberg C, Frohlich T, Hofman E, Schief MD. Transcranial color-coded real time sonography of intracranial veins. Normal values of blood flow velocities and findings in superior sagittal sinus thrombosis. *J. Neuroimaging* 1995; 5: 87-94.

[22] Benamer HTS, Bone I. Cerebral venous thrombosis: anticoagulants or thrombolytic therapy? *J. Neurol. Neurosurg. Psychiatry* 2000;69: 427-430.

[23] Bergui M, Bradac GB, Daniele D. Brain lesions due to cerebral venous thrombosis do not correlate with sinus involvement. *Neuroradiology* 1999;41: 419-424.

[24] Bering EAJ, Salibi B. Production of hydrocephalus by increased cephalic-venous pressure. *AMA Arch. Neurol. Psychiatry* 1959; 81: 47/693-52/698.

[25] Bisaria KK. Anatomic variations of venous sinuses in the region of the torcular Herophili. *J. Neurosurg.* 1985; 62: 90-95.

[26] Bogousslavsky J, Pierre P. Ischaemic stroke in patients under 45. *Neurol. Clin.* 1992;5: 87-94.

[27] Bono F, Lupo MR, Mangone L, Fera F, Pardatscher K, Quattrone A. Cerebral MR venography of transverse sinuses in subjects with normal CSF pressure. *Neurology* 2003; 61:1267-1270.

[28] Bousser MG. Cerebral venous thrombosis: nothing, heparin, or local thrombolysis? *Stroke* 1999; 30: 481-483.

[29] Bousser MG, Chiras J, Bories J, Castaigne P. Cerebral venous thrombosis: a review of 38 cases. *Stroke* 1993; 16: 199-213.

[30] Bousser MG, Russell RR. *Cerebral venous thrombosis*. London, UK: WB Saunders, 1997.

[31] Braun JP, Tournade A. Venous drainage in the cranio-cervical region. *Neuroradiology* 1977;13: 155-158.

[32] Buonanno FS, Moody DM, Ball TLM. CT scan findings in cerebral sinus venous occlusion. *Neurology* 1982; 12: 288-292.

[33] Buonanno FS, Moody DM, Ball MR, Laster DW. Computed cranial tomographic findings in cerebral sinovenous occlusion. *Journal of Computer Assisted Tomography* 1978; 2: 281-290.

[34] Burdette JH, Elster AD, Ricci PE. Acute cerebral infarction: quantification of spin-density and T2 shine through phenomena on diffusion weighted MR images. *Radiology* 1999; 212:333-339.

[35] Burrows PE, Konez O, Bisdorff. Venous variations of the brain and cranial vault. *Neuroimag. Clin. N. Am.* 2003; 13: 13-26.

[36] Cakmak S, Hermier M, Montavont A et al. T2*weighted MRI in cortical vein thrombosis. *Neurology* 2004; 63: 1698.

[37] Canhao P, Batista P, Ferro JM. Venous transcranial Doppler in acute dural sinus thrombosis. *J. Neurol.* 1998; 245: 276-279.

[38] Canhao P, Falcao F, Ferro JM. Thrombolytiics for cerebral sinus thrombosis: a systematic review. *Cerebrovasc. Dis.* 2003; 15: 159-166.

[39] Cantu C, Barinagarrementeria F. Cerebral venous thrombosis associated with pregnancy and puerperium: a review of 67 cases. *Stroke* 1993;24: 1880-1884.

[40] Casey SO, Alberico RA, Patel M, Jimenez JM, Ozsvath RR, Maguire WM, Taylor ML. Cerebral CT venography. *Radiology* 1996; 198:163-170.

[41] Chang R, Friedman DP. Isolated cortical venous thrombosis presenting as subarachnoid hemorrhage: A report of three cases. *AJNR Am. J. Neuroradiol.* 2004; 25: 1676-1679.

[42] Chin SC, Chen CY, Lee CC, Chen FH, Lee KW, Hsiao HS, Zimmerman RA. Giant arachnoid granulation mimicking dural sinus thrombosis in a boy with headache: MRI. *Neuroradiology* 1998; 40:181-183.

[43] Chiras J, Dubs M, Bories J. Venous infarctions. Neuroradiology 1985; 27: 593-600.

[44] Connor SEJ, Jarosz JM. Magnetic resonance imaging of cerebral venous sinus thrombosis. *Clinical Radiology* 2002; 57: 449-461.

[45] Corvol JC, Oppenheim C, Manai R et al. Diffusion-weighted magnetic resonance imaging in a case of cerebral venous thrombosis. *Stroke* 1998; 29:2649-2652.

[46] Crain MR, Yuh WTC, Greene GM et al. Cerebral ischaemia: evaluation with contrast enhanced MR imaging. *AJNR Am. J. Neuroradiol* 1991; 12:631-639.

[47] Cure JK, Van Tassel P, Smith MT. *Normal and variant anatomy of the dural venous sinuses*. Semin Ultrasound CT MR 1994;15: 499-519.

[48] Curnes JT, Creasy JL, Whaley RL, Scatliff JH. Air in the cavernous sinus: a new sign of septic cavernous sinus thrombosis. *AJNR Am. J. Neuroradiol* 1987; 8: 176-177.

[49] Daniels DL, Czervionke LF, Hendrix LE et al. Gradient recalled echo MR imaging of superior sagittal sinus occlusion. *Neuroradiology* 1989; 134-136.

[50] Davis WL, Warnock SH, Harnsberger HR, Parker DL, Chen CX. Intracranial MRA: single volume vs multiple thin slab 3D time-of-flight acquisition. *J. Comput. Assist. Tomogr.* 1993; 17:15-21.

[51] De Bruijn SFTM, deHaan RJ, Stam J, for the Cerebral Venous Sinus Thrombosis Study Group. Clinical features and prognostic factors of cerebral venous sinus thrombosis in a prospective series of 59 patients. *J. Neurol. Neurosurg. Psychiatry* 2001; 70: 105-108.

[52] de Brujn SFTM, Stam J. Randomized, placebo controlled trial of anticoagulant treatment with low molecular weight heparin for cerebral sinus thrombosis. *Stroke* 1999; 30: 484-488.

[53] Derdeyn CP, Powers WJ. Isolated cortical venous thrombosis and ulcerative colitis. *AJNR Am. J. Neuroradiol.* 1998; 19: 488-490.

[54] Deschiens MA, Conard J, Horellou MH et al. Coagulation studies, factor V Lieden, and anticardiolipin antibodies in 40 cases of cerebral venous thrombosis. *Stroke* 1996; 27: 1724-1730.

[55] deVeber G, Andrew M. Cerebral sinovenous thrombosis in children. *N. Engl. J. Med.* 2001; 345: 417-423.

[56] Dormont D, Anxionnat R, Evrard S, Louaille C, Chiras J, Marsault C. MRI in cerebral venous thrombosis. *J. Neuroradiol.* 1994; 21: 81-99.

[57] Dormont D, Sag K, Biondi A, Wechsler B, Marsault C. Gadolinium enhanced MR of chronic dural sinus thrombosis. *AJNR Am. J. Neuroradiol.* 1995; 16:1347-1352.

[58] Ducreux D, Oppenheim C, Vandamme X, Dormont D, Samson Y, Rancurel G, Cosnard G, Marsault C. Diffusion-weighted imaging patterns of brain damage associated with cerebral venous thrombosis. *AJNR Am. J. Neuroradiol.* 2001; 22:261-268.

[59] Einhaupl KM, Villringer A, Meister W, et al. Heparin treatment for cerebral venous and sinus thrombosis. *Lancet* 1991; 338: 597-600.

[60] Elster AD, Moody DM. Early cerebral infarction: gadopentetate dimeglumine enhancement. *Radiology* 1990; 177:627-632.

[61] Farb RI, Scott JN, Willinsky RA et al. Intracranial venous system: Gadolinium enhanced three dimensional MR venography with auto-triggered elliptic centric-ordered sequence-initial experience. *Radiology* 2003; 226: 203-209.

[62] Farb RI, Vanek I, Scott JN et al. Idiopathic intracranial hypertension. The prevalence and morphology of sinovenous stenosis. *Neurology* 2003; 60: 1418-1424.

[63] Ferro JM, Canhao P, Stam J, Bousser MG, Barinagarrementeria F; ISCVT Investigators. *Stroke* 2004; 35: 664-670.

[64] Ferro JM, Lopes MG, Rosas MJ, Ferro MA, Fontes J; Cerebral venous thrombosis Portugese Collaborative Study Group. Long term prognosis of cerebral vein and dural sinus thrombosis: results of the VENOPORT study. *Cerebrovasc. Dis.* 2002; 13: 272-278.

[65] Forbes KPN, Pipe JG, Heiserman JE. Evidence for cytotoxic oedema in the pathogenesis of cerebral venous infarction. *AJNR Am. J. Neuroradiol.* 2001; 22:450-455.

[66] Frerichs KU, Deckert M, Kempski O, Schurer L, Einhaupl K, Baethmann A. Cerebral sinus and venous thrombosis in rats induces long-term deficits in brain function and

morphology: evidence for a cytotoxic genesis. *J. Cereb. Blood Flow Metab.* 1994; 14:289-300.

[67] Fries G, Wallenfang T, Hennen J et al. Occlusion of the pig superior sagittal sinus, bridging and cortical veins: multistep evolution of sinus vein thrombosis. *J. Neurosurg.* 1992; 77: 127-133.

[68] Furlan A, Higashida R, Wechsler L et al. Intra-arterial prourokinase for acute ischaemic stroke. The PROACT II study: a randomized controlled trial. Prolyse in Acute Cerebral Thromboembolism. *JAMA* 1999; 282: 2003-2011.

[69] Gabrielsen TO, Seeger JF, Knake JE, Stilwil EW. Radiology of cerebral vein occlusion without dural sinus occlusion. *Radiology* 1981; 140: 403-408.

[70] Gebarski SS, Gebarski KS. Inferior petrosal sinus: imaging-anatomic correlation. *Radiology* 1995; 194: 239-247.

[71] Giraud P, Thobois S, Hermier M, Brousolle E, Chazot G. Intravenous hypertrophic Paccioni granulations: differentiation from venous dural thrombosis. *J. Neurol. Neurosurg. Psychiatry* 2001; 70: 700-701.

[72] Goldberg AL, Rosenbaum AE, Wang H, Kim WS, Lewis VL, Hanley DF. Computed tomography of dural sinus thrombosis. *J. Comput. Assist. Tomogr.* 1981; 5: 760-762.

[73] Hacker H. Normal supratentorial veins and dural sinuses. In: Newton TH, Potts DG, Eds. *Radiology of the Skull and Brain*, Angiography. St Louis, Mo: CV Mosby Co; 1974.

[74] Halbach VV, Higashida RT, Hieshima GB, Dowd CF, Barnwell SL. Venography and venous pressure monitoring in dural sinus meningiomas. *AJNR Am. J. Neuroradiol.* 1989; 10:1209-1213.

[75] Harris TM, Smith RR, Koch KJ. Gadolinium-DTPA enhanced MR imaging of septic dural sinus thrombosis. *Journal of Computer Assisted Tomography* 1989; 13: 682-684.

[76] Hasegawa Y, Fisher M, Latour LL, Dardzinski BJ, Sotak CH. MRI diffusion mapping of reversible and irreversible ischaemic injury in focal brain ischaemia. *Neurology* 1994; 44:1484-1490.

[77] Healy JF, Nichols. Polycythemia mimicking venous sinus thrombosis. *AJNR Am. J. Neuroradiol* 2002; 23: 1402-1403.

[78] Higgins JN, Gillard JH, Owler BK, Harkness K, Pickard JD. MR venography in idiopathic intracranial hypertension: unappreciated and misunderstood. *J. Neurol. Neurosurg. Psychiatry* 2004; 75: 621-625.

[79] Ho VB, Rovira MJ, Borke RC, Smirniotopoulos JG. Arachnoid granulations in the transverse sinuses. *IJNR* 1997; 3: 482-489.

[80] Hoffmann O, Klingebeil R, Braun JS, Katchanov J, Valdueza JM. Diagnostic pitfall: Atypical cerebral venous drainage via the vertebral venous system. *AJNR Am. J. Neuroradiol.* 2002; 23: 408-411.

[81] Huang YP. Wolf BS. Veins of the posterior fossa, in Newton TH, Potts eds. *Radiology of the skull and brain*, vol2. St Louis: CV Mosby, 1974, Book 3, p2155-2216.

[82] Hunerbein R, Reuter P, Meyer W, Kuhn FP. CT angiography of cerebral venous circulation: anatomical visualization and diagnostic pitfalls in interpretation. *Rofo* 1997; 167: 612-618.

[83] Huston 111 J, Ehman RL. Comparison of time-of-flight and phase contrast MR neuroangiographic techniques. *Radiographics* 1993; 13: 5-19.
[84] Imakita S, Onishi Y, Hashimoto T et al. Subtraction CT angiography with controlled orbital helical scanning for detection of intracranial aneurysms. *AJNR Am. J. Neuroradiol.* 1998; 19:291-295.
[85] Ingstrup HM, Jorgensen PS. Tentorial changes in sigmoid sinus thrombosis. *Journal of Computer Assisted Tomography* 1981; 5: 760-762.
[86] Ito J, Marmarou A, Barzo P, Fatouros P, Corwin F. Characterization of edema by diffusion weighted imaging in experimental traumatic brain injury. *J. Neurosurg.* 1996; 84: 97-103.
[87] Jaillard AS, Hommel M, Mallaret M. Venous sinus thrombosis associated with androgens in a healthy young man. *Stroke* 1994; 25: 212-213.
[88] Jinkins R J. *Atlas of neuroradiologic embryology, anatomy and variants. Pennsylvannia,* USA: Lippincott Williams and Wilkins, 2000.
[89] Johnson BA, Fram EK. Cerebral venous occlusive disease. *Neuroimag. Clin. N. Am.* 1992; 2: 769-783.
[90] Jung HW, Chang KH, Choi DS, Han MH, Han MC. Contrast enhanced MR angiography for the diagnosis of intracranial vascular disease: optimal dose of gadopentetate dimeglumine. *AJR Am. J. Roentgenol.* 1995; 165:1251-1255.
[91] Kadimi S, Terry JB, Gomez CR. Hyperechoic middle cerebral artery: acute occlusion detected on transcranial duplex ultrasonography. *J. Neuroimaging.* 2000; 10: 228-230.
[92] Kallmes DF, Cloft HJ, Jensen ME, Kaptain GJ, Dion JE, Matsumoto JA. Dural arteriovenous fistula: a pitfall of time-of-flight MR venography for the diagnosis of sinus thrombosis. *Neuroradiology* 1998; 40:242-244.
[93] Kamran S, Bates V, Bakshi R, Wright P, Kinkel W, Miletich R. Significance of hyperintense vessels on FLAIR MRI in acute stroke. *Neurology* 2000; 55: 265-269.
[94] Kanaiwa H, Kuchiwaki H, Inao S et al. Changes in the cerebrocortical capillary network following venous sinus occlusion in cats. *Surg. Neurol.* 1995; 44: 172-179.
[95] Kaplan HA, Browder A, Browder J. Narrow and atretic dural sinuses: clinical significance. *Ann. Otol. Rhinol. Laryngol.* 1973; 82: 351-354.
[96] Kastenbauer S, Pfister HW. Pneumococcal meningitis in adults: spectrum of complications and prognostic factors in a series of 87 cases. *Brain* 2003; 126: 1015-1025.
[97] Kaufmann A, Firlik A, Fukui M, Wechsler L, Jungries C, Yonas H. Ischaemic core and penumbra in human stroke. *Stroke* 1999; 30: 93-99.
[98] Keiper MD, Ng SE, Atlas SW, Grossman RI. Subcortical hemorrhage: marker for radiographically occult cerebral vein thrombosis on CT. *J. Comput. Assist. Tomogr.* 1995; 19: 527-531.
[99] Keller E, Flacke S, Urbach H, Schild HH. Diffusion and perfusion weighted magnetic resonance imaging in deep cerebral venous thrombosis. *Stroke* 1999; 30: 1144 -1146.
[100] Keller PJ. Time-of-flight magnetic resonance angiography. *Neuroimag. Clin. N. Am.* 1992; 2: 639-656.

[101] Kenez J, Barsi P, Majtenyi K et al. Can intravascular lymphomatosis mimic sinus thrombosis? A case report with 8 months follow up and fatal outcome. *Neuroradiology* 200; 42: 436-440.

[102] Keseva PP. Recanalization of the falcine sinus after venous sinus thrombosis. *AJNR Am. J. Neuroradiol.* 1996; 1646-1648.

[103] Kilgore DP, Breger RK, Daniels DL, Pojunas KW, Williams AL, Haughton VM. Cranial tissues: normal MR appearance after intravenous injection of Gd-DTPA. *AJNR Radiology* 1986; 160:757-761.

[104] Kim SY, Suh JH. Direct endovascular thrombolytic therapy for dural sinus thrombosis: Infusion of alteplase. *AJNR Am. J. Neuroradiol.* 1997; 18: 639-645.

[105] Kirchof K, Welzel T, Jansen O, Sartor K. More reliable noninvasive visualization of the cerebral veins and dural sinuses: Comparison of three MR angiographic techniques. *Radiology* 2002; 224:804-810.

[106] Kosinski CM, Mull M, Schwarz M, Koch B, Biniek R, Schlafer J, Milkereit E, Willmes K, Schiefer J. Do normal D-dimer levels reliably exclude cerebral sinus thrombosis? *Stroke* 2004; 35: 2820.

[107] Kriss VM. Hyperdense posterior falx in the neonate. *Pediatr. Radiol.* 1998; 28: 817-819.

[108] Krueger K, Kugel H, Grond M, Thiel A, Maintz D, Lackner K.Late resolution of diffusion weighted MRI changes in a patient with prolonged reversible neurological deficit after thrombolysis. *Stroke* 2000; 31: 2715-2718.

[109] Kudo K, Terae S, Ishii A, Omatsu T, Asano T, Tha KK, Miyasaka K. Physiologic change in flow velocity and direction of dural venous sinuses with respiration: MR venography and flow analysis. *AJNR Am. J. Neuroradiol.* 2004; 25:551-557.

[110] Kuehnen J, Schwartz A, Neff W, Hennerici M. Cranial nerve syndrome in thrombosis of the transverse/sigmoid sinuses. *Brain* 1998; 121: 381-388.

[111] Kuroiwa T, Nagaoka T, Ueki M et al. Different apparent diffusion coefficient: water content correlations of grey and white matter during early ischaemia. *Stroke* 1998; 29: 859-865.

[112] Kurokawa Y, Hashi K, Okuyama T, Uede T. Regional ischaemia in cerebral venous hypertension due to embolic occlusion of the superior sagittal sinus in the rat. *Surg. Neurol.* 1990; 34: 390-395.

[113] Lafitte F, Boukobza M, Guichard JP et al. MRI and MRA for diagnosis and follow up of cerebral venous thrombosis [CVT]. *Clin. Radiol.* 1997; 52: 672-679.

[114] Lafitte F, Boukobza M, Guichard JP, Reizine D, Woimant F, Merland JJ. Deep cerebral venous thrombosis: imaging in eight cases. *Neuroradiology* 1999; 41: 410-418.

[115] Lausjaunias P, Berenstein A, ter Brugge KG et al.Intracranial venous system. IN: Lausjaunias P, Berenstein A, terBrugge KG, eds. *Surgical neuroangiography*. Ed 2. Berlin: Springer-Verlag; 2001. p631-695.

[116] Le Bihan D, Breton E, Lallemand D, Aubin M, Vignaud J, Laval-Jeantet M. Separation of diffusion and perfusion in intravoxel incoherent motion MR imaging. *Radiology* 1988; 168: 497-505.

[117] Lee EJY. The empty delta sign. *Radiology* 2002; 224: 788-789.

[118] Lee S-K, terBrugge KG. Cerebral venous thrombosis in adults: the role of imaging evaluation and management. *Neuroimag. Clin. N. Am.* 2003; 13: 139-152.

[119] Leech JL, Jones BV, Tomsick TA, Stewart CA, Balko MG. Normal appearance of arachnoid granulations on contrast enhanced CT and MR of the brain: Differentiation from dural sinus disease. *AJNR Am. J. Neuroradiol.* 1996; 17: 1523-1532

[120] Leker RR, Steiner I. Features of dural sinus thrombosis simulating pseudotumor cerebri. *Eur. J. Neurol.* 1999; 6: 601-604.

[121] Lewin JS, Laub G. Intracranial MR angiography: a direct comparison of three time-of-flight techniques. *AJNR Am. J. Neuroradiol.* 1991; 12:1133-1139.

[122] Lewin JS, Masaryk TJ, Smith AS, Ruggieri PM, Ross JS. Time of flight intracranial MR venography: evaluation of the sequential oblique section technique. *AJNR Am. J. Neuroradiol.* 1994; 15:1657-1664.

[123] Liang L, Korogi Y, Sugahara T et al. Evaluation of the intracranial dural sinuses with a 3D contrast enhanced MP-RAGEsequence: prospective comparison with 2DTOF MR venography and digital subtraction angiography. *AJNR Am. J. Neuroradiol.* 2001; 22:481-492.

[124] Liauw L, van Buchem MA, de Bruine FT, van den Berg R, Hermans J, Wasser MNJM. MR Angiography of the intracranial venous system. *Radiology* 2000; 214:678-682.

[125] Lovblad KO, Schneider J, Bassetti C, El-Koussy et al. Fast contrast-enhanced MR whole brain venography. *Neuroradiology* 2002; 44:681-688.

[126] Ludemann P, Nabavi DG, Junker R, et al. Factor V Leiden mutation in cerebral venous thrombosis. *Stroke* 1998; 29: 2507-2510.

[127] Macchi PJ, Grossman RI, Gomori JM et al. High field MR imaging of cerebral venous thrombosis. *J. Comput. Assist. Tomogr.* 1986; 10: 10-15.

[128] Majoie CBLM, van Straten M, Venema HW, den Heeten GJ. Multisection CT venography of the dural sinuses and cerebral veins by using matched mask bone elimination. *AJNR Am. J. Neuroradiol.* 2004; 25:787-791.

[129] Manzione J, Newman GC, Shapiro A, Santo-Ocampo R. Diffusion and perfusion weighted MR imaging of dural sinus thrombosis. *AJNR Am. J. Neuroradiol.* 2000; 21:68-73.

[130] Marler JR, Tilley BC, Lu M et al. Early stroke treatment associated with better outcome: the NINDS rt-PA stroke study. *Neurology* 2000; 55: 1649-1655.

[131] Mas JL, Meder JF, Meary E. Dural sinus thrombosis:long term follow up by magnetic resonance imaging. *Cerebrovasc. Dis.* 1992; 2: 137.

[132] Matsushima T, Rhoton AL, de Oliveira E, Peace D. Microsurgical anatomy of the veins of the posterior fossa. *J. Neurosurg* 1983; 59: 63-105.

[133] Mattle HP, Wentz KU, Edelman RR et al. Cerebral venography with MR. *Radiology* 1991; 178:453-458.

[134] Medlock MD, Olivero WC, Hanigan WC, Wright RM, Winek SJ. Children with cerebral venous thrombosis diagnosed with magnetic resonance imaging and magnetic resonance angiography. *Neurosurgery* 1992; 11: 870-876.

[135] Mehraein S, Ortwein H, Busch M, Weih M, Einhaupl K, Masuhr F. Risk of recurrence of cerebral venous and sinus thrombosis during subsequent pregnancy and puerperium. *J. Neurol. Neurosurg. Psychiatry* 2003; 74: 814-816.

[136] Mehta NR, Jones L, Kraut MA, Melhem ER. Physiologic variations in dural venous sinus flow on phase contrast MR imaging. *AJR Am. J. Roentgenol.* 2000; 175:221-225.

[137] Miabi Z, Midia R, Rohrer SE et al. Delineation of lateral tentorial sinus with cointrast enhanced imaging and surgical implications. *AJNR Am. J. Neuroradiol.* 2004; 25: 1181-8.

[138] Miller DL, Doppman JL. Petrosal sinus sampling: technique and rationale. *Radiology* 1991; 178: 37-47.

[139] Minematsu K, Li L, Sotak CH, Davis MA, Fisher M. Reversible focal ischaemic injury demonstrated by diffusion weighted magnetic resonance imaging in rats. *Stroke* 1992; 23:1304-1310.

[140] Mullins ME, Grant PE, Wang B, Gonzalez RG, Schaefer PW. Parenchymal abnormalities associated with cerebral venous sinus thrombosis: Assessment with diffusion weighted MR imaging. *AJNR Am. J. Neuroradiol.* 2004; 25:1666-1675.

[141] Nakase H, Heimann A, Kempski O. Alterations of regional cerebral blood flow and oxygen saturation in a rat sinus-vein thrombosis model. *Stroke* 1996; 27: 720-727.

[142] Nishio A, Takami T, Ohata K et al. Three-dimensional rotation venography using the digital subtraction angiography unit with a flat panel detector:usefulness for the transtemporal/transtentorial approaches. *Neuroradiology* 2004; 11: 876-882.

[143] Nussell F, Huber P. High resolution computed tomography of superior sagittal sinus thrombosis and abnormalities. *Neuroradiology* 1989; 31:307-311.

[144] Ogawa T, Inugami A, Fujita H et al. MR diagnosis of subacute and chronic subarachnoisd haemorrhage: comparison with CT. *AJR Am. J. Roentgenol.* 1995; 165: 1257-1262.

[145] Ono M, Rhoton AL, Peace D, Rodriguez RJ. Microsurgical anatomy of the deep venous system of the brain. *Neurosurgery* 1984; 15: 621-657.

[146] Osborn AG. Craniofacial venous plexuses: angiographic study. *AJNR Am. J. Neuroradiol* 1980; 1: 141-148.

[147] Osborn AG. The cerebral veins. IN: *Diagnostic cerebral angio*graphy. 2nd Ed. Pennsylvannia, USA: Lippincott Williams and Wilkins, 1999. p217-237.

[148] Ouanounou S, Tomsick TA, Heitsman C, Holland CK. Cavernous sinus and inferior petrosal sinus flow signal on three-dimensional time-of –flight MR angiography. *AJNR Am. J. Neuroradiol.* 1999; 20: 1476-1481.

[149] Ozsvath RR, Casey SO, Lustrin ES, Alberico RA, Hassankhani A, Patel M. Cerebral venography: comparison of CT and MR projection venography. *AJR Am. J. Roentgenol.* 1997; 169:1699-1707.

[150] Patel MR, Edelman RR, Warach S. Detection of hyperacute primary intraparenchymal hemorrhage by magnetic resonance imaging. *Stroke* 1996; 27: 2321-2324.

[151] Perl J II, Turski PA, Masaryk TJ. MR angiography. In: Atlas SW, ed. *Magnetic resonance imaging of the brain and spine.* 2nd ed. Philadelphia, Pa: Lippincott-Raven, 1996; 1548-1549, 1552-1563.

[152] Preter M, Tzourio C, Ameri A, Bousser MG. Long-term prognosis in cerebral venous thrombosis: follow up of 77 patients. *Stroke* 1996; 27:243-249.

[153] Provenzale JM. CT and MR imaging of non-traumatic neurologic emergencies. *AJR Am. J. Roentgenol.* 2000; 174: 289-299.

[154] Provenzale JM, Joseph GJ, Barboriak DP. Dural sinus thrombosis: Findings on CT and MR imaging and diagnostic pitfalls. *AJR* 1998; 170: 177-183.

[155] Ra CS, Lui CC, Liang CL, Chen HJ, Kuo YL, Chen WF. Superior sagittal sinus thrombosis induced by thyrotoxicosis. Case report. *J. Neurosurg.* 2001; 94: 130-132.

[156] Rao KC, Knipp HC, Wagner EJ. Computed tomographic findings in cerebral sinus and venous sinus thrombosis. *Radiology* 1981; 140:391-398.

[157] Ray BS, Dunbar HS. Thrombosis of the superior sagittal sinus as a cause of pseudotumor cerebri: Methods of diagnosis and treatment. *Trans Am. Neurol. Assoc.* 1950; 75: 12-17.

[158] Ray BS, Dunbar HS. Thrombosis of the dural venous sinuses as a cause of pseudotumour cerebri. *Ann. Surg.* 1951; 134: 376-386.

[159] Reichenbach JR, Essig M, Haacke EM et al. High-resolution venography of the brain using magnetic resonance imaging. *MAGMA* 1998; 6: 62-69.

[160] Remonda L, Heid O, Schroth G. Carotid artery stenosis, occlusion and pseudo-occlusion: first pass, gadolinium enhanced, three-dimensional MR angiography-preliminary results. *Radiology* 1998; 209: 95-102.

[161] Ries S, Steinke W, Neff KW, Hennerici MD. Echocontrast enhanced color-coded sonography for the diagnosis of transverse sinus venous thrombosis. *Stroke* 1997;28: 696-700.

[162] Roland EH, Flodmark O, Hill A. Thalamic hemorrhage with intraventricular hemorrhage in the full term new born. *Pediatrics* 1990; 85: 737-742.

[163] Rollins N, Ison C, Booth T, Chia J. MR venography in the pediatric patient. AJNR AM *J. Neuroradiol.* 2005; 26: 50-55.

[164] Rother J, Waggie K, van Bruggen N, de Crespigny AJ, Moseley ME. Experimental cerebral venous thrombosis: evaluation using magnetic resonance imaging. *J. Cereb. Blood Flow Metab.* 1996; 16:1353-1361.

[165] Saito Y, Kobayashi N. Cerebral venous angiomas: clinical evaluation and possible etiology. *Radiology* 1981; 139: 87-94.

[166] San Millan Ruiz D, Fasel JH, Rufenacht DA, Gailloud P. The sphenoparietal sinus of breschet: does it exist? An anatomical study. *AJNR Am. J. Neuroradiol.* 2004; 25: 112-120.

[167] Sarma D, Farb RI, Mikulis DJ, terBrugge KG. Reversal of restricted diffusion in cerebral venous thrombosis: case report. *Neuroradiology* 2004; 46: 118-121.

[168] Schaefer PW, Buonanno FS, Gonzalez RG, Schwamm LH. Diffusion-weighted imaging discriminates between cytotoxic and vasogenic oedema in a patient with eclampsia. *Stroke* 1997; 28:1082-1085.

[169] Schuknecht B. Latest techniques in head and neck CT angiography. *Neuroradiology* 2004; 46: s208-213.

[170] Schuknecht B, Simmen D, Uksel C, Valavanis A. Tributary venosinus occlusion and septic cavernous sinus thrombosis: CT and MR finfings. *AJNR Am. J. Neuroradiol.* 1998; 19: 617-626.

[171] Scott JN, Farb RI. Imaging and anatomy of the normal intracranial venous system. *Nuroimag. Clin. N. Am.* 2003; 13: 1-12.

[172] Sener RN. The occipitotemporal vein: a cadaver, MRI and CT study. *Neuroradiology* 1994; 36: 117-120.

[173] Sevick RJ, Kanda F, Mintorovitch J et al. Cytotoxic brain oedema: assessment with diffusion-weighted MR imaging. *Radiology* 185: 687-690.

[174] Shinohara Y, Yoshitoshi M, Yoshii F. Appearance and disappearance of empty delta sign in superior sagittal sinus thrombosis. *Stroke* 1986; 17: 1282-1284.

[175] Shroff M, deVeber G. Sinovenous thrombosis in children. *Neuroimag. Clin. N. Am.* 2003; 13: 115-138.

[176] Sohn CH, Sevick RJ, Frayne R. Contrast- enhanced MR angiography of the intracranial circulation. *Magn. Reson. Imaging Clin. N. Am.* 2003; 11: 599-614.

[177] Sorensen A, Buonanno F, Gonzalez G, Schwamm L, Lev M et al. Hyperacute stroke: evaluation with combined multisection diffusion weighted and haemodynamically weighted echo-planar MR imaging. *Radiology* 1996; 199:391-401.

[178] Stolz E, Trittmacher S, Rahimi A, Gerriets T, Rottger C, Siekmann R, Kaps M. Influence of recanalisation on outcome in dural sinus thrombosis. *Stroke* 2004; 35: 544-510.

[179] Stolz E, Kaps M, Dorndorf W. Assessment of intracranial venous haemodynamics in normal individuals and patients with cerebral venous thrombosis. *Stroke* 1999; 30: 70-75.

[180] Suzuki Y, Ikeda H, Shimadu M, Ikeda Y, Matsumoto K. Variations of the basal vein: identification using three-dimensional CT angiography. *AJNR Am. J. Neuroradiol.* 2001; 22: 670-676.

[181] Szajzel R, Coeytaux A, Dehdashti AR, Delavelle J, Sinnreich M. Subarachnoid haemorrhage: a rare presentation of cerebral venous thrombosis. *Headache* 2001; 41: 889-892.

[182] Sze G, Simmons B, Krol G, Walker R, Zimmerman RD, Deck MDF. Dural sinus thrombosis: verification with spin-echo techniques. *AJNR Am. J. Neuroradiol.* 1988; 9:679-686.

[183] Takahashi S, Higano S, Kurihara N, Kayama T, Sakamoto K. Contrast enhanced MR imaging of dural sinus thrombosis: Demonstration of the thrombosis and collateral venous channels. *Clinical Radiology* 1994; 639-644.

[184] Teasdale E. Cerebral venous thrombosis: making the most of imaging. *J. R. Soc. Med.* 2000; 93: 234-237.

[185] Tehindrazanarivelo A, Evrard S, Schaison M, Mas JL, Dormont D, Bousser MG. Prospective study of cerebral venous sinus thrombosis in patients presenting with benign intracranial hypertension. *Cerebrovasc. Dis.* 1992;2: 22-27.

[186] Teksam M, Casey S, McKinney A, Michel E, Truwit CL. Anatomy and frequency of large pontomesencephalic veins CT angiograms of the circle of Willis. *AJNR Am. J. Neuroradiol.* 2003; 24: 1598-1601.

[187] Tomilov II. Otogenic thrombosis of the sigmoid sinus and the bulb of the jugular vein affecting the glossopharyngeal, vagus and accessory nerves. *Vestn. Otorinolaringol.* 1994;100-101.

[188] Trowbin A. *The syndrome of latent cerebral venous thrombosis*: its frequency and relation to age and congestive heart failure 1973; 4: 419-430.

[189] Tsai FY, Higashida RT, Matovich V et al. Acute thrombosis of the intracranial dural sinus:direct thrombolytic treatment. *AJNR Am. J. Neuroradiol.* 1992; 13:1137-1141.

[190] Tsai FY, Wang AM, Matovich VB, et al. MR staging of acute dural sinus thrombosis. Correlation with venous pressure measurements and implications for treatment and prognosis. *AJNR Am. J. Neuroradiol.* 1995; 16:1021-1029.

[191] Tsao PN, Lee WT, Peng SF, Lin JH, Yau KI. Power Doppler ultrasound imaging in neonatal cerebral venous thrombosis. *Pediatr. Neurol.* 1999; 21: 652-655.

[192] Tsuruda JS, Shimakawa A, Pelc NJ, Saloner D. Dural sinus occlusion: evaluation with phase sensitive gradient echo MR imaging. *AJNR Am. J. Neuroradiol.* 1991; 12:481-488.

[193] Ture U, Yasargil MG, Al-Mefty O. The transcallosal-transforaminal approach to the third ventricle with regard to the venous variations in this region. *J. Neurosurg.* 1997; 87: 706-715.

[194] Tuzgen S, Canbaz B, Kaya AH, Sanus GZ, Kuday C, Memis M, Oz B. Experimental study of rapid versus slow sagittal sinus occlusion in dogs. *Neurol. India* 2003;51: 482-486.

[195] Ungersbock K, Heimann A, Kempski O. Cerebral blood flow alterations in a rat model of cerebral sinus thrombosis. *Stroke* 1993;24 [4]: 563-569.

[196] Valdueza JM, Schultz M, Harms L, Einhaupl KM. Venous trancranial Doppler ultrasound monitoring in acute dural sinus thrombosis. Report of two cases. *Stroke* 1995; 26: 1196-9.

[197] Valdueza JM, von Munster T, Hoffmann O, Schreiber S, Einhaupl KM. Postural dependency of the cerebral venous outflow. *Lancet* 2000; 355: 200-201.

[198] van Gijn J. Cerebral venous thrombosis: pathogenesis, presentation and prognosis. *J. R. Soc. Med.* 2000; 93: 230-233.

[199] Venema HW, Hulsmans FJH, den Heeten GJ. CT angiography of the circle of Willis and the intracranial carotid arteries: maximum intensity projection with matched mask bone elimination. *Radiology* 2001; 218:893-898.

[200] Vieregge P, Schwieder G, Kompf D. Cerebral venous thrombosis in hereditary protein C deficiency. *J. Neurol. Neurosurg. Psychiatry* 1989; 52: 135-137.

[201] Villringer A, Mehraen S, Einhaupl KM. Pathophysiological aspects of cerebral sinus venous thrombosis. *J. Neuroradiol.* 1994; 21: 72-80.

[202] Virapongse C, Cazenave C, Quisling R, Sarwar M, Hunter S. The empty delta sign: Frequency and significance in 76 cases of dural sinus thrombosis. *Radiology* 1987; 162: 779-785.

[203] Vogl TJ, Bergman C, Villringer A et al. Dural sinus thrombosis: value of venous MR angiography for diagnosis and follow up. *AJR* 1994; 162: 1191-1198.

[204] Von Mering M, Stiefel M, Brockmann K, Nau R. Deep cerebral venous sinus thrombosis often presents with neuropsychological symptoms. *J. Clin. Neurosci.* 2003; 10: 310-312.

[205] Wasay M, Bakshi R, Bobustuc G, Dubey N, Chhema Z, Dai A. Diffusion-Weighted magnetic resonance imaging in superior sagittal sinus thrombosis. *J. Neuroimaging.* 2002; 12: 267-269.

[206] Wetzel SG, Kirsch E, Stock KW, Kolbe M, Kaim A, Radue EW. Cerebral Veins: *Comparative study of CT venography with intraarterial digital subtraction angiography. AJNR Am. J. Neuroradiol.* 1999; 20:249-255.

[207] Wetzel SG, Law M, Lee VS, Cha S, Johnson G, Nelson K. Imaging of the intracranial venous system with a contrast enhanced volumetric interpolated examination. *Eur. Radiol.* 2003; 13: 1010-1018.

[208] Willinsky R, Goyal M, Terbrugge K et al. Tortuous engorged pial veins in intracranial dural arteriovenous fistulas: correlations with presentation, location, and MR findings in 122 patients. *AJNR Am. J. Neuroradiol.* 1999; 20:1031-1036.

[209] Wingerchuk DM, Dijdicks EF, Fulgham JR. Cerebral venous thrombosis complicated by hemorrhagic infarction: factors affecting the initiation and safety of anticoagulation.

[210] Yano T, Kodama T, Suzuki Y, Watanabe K. Gadolinium enhanced 3D time-of-flight MR angiography: experimental and clinical evaluation. *Acta Radiol.* 1997; 38:47-54.

[211] Yoshikawa T, Abe O, Tsuchiya K, Okubo T, Tobe K et al. Diffusion weighted magnetic resonance imaging of dural sinus thrombosis. *Neuroradiology* 2002; 44:481-488.

[212] Yousem DM, Balakrishnan J, Debrun GM, Bryan RN. Hyperintense thrombus on GRASS MR images: potential pitfall in flow evaluation. *AJNR Am. J. Neuroradiol.* 1990; 11:51-58.

[213] Yuh WTC, Crain MR, Loes DJ et al. MR imaging of cerebral ischaemia: findings in the first 24 hours. *AJNR Am. J. Neuroradiol.* 1991; 12:621-629.

[214] Yuh WTC, Simonson TM, Wang AM, Koci TM, Tali ET, Fisher DJ, Simon JH, Jinkins JR, Tsai F. Venous sinus occlusive disease: MR findings. *AJNR Am. J. Neuroradiol.* 1994; 15:309-316.

[215] Zouaoui A. Cerebral venous sinuses: anatomical variants or thrombosis? *Acta. Anat.* [Basel] 1998; 133: 318-324.

[216] Zuber M, Toulon P, Marnet L et al. Factor V Leiden mutation in cerebral venous thrombosis. *Stroke* 1996; 27: 1721-1723.

In: State-of-the-Art Imaging in Stroke, Volume 2
Editor: Bernhard Schaller, pp. 245-264
ISBN 978-1-60021-499-8


*Chapter VIII*

# Imaging of Ischemic Tolerance in the Brain

***Raymond T. F. Cheung***
Division of Neurology, University Department of Medicine,
The University of Hong Kong, Pokfulam, Hong Kong

## A. Introduction

An adult human brain only weighs about 2% of the total body weight but receives as much as 15% of the total cardiac output and consumes approximately 20% of the total oxygen intake [1]. Brain cells, especially neurons, have a high metabolic demand on energy in the form of adenosine triphosphate (ATP) to maintain their transmembrane ionic gradients, electrical activities, synaptic transmission, macromolecular synthesis, efficient intracellular transport, and cytoskeletal integrity [1, 2]. ATP is derived from oxidative metabolism of glucose under normal circumstances; anaerobic glycolysis generates only one-sixteenth the amount of ATP from oxidative metabolism and also leads to lactic acidosis. As the brain does not have a significant storage of oxygen and glucose, the brain needs a continuous and uninterrupted supply of these substrates via the cerebral circulation. Thus, the brain is very intolerant to ischemia or hypoxia.

The oxygen pressure gradient between the arterial blood (above 70 to 80 mmHg) and venous blood (about 15 to 25 mmHg) is steep in the brain [3]. Hypoxia is a decrease in tissue or ambient oxygen pressure below normal, and this can lead to unconsciousness, brain damage, and death. Cerebral blood flow (CBF) does not change in response to small fluctuations in arterial oxygen pressure [3]. When the arterial oxygen pressure falls below 50 mmHg, the CBF rises steeply. Carbon dioxide is a product of oxidative metabolism of glucose. CBF is very sensitive to small changes in arterial carbon dioxide pressure; vasodilatation and vasoconstriction occur with hypercapnia and hypocapnia, respectively.

Autoregulation of blood flow is a regulatory mechanism that maintains a relatively constant blood flow despite variations of arterial pressure [4]. Autoregulation of CBF is particularly well developed so that fluctuations of systemic arterial pressure are tolerated without development of cerebral ischemia or edema. Mechanisms of cerebral autoregulation are incompletely known and involve neurogenic, myogenic, endothelial and metabolic factors. Cerebral perfusion pressure equals the difference between mean arterial pressure and intracranial pressure. Cerebral resistance arteries dilate and constrict during falls and rises in cerebral perfusion pressure, respectively. At normal human cerebral perfusion pressures between 50 and 110 mmHg, average CBF is approximately 50 mL/min/100 g of brain tissue [4]; the corresponding mean arterial pressures are between 60 and 150 mmHg during this autoregulatory plateau. Ischemia refers to a low blood flow inadequate for delivery of oxygen, glucose and other nutrients as well as removal of metabolic waste products.

Ten per cents of the 55 million annual deaths in the world are attributed to stroke, making it the second leading cause of death (www.who.int/entity/ncd_surveillance /steps/stroke/en/flyerStroke2.pdf). Stroke is the third leading cause of death in United States of America and other developed countries. For every stroke death there are also three to four stroke survivors with variable degrees of neurologic disability. Owing to global aging of populations, the burden of stroke will escalate further; this is especially serious in developing countries. Ischemic stroke, or cerebral infarction, constitutes 85 to 90% of all strokes [5]. Focal ischemia can be due to thrombosis and/or embolism. Cardiac arrest, near drowning, carbon monoxide poisoning, massive hemorrhage, and shock are examples of global ischemia.

Despite decades of effort and billions of dollars spent on research, effective therapies of stroke are limited to intravenous thrombolysis using recombinant human tissue plasminogen activator within 3 hours of onset and intra-arterial thrombolysis using prourokinase within 6 hours of onset [5]. Acute thrombolysis is only feasible in a few percent of stroke patients, and there is also a substantial risk of life-threatening hemorrhagic transformation of the acute infarction. Neuroprotection against ischemia, i.e. enhancement of tolerance of cerebral tissue to ischemic injury, is conceptually very desirable [1]. Although there have been major advances in knowledge of ischemic pathophysiology and positive results have been obtained from experimental studies, neuroprotective chemical strategies have failed in more than 50 clinical trials (www.strokecenter.org/trials/index.htm).

Recent attention is on ischemic tolerance, also termed ischemic preconditioning. Ischemic tolerance is a natural phenomenon of evolutionary significance [6, 7]. All living organisms die upon exposure to a sufficiently toxic environment, such as ischemia or hypoxia. If the insult is not lethal, however, cells survive and, for a finite duration after a latent period, transiently develop relative tolerance to potentially lethal insults of the same as well as different nature. Thus, ischemic tolerance refers to this state of relative resistance to ischemia with much reduced cell death [8]. Ischemic tolerance is a form of endogenous neuroprotection and, potentially, one can augment the underlying mechanisms to lessen the severity of an impending or ongoing stroke. This review will cover ischemic pathophysiology, experimental evidence of ischemic tolerance, mechanisms of ischemic tolerance, clinical knowledge of ischemic tolerance, role of imaging in ischemic tolerance, and future perspectives.

## B. Ischemic Pathophysiology

During focal ischemia, reduction in CBF is severe at the center (ischemic core) and milder in the surrounding peripheral zone (ischemic penumbra) [9]. Middle cerebral artery occlusion is the most popular experimental model of focal ischemia. On the other hand, global ischemia is often achieved experimentally by occlusion of both common carotid arteries [1]. Following global ischemia, selective ischemic neuronal loss via apoptosis develops over next 7 days. Oxygen-glucose deprivation or hypoxia alone is commonly used in the *in vitro* stroke model [10, 11].

An acute occlusion of a cerebral artery usually results in severe cerebral ischemia and tissue infarction within the perfusion territory of the affected artery, unless the occlusion is rapidly reversed or there is adequate collateral circulation [2]. Neurons are rarely replaced after their death, rendering permanency of brain damage. The neurologic outcome is determined by the site and volume of the cerebral infarction. Cerebral autoregulation cannot cope with moderate to severe ischemia. When CBF is reduced to around 20 mL/100 g/min, the oxygen extraction fraction becomes maximal, the cerebral metabolic rate for oxygen begins to fall, normal neuronal functions are impaired, and cortical electroencephalographic activity ceases. This degree of ischemia represents a threshold of loss of neuronal electrical functions. When CBF falls below 10 mL/100 g/min, oxidative metabolism ceases, lactic acidosis develops from anaerobic glycolysis, ionic homeostasis fails, and irreversible cellular and tissue injury rapidly occurs [12].

The fundamental problem of ischemia is inability in maintaining an adequate cellular level of ATP required for various energy-consuming metabolic processes (Figure 1). Owing to a high rate of ATP consumption and an inherent inefficiency of anaerobic glycolysis, neuronal ATP concentrations typically fall to $<10\%$ within 5 minutes of severe ischemia (or hypoxia) [13]. Depletion of cellular ATP causes membrane depolarization plus uptake of sodium and water. Activation of voltage-gated calcium channels leads to calcium ion influx. Reversal of sodium-glutamate co-transportation causes spilling of glutamate into the extracellular space. The latter process is responsible for excessive stimulation of different types of glutamate receptors, leading to excitotoxicity [14]. Activation of the $\alpha$-amino-3-hydroxy-5-methyl-4-isoxazole-4-propionic acid (AMPA) type glutamate receptor leads to influx of sodium ion and water as well as efflux of potassium ion, contributing to depolarization and calcium ion influx via voltage-gated channels. Activation of the N-methyl-D-aspartate (NMDA) type glutamate receptor leads to influx of calcium ion, calcium ion overload and further depolarization. Activation of metabotropic glutamate receptors releases calcium ion from intracellular stores [15]. Elevated intracellular calcium ion concentration causes cellular oxidative stress as well as activation of lipases, proteases and endonucleases, leading to damage of DNA, cell proteins and lipids, and cellular membrane [16].

Nitric oxide (NO), a reactive gaseous free radical, is synthesized from L-arginine by the NO synthase (NOS). Type I or neuronal NOS (nNOS), type II or inducible NOS (iNOS), and type III or endothelial NOS (eNOS) are encoded on chromosome 12, 17, and 7, respectively [17, 18].

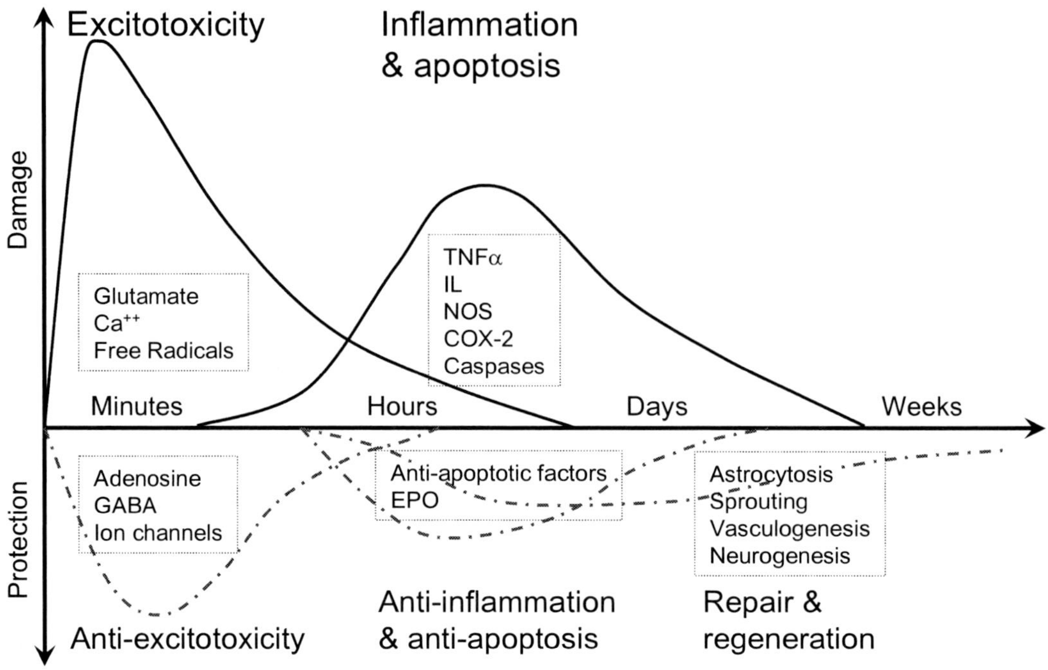


Figure 1. A schematic diagram showing the complex pathophysiology of cerebral ischemia and hypoxia (modified from reference [1]). A reduction in cellular ATP will lead to spreading depolarization, anerobic glycolysis, and failure of sodium-potassium pumps. Major mechanisms of injury include excitotoxicity, disturbed calcium ion homeostasis, mitochondrial dysfunctions, overproduction of nitric oxide and other free radicals, and inflammation. The final results include necrosis and apoptosis. See text for a more detailed description. AMPAR, α-amino-3-hydroxy-5-methyl-4-isoxazole-4-propionic acid type receptor; ATP, adenosine triphosphate; $Ca^{++}$, calcium ion; ER, endoplasmic reticulum; $Na^{+}$, sodium ion; $Na^{+}/K^{+}$, sodium-potassium ionic pump; NMDAR, N-methyl-D-aspartate type receptor; NO, nitric oxide; NOS, nitric oxide synthase; VGCC, voltage-gated calcium channel.

Excessive concentrations of NO cause lipid peroxidation and deplete cellular energy via disruption of mitochondrial enzymes and nucleic acids, react with superoxide anion to form peroxynitrite, a highly toxic and reactive nitrogen-based free radical, and trigger apoptotic cell death.

Depletion of calcium ion stores in the endoplasmic reticulum suppresses protein synthesis [16]. Massive influx of calcium ion into mitochondria causes free radical production from the mitochondrial respiratory chain, opening of the mitochondrial permeability transition pore, and secondary failure of mitochondrial functions. Superoxide anion can also be produced by cytosolic enzymes such as xanthine oxidase [19]. The highly toxic hydroxyl radical is readily generated via the metal-mediated Haber-Weiss reaction. The brain is very vulnerable to oxidative damage because of its relatively low antioxidant capacity, low activity of repair mechanisms, and high membrane surface to cytoplasm ratio [1].

Inflammation is capable of producing secondary damages [20]. There is activation and secretion of inflammatory cytokines such as tumor necrosis factor alpha, interleukin-1, and interleukin-6 [21]. Induction and expression of iNOS and cyclo-oxygenase (COX)-2, which is partly via activation of nuclear factor kappa B, also play a critical role in inflammatory reactions [20-22]. Polymorphonuclear leukocytes secrete toxic enzymes such as myeloperoxidase to produce further tissue and cellular damage [21]. Free radicals are important mediators of inflammatory tissue damage [1].

Apart from necrosis, cell death also occurs via apoptosis, or programmed cell death. Following ischemic injury, apoptosis may be responsible for half of the cellular loss. Free radicals and calcium ion activate pro-apoptotic proteins Bax and Bak, which oligomerize to form mitochondrial pores [23]. Mitochondrial release of cytochrome C provides an intrinsic signal for apoptosis, whereas activation of the tumor necrosis factor superfamily receptors constitutes an extrinsic signal for apoptosis. Upstream mechanisms of apoptosis include nuclear factor kappa B-dependent pathway, P53-dependent pathway, and pro-apoptotic members of the bcl family [21]. Activation of caspases is the downstream mechanism [24]; caspase 3 activates DNA breaking enzymes and energy consuming DNA repair enzymes, leading to DNA breakdown, energy wastage and cell death.

## Experimental Evidence of Ischemic Tolerance

Different types of preconditioning have been investigated in the brain, heart, retina, liver, kidney, and other organs [8, 25-27]. Toxic insults (preconditioning stimuli) used in the studies include ischemia, hypoxia or hyperoxia, hyperthermia or hypothermia, excitotoxicity, depolarization or seizures, and various chemicals.

Kitagawa and colleagues first reported in the gerbil global ischemic model that a brief period of ischemia for 2 min as the preconditioning stimulus plus an interval of 2 days would protect against subsequent damage from 5 to 10 min of global ischemia with reduced hippocampal neuronal loss [28, 29]. Similar results were replicated in the rat global ischemic stroke model [30]. Subsequent studies using rats or gerbils have shown that transient focal ischemia is capable of inducing local and remote ischemic tolerance against global ischemia [31, 32]. Ischemic tolerance against focal ischemia can be induced in rats or gerbils by either a brief episode of global or focal ischemia [33-37]. The aforementioned scenarios constitute the global-global, focal-global, global-focal, and focal-focal paradigms of ischemic tolerance, respectively. In general, ischemic tolerance is observed 24 hours or more after the preconditioning ischemic stimulus and lasts for 5 to 7 days [38]. Ischemic preconditioning also reduces susceptibility to damage due to seizures [39-41]. Epileptic tolerance is a related phenomenon in which prior brief periods of seizures would protect against subsequent neuronal injury due to severe or prolonged seizures [42].

Gidday and colleagues first reported in neonatal rat pups that a prior exposure to hypoxia (8% oxygen) for 3 hours at 1 day ago protected against combined hypoxia/ischemia [43]. A prior sub-lethal hypoxic stimulus also induces protection against the murine model of focal ischemia [44-46]. In addition, hypoxic preconditioning protects against subsequent lethal hypoxia or status epilepticus [47, 48]. Paradoxically, breathing pure oxygen at normal atmospheric pressure for 24 hours or hyperbaric oxygen for 1 hour induces tolerance against focal or global ischemia in the rats and gerbils [49, 50].

Cortical spreading depression (depolarization) is capable of producing ischemic tolerance in the rat brain [51, 52]. Transient hyperthermia or hypothermia can also act as a preconditioning stimulus for ischemic tolerance in both adult and neonatal rats [53, 54]. Chemical preconditioning refers to induction of ischemic tolerance by chemicals; this can be achieved by a mitochondrial inhibitor (e.g. 3-nitropropionic acid), kainic acid, thrombin, lipopolysaccharide, tumor necrosis factor alpha, E-selectin, linoleic acid, myelin basic protein, isoflurance, erythropoietin, ceramide, and desferrioxamine [55-66].

## Mechanisms of Ischemic Tolerance

Paradoxically, many mediators of ischemic pathophysiology (Figure 1) are also important or even required for the establishment of ischemic tolerance. It can be envisaged that ischemic tolerance is a form of endogenous adaptive neuroprotection developed in all living organisms from evolution in order to enhance survival against recurrent environmental hardships [6-8]. Thus, sub-lethal ischemic and non-ischemic insults can induce ischemic tolerance in the brain in which the acquired neuroprotection works well for subsequent ischemic and non-ischemic injury (i.e. cross tolerance). In addition, the same insults can induce ischemic tolerance in other organs. Furthermore, induced tolerance in one organ can spread to other organs (i.e. remote tolerance) [8]. Theoretically, induction of ischemic tolerance can be a useful clinical strategy to protect the brain against anticipated ischemia. These situations include operations on the heart and brain or their vascular supply as well as other high risk settings. There is a greater potential of clinical implications from elucidating the mechanisms of endogenous neuroprotection. Augmenting these endogenous neuroprotective mechanisms within a time window after onset of ischemia could greatly lessen the final volume of infarction.

As an example, focal cerebral ischemia not only induces a complex series of destructive mechanisms such as excitotoxicity, inflammation, and apoptosis but also, at the same time, activates rapid and delayed protective mechanisms, including anti-excitotoxicity, anti-inflammation and anti-apoptosis, and repair and regeneration (Figure 2) [8]. When the destructive effects prevail and exceed the rapid protective actions, ischemic infarction will appear. In contrast, a moderate ischemic insult does not cause tissue damage because the rapid protective actions equal or exceed the destructive effects. At the same time, the delayed protective actions, which involve de novo protein synthesis and outlast the ischemic insult, manifest as ischemic tolerance [8].

Numerous in vivo and in vitro studies have addressed the signaling mechanisms of ischemic tolerance. First, the state of ischemic tolerance is characterized by improved preservation of cellular energy metabolism despite ischemia. Successful adaptation to extreme habitats for a variety of vertebrates (e.g. fish, frog, turtles, snakes, diving seals and squirrels) illustrates that different animals have acquired during evolution different strategies to cope with brain anoxia (i.e. anoxia tolerant) or hibernation [6, 7]. The various mechanisms include suppression of metabolism, up or down regulation of key glycolytic enzymes, reduced conductance of ion channels, suppression of neural activity, expression of heat shock protein, adaptations in blood rheology, and increased level of antioxidants. Some but not all of these mechanisms were found in models of ischemic tolerance. For example, the response to hypoxia is highly conserved.

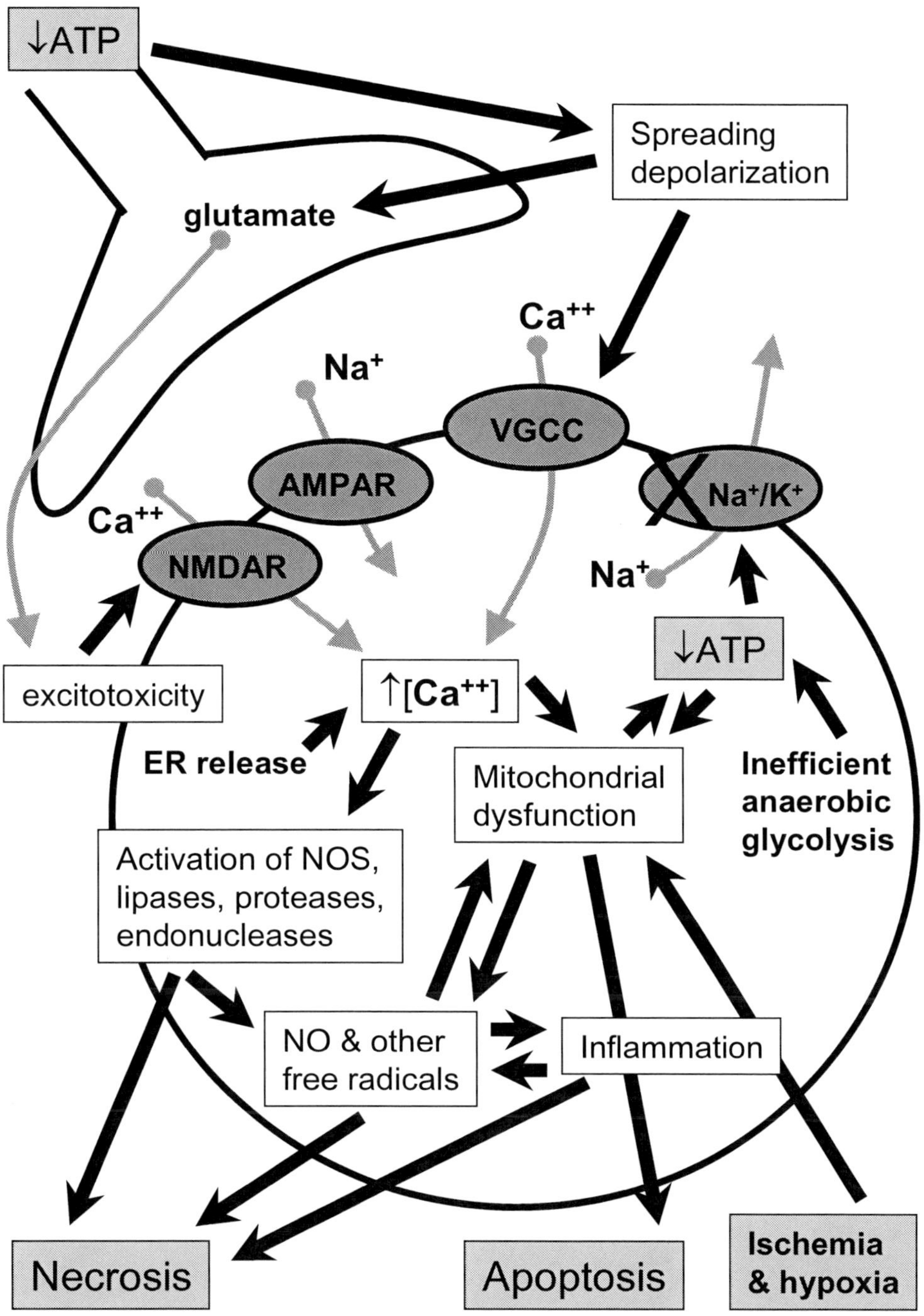


Figure 2. A schematic diagram summarizing the concept of ischemic tolerance (adapted from reference [6]). A noxious stimulus will simultaneously initiate both destructive and protective mechanisms. Excitotoxicity and anti-excitotoxicity represent immediate mechanisms. Inflammation and apoptosis as well as anti-inflammation and anti-apoptosis are early mechanisms. Repair and regeneration belong to late mechanisms. Conceptually, the final infarct will be determined by the balance of the destructive and protective mechanisms. $Ca^{++}$, calcium ion; COX-2, cyclo-oxygenase 2; EPO, erythropoietin; gaba, gama-amino-butyric acid; IL, interleukin; NOS, nitric oxide synthase; TNFα, tumor necrosis fator; and NOS, nitric oxide synthase.

Hypoxia activates the transcription factor hypoxia-inducible factor-1 which, in turn, up-regulates the activity of glucose transporter-1, phosphofructokinase and lactate dehydroxygenase [67, 68].

Adenosine, a breakdown product of ATP, adenosine A1 receptor and ATP-sensitive potassium ion channels play a key role in antagonizing the early events of ischemic pathophysiology [69]. In addition, adenosine is implicated in induction of ischemic tolerance. Thus, inhibition of adenosine receptors can block ischemic tolerance [70].

Many ischemic preconditioning models have shown the requirement of NMDA-receptor activation, modification of subunit composition of glutamate receptors, and/or up-regulation of inhibitory neurotransmitters [71]. Thus, exposure of cultured neuronal cells to low levels of glutamate or NMDA can induce ischemic tolerance. In addition, an NMDA antagonist can block the induction of ischemic tolerance by oxygen-glucose deprivation [72]. In preconditioned tissues, the expression of AMPA and metabotropic glutamate receptors is reduced [73, 74]. Furthermore, down-regulation of glutamate transporters on glial cells following cortical spreading depression may lessen the degree of excitotoxicity due to reversal of sodium-glutamate co-transportation during ischemia [75].

Dysregulated intracellular calcium ion concentrations mediate both ischemic pathophysiology and ischemic tolerance. The role of calcium ion in the mechanism of ischemic tolerance is multifactorial. It has a stimulatory role for the sublethal stimulus. During ischemic tolerance, calcium ion-dependent neurotoxic signaling to normally lethal ischemia is suppressed [71]. Genomics-based studies have shown pronounced up-regulation of gene expression in ischemic tolerance. This is partly via calcium-dependent phosphorylation of cAMP-response-element-binding protein (CREB). Increased CREB phosphorylation activates a number of genes [76]. NO can activate Ras and subsequently Erk; this pathway is required in the induction of ischemic tolerance by oxygen-glucose deprivation [77]. CREB is a potential target of Erk. Upon repeated exposure to hypoxia to induce ischemic tolerance, brain NO levels are reduced [78].

Chemical preconditioning from lipopolysaccharide involves an increased activity of superoxide dismutase and eNOS [58]. Interleukin-1 and tumor necrosis factor-alpha are also up-regulated [79]. Chemical preconditioning from tumor necrosis factor-alpha or its downstream mediator, ceramide, blocks recruitment of a calcium-binding protein to the p65 nuclear factor kappa B binding sites on DNA, which in turn, modifies nuclear factor kappa B expression. The latter effect lessens expression of pro-inflammatory intercellular-adhesion molecule 1 but preserves expression of manganese superoxide dismutase [80]. Inhibition of nuclear factor kappa B activity can block ischemic tolerance [81].

Ischemia activates genes for both apoptosis (e.g. bax) and also anti-apoptosis (e.g. bcl2) [82]. Phosphorylation of CREB is a driving factor for bcl2 induction during ischemic tolerance, and bcl2 up-regulates mitochondrial base-excision repair capability [83].

Ischemia or hypoxia also leads to induction of heat shock proteins. These proteins function as 'molecular chaperones' to assist protein conformation, degradation or reactivation of damaged proteins, intracellular trafficking, and nuclear receptor binding. [84]. Thus, the beneficial effects of heat shock proteins may derive from stabilization of anti-oxidative enzymes, reduction of calcium ion influx, attenuation of activity of destructive enzymes, and inhibition of caspase [85-87].

Although there is much information on the signaling cascades and important factors of many models of ischemic tolerance, the underlying mechanisms of ischemic tolerance have not been fully elucidated. It is possible that some mechanisms are organ/tissue specific and/or species specific. More experimental studies are required for this aspect.

# C. Clinical Knowledge

Efficacy and safety of ischemic tolerance in the brain have not been addressed by prospective randomized control trials. Nevertheless, the clinical scenario of a transient ischemic attack (TIA) followed by a ischemic stroke raises the intriguing debate of whether the prodromal TIA can induce a state of ischemic tolerance and lessen the severity of the subsequent stroke. Weih and colleagues conducted a retrospective case-control study in 148 stroke patients with or without a preceding TIA. Their results indicated that a preceding TIA was an independent predictor of milder strokes in multivariate models and supported the existence of ischemic tolerance in the human brain [88].

In a larger retrospective review of 2,490 stroke patients in a prospective database, Moncayo and colleagues confirmed that patients with prior ipsilateral TIAs before their ischemic strokes had less severe strokes and a more favorable outcome. The additional characteristics of a 'protective' TIA include duration between 10 and 20 minutes and an interval within one week of the presenting ischemic strokes [89].

Paradoxically, there is strong evidence that early risk of stroke after TIA is higher than after ischemic stroke. The reported risks of stroke after a stroke range from 2% to 7% at 3-month follow-up [90-92]. An early study on short-term prognosis of TIA from a retrospective chart review of 199 patients with a diagnosis of TIA in Rochester, Minnesota reported an 8% risk of stroke in the first month after a TIA [93]. A more recent study of 1,707 patients from 16 hospitals in a health maintenance organization in Northern California reported a 90-day stroke risk of 10.5%, and 50% of the strokes occurred within the first 2 days of the TIA [94]. Repeat analysis of the population-based study from the Oxfordshire Community Stroke Project in England including 209 first-ever TIA patients noted a 7-day stroke risk of 8.6% and a 30-day stroke risk of 12% [95]. Another recent but small study of 87 TIA patients in Oxfordshire reported an 8.0% risk of recurrent stroke at 7 days, 11.5% at 30 days, and 17.3% at 90 days [96].

## Role of Imaging in Ischemic Tolerance

Unlike experimental studies in which the inducing stimulus and the otherwise lethal ischemia can be tightly regulated plus quantitative measurement of the ischemic damage and functional impairment, most clinical studies measure neurologic deficits and report clinical outcomes. Perfusion imaging of cerebral ischemia can greatly assist clinical studies of novel neuroprotective therapies, including ischemic tolerance. The concept of ischemic tolerance is that the brain tissue is more resistant to ischemia. Measuring the CBF can quantify the degree and extent of ischemia, and ischemic tolerance is revealed by brain regions surviving with low CBF which would otherwise become infarcted.

A recent retrospective case-control study of 65 stroke patients of a prospective database who received diffusion- and perfusion-weighted magnetic resonance imaging within 12 hours of symptom onset serves as an example. In this study, Wegener and colleagues noted that patients with a prior TIA had similar perfusion deficits as in others without a prior TIA. Nevertheless, a prior TIA is associated with smaller initial diffusion lesions and final infarct volumes as well as a better clinical outcome. The optimal interval between the TIA and stroke should be within 4 weeks [97]. Without documenting similar perfusion deficits at baseline, Wegener and colleagues would not be able to conclude from a relatively small number of patients that a prior TIA may induce ischemic tolerance in the human brain.

Several imaging techniques are available for CBF measurement [98]. Radioactive xenon ($^{133}Xe$) is lipophilic, permitting diffusion through the blood-brain barrier; this is the oldest used tracer. Following inhalation or injection, probes placed over the scalp can measure perfusion to the cerebral cortex [99]. Using a number of radioisotopes, positron emission tomography (PET) can measure CBF and various metabolic processes [100]. Nevertheless, PET remains an expensive research tool with limited availability. Stable xenon is utilized as a perfusion tracer in xenon-enhanced computed tomography (CT) [101]. Compounds metabolized by the brain cells can be tagged to radioisotopes to generate perfusion imaging in single photon emission CT [102].

Perfusion-weighted magnetic resonance imaging can be based on the first pass bolus tracking technique or the arterial spin-labelling method [103-105]. Finally, availability of helical and spiral multislice CT technology has permitted CT perfusion imaging methods. The latter include a slow-infusion/whole-brain non-quantative technique, a fast-injection (10 to 20 mL/s) first-pass bolus-tracking quantitative method, and a slow-injection (3 to 4 mL/s) first-pass bolus tracking quantitative technique (Figure 3) [106-109]. A recent review from the American Heart Association on perfusion imaging in cerebral ischemia outlines the basic principles, the published data, the advantages and disadvantages of commonly available imaging techniques (Table 1), and calls for more studies [98].

## D. Future Perspectives

The fact that the brain's resistance to ischemic injury can be significantly enhanced by a preconditioning stimulus in the form of ischemic tolerance is both exciting and attractive. Existence of anoxia tolerant brains in some vertebrates has clearly shown that different natural forms of ischemic tolerance are independently derived from evolution. Demonstration of ischemic tolerance in various models involving different organs further illustrates its physiological nature. Although the mechanisms of ischemic tolerance have been investigated in many experimental studies, there is no unified theory on the cellular mechanisms. Whereas TIA may be the clinical counterpart of the conditioning stimulus, TIA is itself a high risk condition and cannot be used as a preconditioning stimulus for ischemic tolerance. Of all inducing stimuli, chemical preconditioning appears to have some therapeutic potential. Clinically approved drugs like erythropoietin, isoflurane and ATP-sensitive potassium ion channel-openers may be suitable as inducers. In addition, small molecules capable of activating specific transcription factors may mediate endogenous neuroprotection.

A more complete understanding of the cellular mechanisms of ischemic tolerance is required to identify or produce more precisely targeted preconditioning drugs. Next, well-designed randomized control trials are awaited to show the clinical relevance of ischemic tolerance. Ability to quantify the CBF is required to reveal the existence of ischemic tolerance in clinical studies as regions with low CBF which would otherwise become infarcted. Nevertheless, two fundamental properties of ischemic tolerance may hinder its therapeutic potential: delayed in onset and transient nature. Thus, the effective time window of using this form of treatment is uncertain. It is also unknown whether ischemic tolerance can be persistently induced and if prolonged ischemic tolerance has any negative effect on the brain and rest of the body.

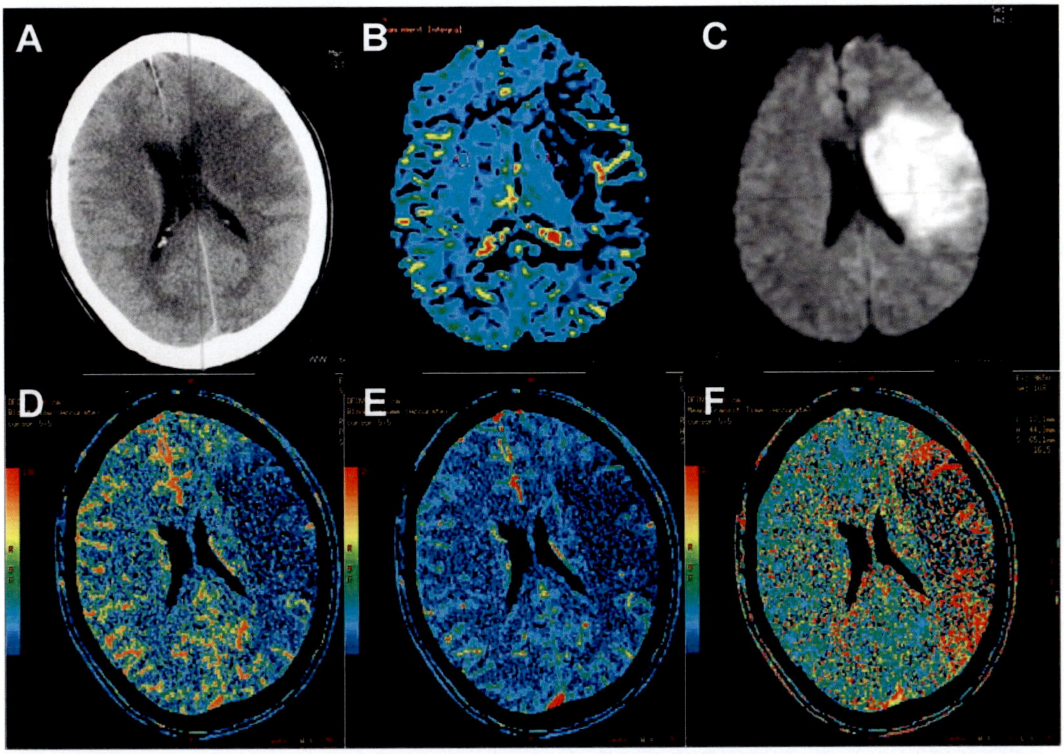


Figure 3. A 51-year-old with acute left middle cerebral artery (MCA) territory infarction presented with right hemiplegia and aphasia. Computed tomography (CT) and magnetic resonance imaging (MRI) were performed at about 15 hours of onset. Plain CT (A) reveals hypodensity over left MCA territory. Perfusion-weighted MRI (B) reveals marked hypoperfusion over entire left MCA territory which is larger than the acute infarction as shown by diffusion-weighted MRI (C). A dynamic CT perfusion study using intravenous injection of 40 mL of contrast at 4 mL/s revealed a marked decrease in cerebral blood flow (CBF; D) and cerebral blood volume (CBV; E) with low value of mean transient time (MTT; F). The regions with perfusion-diffusion mismatch (B, C) represent ischemic penumbra where CBV is maintained, CBF is low, and MTT is prolonged. Therapeutic use of ischemic tolerance in acute stroke treatment is expected to salvage the ischemic penumbra plus parts of the brain tissue undergoing infarction.

**Table 1. Advantages and disadvantages of commonly available perfusion technologies (adapted from [98])**

| Perfusion techniques | Relative advantages | Relative disadvantages |
|---|---|---|
| Xenon CT | CT widely available<br>Additional complementary data from plain CT, CT angiography<br>Quantitative CBF data obtainable<br>Hardware and software relatively non-expensive<br>Standardization between different systems feasible<br>Challenge tests available for cerebrovascular reserve<br>Ample animal and human data from the literature | Sedative effect<br>Susceptible to motion artifacts<br>Data on CBF only<br>Cell/tissue viability not assessed |
| Single photon emission CT | Easy to perform<br>Widely available in large radiology departments<br>Generating 3 orthogonal views of CBF<br>Semi-quantitative data obtainable | Required a short time to make the injected radioisotope<br>Non-anatomic data requiring tedious co-registration with the CT or MRI image<br>Low spatial resolution<br>Semi-quantitative data only<br>Comparisons between repeated studies, among different patients, or between different systems difficult and misleading<br>Limited ability to perform challenge tests on cerebrovascular reserve |

**Table 1. (Continued)**

| Perfusion techniques | Relative advantages | Relative disadvantages |
|---|---|---|
| Perfusion CT | Helical and spiral CT scanners widely available | Limited coverage of brain tissue |
| | Additional complementary data from plain CT, CT angiography | Radiation dose |
| | Rapid methodology | Infarcted tissue not readily visualized |
| | Quantitative CBF data obtainable | Required a robust measurement of arterial input function for quantification |
| | Additional data on CBV and MTT | Accuracy affected by breakdown of blood-brain-barrier |
| | Software relatively non-expensive | Uncertain role in chronic ischemia, vasospasm, head injury, and risk of hemorrhagic transformation |
| | Challenge tests available for cerebrovascular reserve | Number of repeated examinations limited by total amount of tolerable contrast |
| | Available animal and human data from the literature | |
| Perfusion MRI | Additional complementary data from anatomical MRI, MR angiography | Expensive equipment |
| | Infarct revealed by diffusion-weighted MRI | Total time of examination being long |
| | Rapid methodology for a whole brain examination | Non-quantitative CBF and MTT data |
| | Available human data from the literature | Comparisons between different systems impossible |
| | | Limited ability to perform challenge tests on cerebrovascular reserve |
| | | Uncertain role in chronic ischemia, vasospasm, head injury, and risk of hemorrhagic transformation |

CBF, cerebral blood flow; CBV, cerebral blood volume; CT, computed tomography; MR, magnetic resonance; MRI, magnetic resonance imaging; MTT, mean transient time.

# E. Take-Home-Message

The human brain is very sensitive to ischemia, and stroke is a major global disease with high mortality and morbidity. Ischemic tolerance, a natural phenomenon seen in many organs, may be utilized for neuroprotection against stroke. A sub-lethal noxious stimulus will activate a complex and interacted processes, including both damaging and protective mechanisms. Protective mechanisms, which involve new protein synthesis, outlast the stimulus and manifest as ischemic tolerance. TIA is the clinical equivalence of preconditioning stimulus. However, more work is required to identify the most important cellular mechanism and the promising chemical agents for further evaluation in clinical trials. Direct visualization of severity and extent of ischemia by quantitative imaging of CBF will facilitate clinical studies on the therapeutic potential of ischemic tolerance. Unless it is possible and safe to repeatedly or persistently induce ischemic tolerance, however, this therapy may not overcome the problem of short therapeutic time window when used as an acute treatment and may not be safe when adopted as a preventive measure.

# References

[1] Cheung RT. The utility of melatonin in reducing cerebral damage resulting from ischemia and reperfusion. *J. Pineal. Res.* 2003; 34: 153-160.

[2] Schaller B, Graf R. Cerebral ischemia and reperfusion: the pathophysiologic concept as a basis for clinical therapy. *J. Cereb. Blood Flow Metab.* 2004; 24: 351-371.

[3] Golanov EV, Reis DJ. Oxygen and cerebral blood flow. In Welch KM, Caplan LR, Reis DJ, Siesjo BK, Weir B (eds.): *Primer on Cerebrovascular Diseases*, Academic Press, New York, 1997; Chp. 15: 58-60.

[4] Chillon JM, Baumbach GL. Autoregulation of cerebral blood flow. In Welch KM, Caplan LR, Reis DJ, Siesjo BK, Weir B (eds.): *Primer on Cerebrovascular Diseases*, Academic Press, New York, 1997; Chp. 13: 51-54.

[5] Cheung RT. Cerebrovascular disease - advances in management. *Hong Kong Med. J.* 2001; 7: 58-66.

[6] Bickler PE, Donohoe PH, Buck LT. Molecular adaptations for survival during anoxia: lessons from lower vertebrates. *Neuroscientist* 2002; 8: 234-242.

[7] Nilsson GE, Lutz PL. Anoxia tolerant brains. *J. Cereb. Blood Flow Metab.* 2004; 24: 475-486.

[8] Dirnagl U, Simon RP, Hallenbeck JM. Ischemic tolerance and endogenous neuroprotection. *Trend Neurosci.* 2003; 26: 248-254.

[9] Hossmann KA. Viability thresholds and the penumbra of focal ischemia. *Ann. Neurol.* 1994; 36: 557-565.

[10] Lipton P. Ischemic cell death in brain neurons. *Physiol. Rev.* 1999; 79: 1431-1568.

[11] Pei Z, Cheung RT. Melatonin protects SHSY5Y neuronal cells but not cultured astrocytes from ischemia due to oxygen and glucose deprivation. *J. Pineal. Res.* 2003; 34: 194-201.

[12] Hakim AM. The cerebral ischemic penumbra. *Can. J. Neurol. Sci.* 1987; 14:557-559.

[13] Siesjo BK. Pathophysiology and treatment of focal cerebral ischemia: Part I. Pathophysiology. *J. Neurosurg.* 1992; 77: 169-184.

[14] Ikonomidou C, Turski L. Excitotoxicity and neurodegenerative diseases. *Curr. Opin. Neurol.* 1995; 8: 487-497.

[15] Lee JM, Zipfel GJ, Choi DW. The changing landscape of ischaemic brain injury mechanisms. *Nature* 1999; 399(suppl): A7-A14.

[16] Paschen W. Role of calcium in neuronal cell injury: which subcellular compartment is involved? *Brain Res. Bull.* 2000; 53:409-413.

[17] Chen SH, Fung PC, Cheung RT. Neuropeptide Y-Y1 receptor modulates nitric oxide level during stroke in the rat. *Free Rad. Biol. Med.* 2002; 32: 776-784.

[18] Pei Z, Fung PC, Cheung RT. Melatonin reduces nitric oxide level during ischemia but not blood-brain-barrier breakdown during reperfusion in a rat middle cerebral artery occlusion stroke model. *J. Pineal. Res.* 2003; 34: 110-118.

[19] Chan PH. Reactive oxygen radicals in signaling and damage in the ischemic brain. *J. Cereb. Blood Flow Metab.* 2001; 21: 2-14.

[20] Iadecola C, Alexander M. Cerebral ischemia and inflammation. *Curr. Opin. Neurol.* 2001; 14: 89-94.

[21] Leker RR, Shohami E. Cerebral ischemia and trauma – different etiologies yet similar mechanisms: neuroprotective opportunities. Brain *Res. Rev.* 2002; 39: 55-73.

[22] Cheung RT, Pei Z, Feng ZH, et al. Cyclooxygenase-1-gene knockout does not alter middle cerebral artery occlusion in a mouse stroke model. *Neurosci. Lett.* 2002; 330: 57-60.

[23] Mattson MP, Kroemer G. Mitochondria in cell death: novel targets for neuroprotection and cardioprotection. *Trends Mol. Med.* 2003; 9: 196-205.

[24] Snider BJ, Gottron FJ, Choi DW. Apoptosis and necrosis in cerebrovascular disease. *Ann. NY Acad. Sci.* 1999; 893: 243-253.

[25] Rejdak R, Rejdak K, Sieklucke-Dziuba M, et al. Brain tolerance and preconditioning. *Pol. J. Pharmacol.* 2001; 53: 73-79.

[26] Sharp FR, Ran R, Lu A, et al. Hypoxic preconditioning protects against ischemic brain injury. *Neurorx* 2004; 1: 26-35.

[27] Zemke D, Smith JL, Reeves MJ, et al. Ischemia and ischemic tolerance in the brain: an overview. *Neurotoxicology* 2004; 25: 895-904.

[28] Kitagawa K, Matsumoto M, Tagaya M, et al. 'Ischemic tolerance' phenomenon found in the brain. Brain Res 1990; 528: 21-24.

[29] Kitagawa K, Matsumoto M, Kuwabara K, et al. 'Ischemic tolerance' phenomenon detected in various brain regions. *Brain Res.* 1991; 561: 203-211.

[30] Nishi S, Taki W, Uemura Y, et al. Ischemic tolerance due to the induction of HSP70 in a rat ischemic recirculation model. *Brain Res.* 1993; 615: 281-288.

[31] Glazier SS, O'Rourke DM, Graham DI, et al. Induction of ischemic tolerance following brief focal ischemia in rat brain. *J. Cereb. Blood Flow Metab.* 1994; 14: 545-553.

[32] Miyashita K, Abe H, Nakajima T. Induction of ischaemic tolerance in gerbil hippocampus by pretreatment with focal ischaemia. *Neuroreport* 1994; 6: 46-48.

[33] Barone FC, White RF, Spera PA, et al. Ischemic preconditioning and brain tolerance: temporal histological and functional outcomes, protein synthesis requirement, and

interleukin-1 receptor antagonist and early gene expression. *Stroke* 1998; 29: 1937-1950.

[34] Simon RP, Niiro M, Gwinn R. Prior ischemic stress protects against experimental stroke. *Neurosci. Lett.* 1993; 163: 135-137.

[35] Chen J, Graham SH, Zhu RL, et al. Stress proteins and tolerance to focal cerebral ischemia. *J. Cereb. Blood Flow Metab.* 1996; 16: 566-577.

[36] Kitagawa K, Matsumoto M, Matsushita K, et al. Ischemic tolerance in moderately symptomatic gerbils after unilateral carotid occlusion. *Brain Res.* 1996; 716: 39-46.

[37] Kitagawa K, Matsumoto M, Mabuchi T, et al. Ischemic tolerance in hippocampal CA1 neurons studied using contralateral controls. *Neuroscience* 1997; 81: 989-998.

[38] Chen J, Simon R. Ischemic tolerance in the brain. *Neurology* 1997; 48: 306-311.

[39] Bortolotto ZA, Heim C, Sieklucka M, et al. Effects of bilateral clamping of carotid arteries on hippocampal kindling in rats. *Physiol. Behav.* 1991; 49: 667-671.

[40] Heim C, Bortolotto ZA, Cavalheiro EA, et al. Transient occlusion of rat carotid arteries decreases susceptibility to pilocarpine seizures. *Brain Res.* 1991; 18: 253-259.

[41] Sieklucka M, Bortolotto ZA, Heim C, et al. Decreased susceptibility to seizures induced by bicuculline after transient bilateral clamping of carotid arteries in rats. *J. Neural. Transm.* 1991; 83: 127-137.

[42] Sasahira M, Lowry T, Simon RP, et al. Epileptic tolerance: prior seizures protect against seizure-induced neuronal injury. *Neurosci. Lett.* 1995; 185: 95-98.

[43] Gidday JM, Shah AR, Maceren RG, et al. Nitric oxide mediates cerebral ischemic tolerance in a neonatal rat model of hypoxic preconditioning. *J. Cereb. Blood Flow Metab.* 1999; 19: 331-340.

[44] Miller BA, Perez RS, Shah AR, et al. Cerebral protection by hypoxic preconditioning in a murine model of focal ischemia-reperfusion. *Neuroreport* 2001; 12: 1663-1669.

[45] Bernaudin M, Nedelec AS, Divoux D, et al. Normobaric hypoxia induces tolerance to focal permanent cerebral ischemia in association with an increased expression of hypoxia-inducible factor-1 and its target genes, erythropoietin and VEGF, in the adult mouse brain. *J. Cereb. Blood Flow Metab.* 2002; 22: 393-403.

[46] Prass K, Scharff A, Ruscher K, et al. Hypoxia-induced stroke tolerance in the mouse is mediated by erythropoietin. *Stroke* 2003; 34: 1981-1986.

[47] Stroev SA, Gluschenko TS, Tjulkova EI, et al. Preconditioning enhances the expression of mitochondrial antioxidant thioredoxin-2 in the forebrain of rats exposed to severe hypobaric hypoxia. *J. Neurosci. Res.* 2004; 78: 563-569.

[48] Emerson MR, Nelson SR, Samson FE, et al. Hypoxia preconditioning attenuates brain edema associated with kainic acid-induced status epilepticus in rats. *Brain Res.* 1999; 825: 189-193.

[49] Wada K, Ito M, Miyazawa T, et al. Repeated hyperbaric oxygen induces ischemic tolerance in gerbil hippocampus. *Brain Res.* 1996; 740: 15-20.

[50] Zhang X, Xiong L, Hu W, et al. Preconditioning with prolonged oxygen exposure induces ischemic tolerance in the brain via oxygen free radical formation. *Can. J. Anaesth.* 2004; 51: 258-263.

[51] Kobayashi S, Harris VA, Welsh FA. Spreading depression induces tolerance of cortical neurons to ischemia in rat brain. *J. Cereb. Blood Flow Metab.* 1995; 15: 721-727.

[52] Matsushima K, Hogan MJ, Hakim AM. Cortical spreading depression protects against subsequent focal cerebral ischemia in rats. *J. Cereb. Blood Flow Meatb.* 1996; 16: 221-226.
[53] Chopp M, Chen H, Ho KL. Transient hyperthermia protects against subsequent forebrain ischemic cell damage in the rat. *Neurology* 1989; 39: 1396-1398.
[54] Nishio S, Yunoki M, Chen ZF, et al. Ischemic tolerance in the rat neocortex following hypothermic preconditioning. *J. Neurosurg.* 2000; 93: 845-851.
[55] Nakase H, Heimann A, Uranishi R, et al. Early-onset tolerance in rat global cerebral ischemia induced by a mitochondrial inhibitor. *Neurosci. Lett.* 2000; 290: 105-118.
[56] Plamondon H, Blondeau N, Heurteaux C, et al. Mutually protective actions of kainic acid epileptic preconditioning and sublethal global ischemia on hippocampal neuronal death: involvement of adenosine A1 receptors and K(ATP) channels. *J. Cereb. Blood Flow Metab.* 1999; 19: 1296-1308.
[57] Striggow F, Riek M, Breder J, et al. The protease thrombin is an endogenous mediator of hippocampal neuroprotection against ischemia at low concentrations but causes degeneration at high concentrations. *Proc. Natl. Acad. Sci. USA* 2000; 97: 2264-2269.
[58] Bordet R, Deplanque D, Maboudou P, et al. Increase in endogenous brain superoxide dismutase as a potential mechanism of lipopolysaccharide-induced brain ischemic tolerance. *J. Cereb. Blood Flow Metab.* 2000; 20: 1190-1196.
[59] Nawashiro H, Tasaki K, Ruetzler CA, et al. TNF-alpha pretreatment induces protective effects against focal cerebral ischemia in mice. *J. Cereb Blood Flow Metab.* 1997; 17: 483-490.
[60] Takeda H, Spatz M, Ruetzler C, et al. Induction of mucosal tolerance to E-selectin prevents ischemic and hemorrhagic stroke in spontaneously hypertensive genetically stroke-prone rats. *Stroke* 2002; 33: 2156-2163.
[61] Blondeau N, Widmann C, Lazdunski M, et al. Polyunsaturated fatty acids induce ischemic and epileptic tolerance. *Neuroscience* 2002; 109: 231-241.
[62] Becker KJ, McCarron RM, Ruetzler C, et al. Immunologic tolerance to myelin basic protein decreases stroke size after transient focal cerebral ischemia. *Proc. Natl. Acad. Sci. USA* 1997; 94: 10873-10878.
[63] Xiong L, Zheng Y, Wu M, et al. Preconditioning with isoflurane produces dose-dependent neuroprotection via activation of adenosine triphosphate-regulated potassium channels after focal cerebral ischemia in rats. *Anesth. Analg.* 2003; 96: 233-237.
[64] Digicaylioglu M, Lipton SA. Erythropoietin-mediated neuroprotection involves cross-talk between Jak2 and NF-κB signaling cascades. *Nature* 2001; 412: 641-647.
[65] Furuya K, Ginis I, Takeda H, et al. Cell permeable exogenous ceramide reduces infarct size in spontaneously hypertensive rats supporting in vitro studies that have implicated ceramide in induction of tolerance to ischemia. *J. Cereb. Blood Flow Metab.* 2001; 21: 226-232.
[66] Prass K, Ruscher K, Karsch M, et al. Desferrioxamine induces delayed tolerance against cerebral ischemia in vivo and in vitro. *J. Cereb. Blood Flow Metab.* 2002; 22: 520-525.

[67] Jones NM, Bergeron M. Hypoxic preconditioning induces changes in HIF-1 target genes in neonatal rat brain. *J. Cereb. Blood Flow Metab.* 2001; 21: 1105-1114.
[68] Bernaudin M, Nedelec AS, Divoux D, et al. Normobaric hypoxia induces tolerance to focal permanent cerebral ischemia in association with an increased expression of hypoxia-inducible factor-1 and its target genes, erythropoietin and VEGF, in the adult mouse brain. *J. Cereb. Blood Flow Metab.* 2002; 22: 393-403.
[69] Heurteaux C, Lauritzen I, Widmann C, et al. Essential role of adenosine, adenosine A1 receptors, and ATP-sensitive $K^+$ channels in cerebral ischemic preconditioning. *Proc. Natl. Acad. Sci. USA* 1995; 92: 4666-4670.
[70] Hiraide T, Katsura K, Muramatsu H, et al. Adenosine receptor antagonists cancelled the ischemic tolerance phenomenon in gerbils. *Brain Res.* 2001; 910: 94-98.
[71] Tauskela JS, Morley P. On the role of $Ca^{2+}$ in cerebral ischemic preconditioning. *Cell Calcium.* 2004; 36: 313-322.
[72] Grabb MC, Choi DW. Ischemic tolerance in murine cortical cell culture: critical role for NMDA receptors. *J. Neurosci.* 1999; 19: 1657-1662.
[73] Sommer C, Roth SU, Kuhn R, et al. Metabotropic glutamate receptor subtypes are differentially expressed after transient cerebral ischemia without, during and after tolerance induction in the gerbil hippocampus. *Brain Res.* 2000; 872: 172-180.
[74] Deng W, Rosenberg PA, Volpe JJ, et al. Calcium-permeable AMPA/kainite receptors mediate toxicity and preconditioning by oxygen-glucose deprivation in oligodendrocyte precursors. *Proc. Natl. Acad. Sci. USA* 2003; 100: 6801-6806.
[75] Douen AG, Akiyama K, Hogan MJ, et al. Preconditioning with cortical spreading depression decreases intraischemic cerebral glutamate levels and down-regulates excitatory amino acid transporters EAAT1 and EAAT2 from rat cerebal cortex plasma membranes. *J. Neurochem.* 2000; 75: 812-818.
[76] Hara T, Hamada J, Yano S, et al. CREB is required for acquisition of ischemic tolerance in gerbil hippocampal CA1 region. *J. Neurochem.* 2003; 86: 805-814.
[77] Gonzalez-Zulueta M, Feldman AB, Klesse LJ, et al. Requirement for nitric oxide activation of p21(ras)/extracellular regulated kinase in neuronal ischemic preconditioning. *Proc. Natl. Acad. Sci. USA* 2000; 97: 436-441.
[78] Lu GW, Liu HY. Downregulation of nitric oxide in the brain of mice during their hypoxic preconditioning. *J. Appl. Physiol.* 2001; 91: 1193-1198.
[79] Ohtsuki T, Ruetzler CA, Tasaki K, et al. Interleukin-1 mediates induction of tolerance to global ischemia in gerbil hippocampal CA1 neurons. *J. Cereb. Blood Flow Metab.* 1996; 16: 1137-1142.
[80] Ginis I, Jaiswal R, Klimanis D, et al. TNF-alpha-induced tolerance to ischemic injury involves differential control of NF-kappaB transactivation: the role of NF-kappaB association with p300 adaptor. *J. Cereb. Blood Flow Metab.* 2002; 22: 142-152.
[81] Blondeau N, Widmann C, Lazdunski M, et al. Activation of the nuclear factor-kappaB is a key event in brain tolerance. *J. Neurosci.* 2001; 21: 4668-4677.
[82] Shimizu S, Nagayama T, Jin KL, et al. bcl-2 Antisense treatment prevents induction of tolerance to focal ischemia in the rat brain. *J. Cereb. Blood Flow Metab.* 2001; 21: 233-243.

[83] Walton MR, Dragunow I. Is CREB a key to neuronal survival? *Trends Neurosci.* 2000; 23: 48-53.
[84] Tanaka H, Calderone A, Jover T, et al. Ischemic preconditioning acts upstream of GluR2 down-regulation to afford neuroprotection in the hippocampal CA1. *Proc. Natl. Acad. Sci. USA* 2002; 99: 2362-2367.
[85] Koroshetz WJ, Bonventre JV. Heat shock response in the central nervous system. *Experientia* 1994; 50: 1085-1091.
[86] Mosser DD, Caron AW, Bourget L, et al. Role of the human heat shock protein hsp70 in protection against stress-induced apoptosis. *Mol. Cell Biol.* 1997; 17: 5317-5327.
[87] Yenari MA, Giffard RG, Sapolsky RM, et al. The neuroprotective potential of heat shock protein 70 (HSP70). *Mol. Med. Today* 1999; 5: 525-531.
[88] Weih M, Kallenberg K, Bergk A, et al. *Attenuated stroke severity after prodromal TIA*: a role for ischemic tolerance in the brain?
[89] Moncayo J, de Freitas GR, Bogousslavsky J, et al. Do transient ischemic attacks have a neuroprotective effect? *Neurology* 2000;54:2089-2094.
[90] Burn J, Dennis M, Bamford J, et al. Long-term risk of recurrent stroke after a first-ever stroke. The Oxfordshire Community Stroke Project. *Stroke* 1994; 25: 333-337.
[91] Sacco RL, Shi T, Zamanillo MC, et al. Predictors of mortality and recurrence after hospitalized cerebral infarction in an urban community: the Northern Manhattan Stroke Study. *Neurology* 1994; 44: 626-634.
[92] Petty GW, Brown RD Jr, Whisnant JP, et al. Survival and recurrence after first cerebral infarction: a population-based study in Rochester, Minnesota, 1975 through 1989. *Neurology* 1998; 50: 208-216.
[93] Whisnant JP, Matsumoto N, Elveback LR. Transient cerebral ischemic attacks in a community. Rochester, Minnesota, 1955 through 1969. *Mayo Clin. Proc.* 1973; 48: 194-198.
[94] Johnston SC, Gress DR, Browner WS, et al. Short-term prognosis after emergency department diagnosis of TIA. *JAMA* 2000; 284: 2901-1906.
[95] Lovett JK, Dennis MS, Sandercock PA, et al. Very early risk of stroke after a first transient ischemic attack. *Stroke* 2003; 34: e138-e140.
[96] Coull AJ, Lovett JK, Rothwell PM; Oxford Vascular Study. Population based study of early risk of stroke after transient ischaemic attack or minor stroke: implications for public education and organisation of services. *BMJ* 2004; 328: 326-328.
[97] Wegener S, Gottschalk B, Jovanovic V, et al. Transient ischemic attacks before ischemic stroke: preconditioning the human brain? A multicenter magnetic resonance imaging study. *Stroke* 2004; 35: 616-621.
[98] Latchaw RE, Yonas H, Hunter GJ, et al. Guidelines and recommendations for perfusion imaging in cerebral ischemia: A scientific statement for healthcare professionals by the writing group on perfusion imaging, from the Council on Cardiovascular Radiology of the American Heart Association. *Stroke* 2003; 34: 1084-1104.
[99] Obrist WD, Thompson HK, Wang HS, et al. Regional cerebral blood flow estimated by 133-xenon inhalation. Stroke 1975; 6: 245-256.

[100] Powers WJ, Grubb RL, Darriet D, et al. Cerebral blood flow and cerebral metabolic rate of oxygen requirements for cerebral function and viability in humans. *J. Cereb. Blood Flow Metab.* 1985; 5: 600-608.

[101] Yonas H, Gur D, Claassen D, et al. Stable xenon enhanced computed tomography in the study of clinical and pathologic correlates of focal ischemia in baboons. *Stroke* 1988; 19: 228-238.

[102] Weir CJ, Bolster AA, Tytler S, Murray GD, Corrigall RS, Adams FG, Lees KR. Prognostic value of single-photon emission tomography in acute ischaemic stroke. *Eur. J. Nucl. Med.* 1997; 24: 21-26.

[103] Kucharczyk J, Mintorovitch J, Asgari H, et al. Diffusion/perfusion MR imaging of acute cerebral ischemia. *Magn. Reson. Med.* 1991; 19: 311-315.

[104] Rother J, Guckel F, Neff W, et al. Assessment of regional cerebral blood volume in acute human stroke by use of single-slice dynamic susceptibility contrast-enhanced magnetic resonance imaging. *Stroke* 1996; 27: 1088-1093.

[105] Chalela JA, Alsop DC, Gonzalez-Atavales JB, et al. Magnetic resonance perfusion imaging in acute ischemic stroke using continuous arterial spin labeling. *Stroke* 2000; 31: 680-687.

[106] Lev MH, Segal AZ, Farkas J, et al. Utility of perfusion-weighted CT imaging in acute middle cerebral artery stroke treated with intra-arterial thrombolysis: prediction of final infarct volume and clinical outcome. *Stroke* 2001; 32: 2021-2028.

[107] Wintermark M, Thiran JP, Maeder P, et al. Simultaneous measurement of regional cerebral blood flow by perfusion CT and stable xenon CT: a validation study. *Am. J. Neuroradiol.* 2001; 22: 905-914.

[108] Cheung RT, Cheng PW, Lui WM, et al. Visualization of ischaemic penumbra using a computed tomography perfusion method. *Cerebrovas. Dis.* 2003; 15: 182-187.

[109] Lee R, Cheung RT, Hung KN, et al. Use of CT perfusion to differentiate between brain tumour and cerebral infarction. *Cerebrovasc. Dis.* 2004; 18: 77-83.

In: State-of-the-Art Imaging in Stroke, Volume 2
Editor: Bernhard Schaller, pp. 265-284
ISBN 978-1-60021-499-8


*Chapter IX*

# Telemedicine in Ischemic Stroke: The Role of Imaging

***Sam Wang and Brent Moister***
Department of Neurology, Medical College of Georgia
Augusta, Georgia, USA

## A. Experimental Knowledge

Rapid computed tomography (CT) and other modes of cranial imaging are critical in determining the status of a stroke patient. Since its inception in the 1970s these digital images have become ubiquitous in providing non-invasive diagnoses. To maintain compatibility, the American College of Radiology (ACR) and the National Electrical Manufacturers Association (NEMA) devised a standard in 1985 that allowed these images to be digitally transferred and stored between multiple devices, regardless of manufacturer [1]. It basically provides a common language to transfer healthcare information between medical imaging equipment, such as modalities, image viewers, and storage systems. To this day, the standard known as the Digital Imaging and Communications in Medicine (DICOM), allows for communication and data transfer in a Transmission Control Protocol/Internet Protocol (TCP/IP) network environment, without specifying a file format or choice of physical media or file system, leaving it up to the audience to specify a storage medium.

Meanwhile, the global proliferation of TCP/IP as the platform-independent protocol of choice allowed for the enormous growth of the Internet, allowing for the exchange of large amounts of data in real time. Internet broadband access has also permeated beyond corporate and institutional settings to become available in urban areas in the United States, Asia and Europe. Though several other factors are involved, the DICOM standard and the proliferation of the TCP/IP standard played key roles in bringing together the role of imaging in telemedicine.

## Hardware and Technical Requirements

To develop a typical telemedicine setup (either real-time or store-and-forward), a capture device, or modality is required which is capable of generating a DICOM Message that encapsulates a DICOM image from radiographic images, and is capable of transmitting it to a Picture Archiving and Communication Systems (PACS). This receiving device is generally a printer or file server, and results in archival of the image in digital or print format. (All requirements to conform to these standards are documented in articles published by NEMA) [1]. The general requirements are a CT or MR scanner capable of generating images that meet DICOM 3.0 standards, and the ability to transmit them over a TCP/IP network to a receiving PACS.

As the DICOM standard does not dictate the implementation or role of any PACS system, manufacturers have developed several variations to this solution, with availability ranging from open-source to commercial alternatives, which dictate the level of sophistication in the software package. This open architecture as designed by NEMA allows the software development community the ability to scale to the needs of its audience. Features in server software can range from a personal PACS that accepts a small number of images per day and stores them to local disk storage for personal user, to large multiprocessor server farms that handle the entire volume of patients for an entire health care facility.

DICOM Messages can be transmitted over TCPI/IP globally via the Internet, and can be done in real time or with store-and-forward methods. However the benefits of this convenience are both its greatest asset and its worst risk. As the TCP/IP network was devised as an open protocol initially used between academic institutions, with implicit trust between the sender and recipient, data transmitted over any IP network is inherently unencrypted and therefore insecure. With the advent of the Health Insurance Privacy and Accountability Act (HIPAA) regulations enacted in 1996, demand for secure communications have become yet another essential component in transmitting confidential patient information between health care sites and professionals. DICOM has incorporated a secure file format – PS 3.10-2003 section 7.4 – that allows for secure data transmission.

An encrypted method of communication known as secure tunneling provides a solution to the issue of private information traveling over the public internet. In this method, two devices are setup at each end of the desired connection. These devices have access to a trusted private domain of information as well as the public internet. They then establish a "tunnel" over the public internet that can be used as a conduit for transmitting encrypted information. Any information passing between the private domains through the encrypted tunnel cannot be accessed as it travels over the public internet. This basic technique is utilized in Virtual Private Networks (VPN), secure hypertext transfer protocol (HTTPS) and many other software and hardware products.

As scanning resolution continues to improve, file sizes become ever increasing. As a result, current requirements for each slice of a head CT requires 500kb of disk space. In a typical 20-30 slice head CT this translates to approximately 2-3Mbs per study. With the addition of a bone study, in a patient involved in a trauma for instance, each patient series can easily weigh in at 5-7Mbs. This places a demand on bandwidth requirements, requiring reasonably robust telecommunications capabilities on both the transmitting and storage facility. Furthermore, digital storage and archiving can quickly become a constraining issue as the volume of patients increases. Lastly, these images need to be promptly presented in a digital manner to the consulting physician. The development of a telemedicine rig will thus need to consider the option of either providing a fixed imaging terminal with high bandwidth to provide full imaging capability, or alternatively providing compressed images at lower resolution that can be better transmitted over lower bandwidth lines such as dialup.

In short summary the infrastructure involved in a basic telemedicine imaging setup consists of a DICOM modality capable of constructing and transmitting DICOM images. These images need to be digitally transmitted in a secure and encrypted manner. Bandwidth requirements need to support these transmissions, and a secure archiving solution needs to accept these images. In turn, these images need to be delivered to the consulting physician without significant compromise in resolution. Let's discuss these logistics in further detail.

## Digital Imaging and Communications in Medicine Modality

The first step in providing imaging in a telemedicine rig is to wrap acquired images obtained from a source such as CT or MRI into a DICOM message and transmit it to a receiving PACS. This is highly dependent on the abilities of the transmitting modality. Generally newer modalities are network capable and can generate DICOM messages directly. Older generation devices simply output to a video monitor and require an upgrade with frame grabbers (another piece of hardware and software) that acquire and digitize the monitor images. This generally results in decreased image quality and limits the image to an 8bit grayscale depth. This image is then typically wrapped in a DICOM message for transmission. As the imaging equipment within the medical institution may be highly customized to the particular facility, this will always include involvement of the manufacturers' technical support staff.

Whether frame grabbed or directly generated, the radiology staff involved will need to be versed in acquiring and transmitting the obtained data. Training involved is minimal, though frame grabbed images will require more expertise in producing images with the appropriate window/level settings. Clearly, though, well trained radiology staff are integral in achieving a successful telemedicine program. Since the DICOM standard allows for seamless communication between all devices involved in generating these images, the staff should be readily familiar with image transmission from the capture modality to their local film printer or local file server. Addition of a remote telemedicine location should ideally appear as an extra modality in the recipient list, and transmission of data should be as easy as switching target modalities from printer to remote site.

Furthermore, as the development of a telemedicine rig will require data transmission outside the site's facilities, it will also be necessary to involve the Information Technology group. As institutions become more and more dependant on the digital medium, it is most likely that the facility is firewalled to the world, and is restricting the type of information into and out of the site. Depending on the solution selected, configuration changes will need to be applied to the firewall in order to allow packets to enter and exit the facility. So let's look at some of the options available.

## Telecommunications and Bandwidth

Assuming the telemedicine consult demands real-time response, typically nowadays within the United States there are three major options to digitally connect a medical facility to a remote telemedicine site: digital subscriber lines (DSL), dedicated lines (typically T1), and entirely private networks. DSL are typically applied in smaller facilities or in places located in more rural locations, and dedicated lines are necessarily used in larger establishments, supporting demand for large staffs that require large and constant amounts of data throughput. Both these options place the site onto the public Internet and allow access to vast worldwide access. Meanwhile private networks are entirely self contained and provide point to point access between the two parties. In contrast to real-time needs, if the telemedicine consultation is not a critical criteria, store-and-forward solutions may also require high bandwidth solutions when large volumes of information are involved.

As always, there are pros and cons to each solution. First and foremost is the cost and time of installation, which also translates directly into cost. The lowest cost solution is to purchase DSL lines, which means a bandwidth cap of usually 1.5Mbits downstream and an upstream rate dependent on carrier (within the United States). This provides for a reasonable bandwidth solution in small to medium sized staffs. Increasing needs within the facility demand that dedicated T1 lines be used. These lines dedicate larger bandwidth options, and as needs arise several lines can be bonded together to achieve greater throughput. In contrast to the aforementioned, both of which place the medical facility onto the public Internet, private networks can be installed which as the name suggests tie the imaging facility transmitting the data to the receiving telemedicine archival site direcly through a central office. This bypasses the public Internet completely, at the expense of comparatively higher costs and lengthier installation times (within the United States, but surely applies worldwide).

Access to the Internet means worldwide availability in configuring your telemedicine topology. It means the transmitting facility can be reasonably located anywhere IP access is achievable. It means the facility can be located in more remote locations, such as rural sites in parts of the country where private networks cannot be established. It means store-and-forward solutions can even be emailed if necessary. It also means the receiving facility can be established in a myriad of locations. It is only constrained by availability of IP access – the transmitting facility can then transmit to fixed DNS name, which can point to a number of variable IPs. DNS names can be changed within 24-48 hours, which precludes the receiving facility from being tied to one hosting solution or telecommunications carrier. In contrast, private networks are somewhat more constrained in their availability. Physical circuits often need to be established with the central office, locking the facilities into fixed locations that may require urban or suburban facilities. There are positive and negative aspects to choosing either configuration, namely the convenience of having the ability to rearrange your topology versus having a fixed location with consistent and reliable connections. However this means locking the telemedicine topology into a fixed point-to-point arrangement that precludes for rearrangement should the need arise.

While using the Internet offers significant cost and access advantages, this approach introduces security and performance issues that are not seen in private networks. Network performance restrictions and bottlenecks can degrade and even prevent the consultation.

Reliable bandwidth availability may be an inconsistent component in the system, as it relies on the availability of the public Internet. Congestion and even blackouts have been known to occur – this may be an unacceptable criteria if timely and real-time consultations are critical. With the advent and exploding popularity of Internet worms, viruses, and trojans, exposure of a facility to these elements may also be an unacceptable risk. The man power and technical challenge of keeping these unwanted elements at bay are serious points to consider when establishing an archival facility responsible for transmitting or maintaining confidential patient records. In larger medical facilities where entire divisions are dedicated to maintenance of data facitilies this is not an issue, but may be a daunting task for smaller sites.

Additionally, developments in internet architecture have complicated the design of distributed internet applications. All computers communicating using IP have a numerical address (IP address). This address has a fixed number of digits, limiting the total number of computers communicating over IP to approximately 4 billion. In an effort to surmount this limitation, individuals devised a system where multiple devices could share a single internet address (Network Address Translation and Private Addressing). Unfortunately, two separate computers utilizing this scheme cannot communicate bi-directionally to each other. This has important implications for telestroke applications implementing TCP/IP, where real time video access is essential. A video stream originating at the patient bedside must pass through an intermediate computer that is not "sharing" an internet address to be bi-directional and accessible to the consulting physician. This can impart significant network overhead. For instance, if a physician at a conference in Charleston, South Carolina delivers a remote consultation to patient located at a rural medical center only 50 miles away, the video stream may have to travel 300 miles round trip through an intermediate computer in Atlanta. The newer Internet protocol version 6 (IPv6) solves these issues, but it will be tens of years before this standard is fully adopted.

Furthermore, the choice of network infrastructure limits the options available in developing an end user client that accesses these data. As previously mentioned, with an open IP configuration there are numerous client softwares that can be developed or purchased for customization with the system.

In telestroke applications, the client is the system component that provides the consulting physician access to the information they require to perform a consultation. When designing distributed systems, there are various types of clients to consider, each with inherent advantages and limitations. In a thick client architecture most of the processing occurs on the client computer, minimizing server and network overhead. Alternatively, thin clients perform minimal processing, simply displaying information that has already been processed and generated on the server side. While decreasing the hardware requirements on the client side, this approach can lead to significant performance bottlenecks on the server side as the number of clients increase. In practice, most applications lie on a continuum between these two extremes.

The difference between thin and thick architectures can be demonstrated with email applications familiar to most users. Users may access email through a dedicated thick client application (Microsoft Outlook, Eudora, Novell Groupwise), but can often access the same email through a web based thin client.

A web browser acts as the client agent in a web based client system. Web browsers can deliver information in the form of hypertext markup language (HTML) pages, and web browser functionality can be extended with small applications such as Java applets or ActiveX controls. The use of these applications is essential to accomplish anything beyond the most rudimentary image manipulation at the client end. ActiveX controls and Java applets are applications that run within the context of the web browser. When developing these applications developers have access to almost all of the programming resources normally available when developing free standing software. This demonstrates the flexibility provided by browser based interface when developing either thick or thin clients.

Additionally, because web based clients operate within the context of a web browser, there is no software for the user to install, and software upgrades can be transparently distributed to users. The web browser provides basic functionality such as image processing and user interface management that would otherwise have to be developed. The application can be accessed at any computer with internet access and adequate bandwidth. Web browser clients have their drawbacks as well. Applications operating within the browser incur processing overhead and cannot utilize system resources as efficiently as free standing applications. Despite these limitations, web browsers provide a powerful tool for developing client applications, as evinced by their widespread use in online banking applications, shopping and auction applications, and news delivery services.

## Encryption and Security

Protecting the privacy and security of the medical information transferred between the patient site and the telemedicine facility can be handled in an innumerable number of methods, and lengthy discussion of each is beyond the scope of this chapter. Experience, however, has led to the use of Secure Socket Layers (SSL), developed by the Netscape Communications Corporation, as the method of encryption in the telemedicine program developed at the author's institution. The SSL protocol was chosen due to its ability to run above the TCP/IP layer but below higher-level protocols such as HTTP or IMAP. It uses TCP/IP on behalf of the higher-level protocols, and in the process allows an SSL-enabled server to authenticate itself to an SSL-enabled client, allows the client to authenticate itself to the server, and allows both machines to establish an encrypted connection. This is the same encryption technology used and endorsed by the banking community within the United States to conduct online banking transactions with an extremely large volume of clients.

The SSL protocol uses a combination of public-key and symmetric-key encryption [2]. Symmetric-key encryption is faster than public-key encryption; however, public-key encryption provides better authentication techniques. An SSL session always begins with an exchange of messages called the SSL handshake. The handshake allows the server to authenticate itself to the client by using public-key techniques, and then allows the client and the server to cooperate in the creation of symmetric keys used for rapid encryption, decryption, and tamper detection during the session that follows. Optionally, the handshake also allows the client to authenticate itself to the server. The SSL handshake is now complete and the session begins. The client and the server use the session keys to encrypt and decrypt the data they send to each other and to validate its integrity. Public key authentication is accomplished with certificates obtained from trusted root certification authorities such as Verisign Corp.

### Picture Archiving and Communications System (PACS)

These server based imaging systems are replacing film based systems throughout the medical community. It is one of the basic components necessary for a successful telemedicine system, and its advantages in image review have been shown convincingly for several imaging techniques [2-5]. Additionally, the usage of digital PACS systems has also been shown to increase sensitivity for stroke detection, from 57% to 71%, without loss of sensitivity [2]. This is accomplished by providing the physician with adjustable window width and center level settings to accentuate the contrast between normal and edematous tissue when viewing radiographic images digitally.

General-purpose systems, designed for review of images by clinicians, have much less rigorous technical requirements and a much greater potential audience than special-purpose systems designed for primary interpretation by radiologists [2, 3]. However, both of these systems share five basic components of a common architectural model: acquisition, storage, display, database management, and a network. PACS systems can be obtained in commercial packages, can be developed inhouse, or can be obtained from open-source projects created within the medical software development community.

## B. Clinical Knowledge

### Remotely Evaluating Stroke at the Medical College of Georgia in Southeast USA

Despite the fact that thrombolytic therapy has been FDA approved for acute stroke treatment since the NINDS study in 1995, use in the US has been limited to only 3% of stroke victims [2]. While public awareness and education are underway via the American Stroke Association and the Ad Council, to get acute stroke patients to an emergency department immediately, many facilities do not have any type of acute stroke pathway in place, so when acute stroke patients do present urgently, essentially nothing happens relevant to tPA consideration. There are over 2100 rural community hospitals in the United States, many which have no neurologists on staff, nor radiologists available to read CT scans in a timely fashion. Moreover, many small hospitals do not even have tPA on their hospital formulary.

The "buckle" of the United States Stroke Belt is reported to be the coastal plain sectors of North Carolina, South Carolina, and Georgia. Although stroke is the third leading cause of death in the country, stroke mortality within the Stroke Belt is twice as high as the national average. Racial factors may contribute to the high incidence of stroke in the Southeast, due to higher rates of hypertension and its related complications. Some evidence also suggests that the quality of rural medical care may contribute to the higher stroke mortality in the Southeast, primarily because rural hospitals are medically underserved.

This lack of dedicated infrastructure for tPA administration demands that patients be transferred to medical centers that have specialists available for emergency patient assessment and tPA intervention. Patients who might qualify for tPA can miss this three hour window due to delays in transport to a higher level medical facility. The problem becomes increasingly difficult in rural areas as transportation distance becomes a time limiting barrier; this limitation contributes to the higher rate of stroke deaths (reported by the CDC [2]) in rural and underserved communities. The disappointing low use of tPA in stroke patients in the United States is partly attributable to the lack of on-site stroke specialist expertise.

To compound matters, all the North American Emergency Medicine Physician organizations, American Academy of Emergency Medicine [2], American College of Emergency Physicians [2], and the Society of Academic Emergency Medicine [2], and the Canadian Association of Emergency Physicians [2] recommend against the widespread use of thrombolytics in stroke, unless neurologic experts are directly involved in reading the CT scan and recommending its use with strict adherence to NINDS criteria. The American College of Emergency Physicians (ACEP) 2002 policy statement on tPA says, "There is insufficient evidence at this time to endorse the use of tPA use in clinical practice when systems are not in place to ensure that the inclusion/exclusion criteria established by the NINDS guidelines for tPA use in acute stroke are followed." Indeed, many patients may have suffered untoward events due to protocol violations both in over and underuse of tPA. Nonetheless, there have been several lawsuits filed against physicians for failing to consider or offer tPA to their acute stroke patients [13].

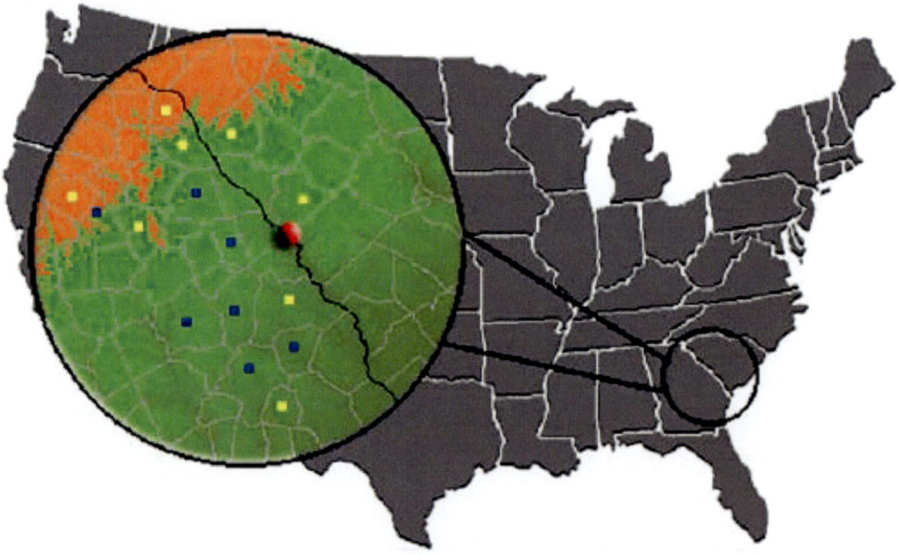

Figure 1.

Although there is an acute stroke module in the American Heart Association (AHA) Advanced Cardiac Life Support (ACLS) course and acute stroke management is described in the major emergency medicine texts, the topics are a relatively minor component in residents' and practicing physicians' education compared to other topics such as acute myocardial infarction. Additionally, when an acute stroke patient presents, there are almost no readily accessible references for physicians to use at the bedside. Screening to determine tPA eligibility requires competence in several areas: establishing all necessary historical elements, meeting all blood pressure criteria, verifying all necessary blood work parameters, correctly reading a head CT scan, and performing an NIH stroke score examination. With little training and no checklists to review for something which they are asked to do relatively infrequently, it is not surprising that physicians are hesitant or even reluctant to make the determination to order tPA for an acute stroke patient.

Patient care efficiency and medical error reduction have shown significant improvement in other sites when medical information is readily available in electronic format [2-5]. Studies have shown that more than half of physicians under the age of 35 now use PDAs in their daily practice [2, 3]. Though usage by EMS staff is not as prevalent [2], usage will only increase with time, and presenting the duties of all levels of providers will allow better integration of services and a more cohesive team approach to provide optimal acute stroke patient care.

The Medical College of Georgia's efforts to deliver quality neurological care to rural community hospitals prompted the author and the Department of Neurology stroke care physicians to examine the hurdles involved in delivering expert neurological consultation to suspected stroke patients. Commonly a stroke patient presenting at a rural site is transferred via ambulance or helicopter to our tertiary center, and evaluated by a consulting neurologist or resident. As the coverage radius exceeds 100 miles, ambulance transfer times are upwards of an hour. Even helicopter transfers have shown roundtrip transport distances of 40, 80, and 120 miles corresponding to transport times of 60, 90, and 120 minutes, respectively [2].

It became apparent that the 1 ½ hour delay to receiving tPA would continue unless a way could be created to deliver the medication at the rural site. Additionally, this order of magnitude in delay of transport made it impossible for patients from rural areas to ever be treated under 2 hours. It has been shown that patients treated with IV tPA in the first 90 minutes after the onset of an acute stroke have a predictably better outcome than patients treated in the last 90 minutes of the three hour window. It would seem intuitive that if patients can be evaluated and treated properly in the first 90 minutes at a rural site, the outcome will be better than delaying the treatment until the patient is transferred to a regional stroke center an average of 90 minutes away. Patients will likely still require transfer from the rural site after receiving tPA; however, it can be done safely after tPA administration, ie after the time urgency has been lifted.

## Hardware and Software Configuration

The joint efforts of the Departments of Neurology and Emergency Medicine at the Medical College of Georgia have developed a unique telestroke approach that allows a consulting physician to sit down at any broadband accessible computer and obtain a patient video feed from the rural hospital, as well the head CT transmitted from the rural hospital radiology room, and relevant clinical labs entered by the bedside staff. They have endeavored to develop a telestroke tool – the Remote Evaluation for Acute Ischemic Stroke (REACH) – that allows community hospitals to easily afford and maintain a small medical cart that is wirelessly connected to the Internet through a hospital DSL line.

The medical staff in the emergency department activates the remote evaluation protocol upon triaging an acute stroke patient who may be eligible for tPA by contacting the tertiary medical center Emergency Communication Center (ECC). The tertiary medical center ECC contacts one of the on-call physicians: Robert Adams, Fenwick Nichols, Hartmut Gross, and David Hess, who log onto the REACH system to conduct the neurological evaluation by performing an NIHSS to determine the level of neurological deficit in the patient, interpret the transmitted CT scan to rule out hemorrhage, and evaluate the patient. The REACH consultant then makes a recommendation for or against tPA treatment as well as any other needed therapy.

The remote evaluation cart is comprised of an MPEG high-resolution Pan/Tilt/Zoom camera, a PC workstation and LCD monitor, wireless bridge, ethernet switch, and Universal Power Supply, all housed on a mobile, ergonomic cart. The computer workstation and camera are connected to the Ethernet switch, which is wirelessly networked to the hospital LAN via a wireless access point. This allows the cart to be maneuvered anywhere in the ED without the need for a wired infrastructure. In fact, the remote evaluation cart is designed to be taken to the patient rather than bringing the patient to the camera, which is customary on most current telemedicine systems.

The cart can be moved easily to the bedside of the emergent stroke patient where the camera is operated remotely by the stroke specialist, with minimal intervention from the busy ED staff. The off-the-shelf Uninterruptible Power Supply and wireless bridge allow the cart to be a remote unit. The UPS battery can power the PC workstation, camera, and wireless bridge for 15-20 minutes, allowing the wireless network connection, established with a wireless bridge, to connect to a 802.11b Wireless Access Point (WAP). The WAP is wired to the remainder of the hospital LAN. The connection established is secured with the Wired Equivalent Privacy (WEP) algorithm, a method that encrypts each 802.11b frame before transmission using an RC4 [3] stream cipher. Though the WEP scheme has been shown to have limitations [3] it is non-trivial to exploit and is the first layer of security used to keep the casual exploiter from accessing the network. Combined with SSL encryption, this architecture forms a secure multi-layered scheme. Heavy emphasis was placed on a design that departed from conventional telemedicine in its cost, ease of use, and accessibility, as depicted in Figure 2.

All active sites signed Memorandums of Understanding (MOU) prior to participating. These MOUs dictated the responsibilities of both parties involved, as well as the technical and logistical requirements necessary to implement, activate, and maintain the REACH system. Eight REACH sites were actived, consisting of McDuffie Regional Medical Center (active 3/2003), Emanuel Hospital (active 3/2003), Jenkins Hospital (active 7/2003), Wills Memorial Hospital (active 5/2003), and Washington County Regional Medical Center (active 8/2003), Jefferson Hospital (active 1/2004), Morgan Memorial Hospital (active 3/2004), and Elbert Memorial Hospital (active 3/2005).

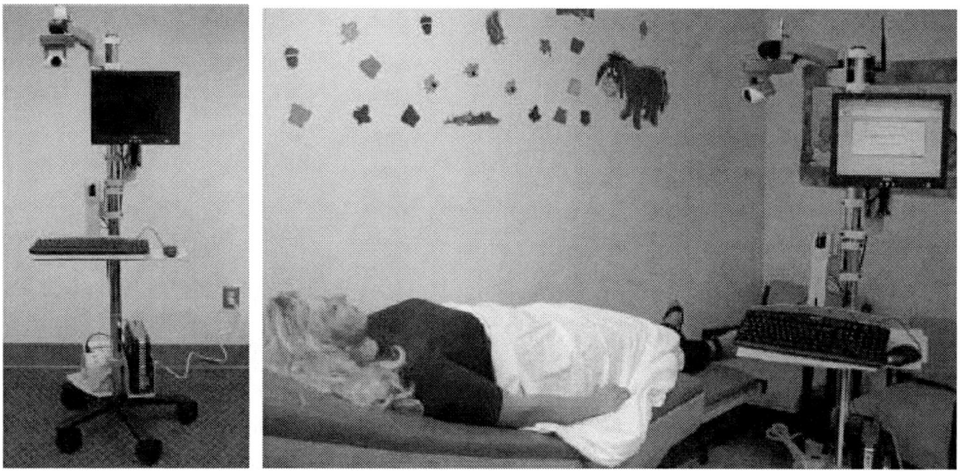

Figure 2. Photographs of REACH cart in use.

## Video Imaging

An imaging method which adds considerable depth to the remote consultation, the video feed, is accomplished in the REACH system by the addition of an IP based ethernet camera that can be remotely controlled by the consulting physician. It is also SSL encrypted to meet HIPAA requirements. The camera provides wide coverage with its ability stream in MPEG-4 and to pan 340 degrees, tilt 100 degrees and zoom in on specific details. Image quality is sufficient to provide details such as observation of pupil dilation and extraocular movement from a distance of 20 to 30 feet away. It also allows the evaluator to perform the NIHSS exam in the evaluation of a suspected stroke, with the additional support of local staff at the patient's bedside.

## National Institutes of Health Stroke Scale - A Telemedicine Approach

The National Institutes of Health Stroke Scale (NIHSS) is a validated [3-5] tool for measuring the severity of stroke. Other studies [3] have shown that the NIHSS remains a reliable clinical instrument when used over interactive video, but it was achieved under controlled conditions with proprietary video conferencing equipment and dedicated bandwidth. To confirm that the NIHSS could be accurately performed over a video image feed, a clinical study was performed using the REACH system in an intranet environment, similar to the study performed by Shaqfat et al, though with lower cost off-the-shelf components.

Twenty patients were recruited. Upon obtaining consent, a neurologist performed a bedside NIHSS evaluation on each patient. Within one hour, using any broadband connected workstation – either office or home PC, and a landline phone to speak with the patient – a second neurologist remotely evaluated the patient through the REACH system. Paired T-tests and Pearson correlation coefficients were used to examine NIHSS reliability performed bedside and remotely. NIHSS scores ranged from 1 to 24. Correlations between bedside and remote locations (r=0. 9552, p=0.0001) was very strong, and t-test indicate that the means were not different. From the results, it was concluded that the NIHSS could be reliably performed over the REACH system [3].

## Radiologic Imaging with REACH

Studies have demonstrated that digital representation of CT scans may be adequately visualized and interpreted by radiologists, provided the computer monitor has sufficient resolution to properly display the image [3]. In the REACH system, waiting on an official reading from a radiologist is impractical and at rural sites oftentimes impossible to obtain until the next working day. At their own institutions, neurologists have long interpreted CT scans and acted upon them independently, only later to review a final radiologists official report. Trained emergency physicians have done the same with plain films and at many sites with head CT scans, only later to later receive and review a radiologists final reading as a QA activity.

Within the REACH system a mini PACS system was incorporated using the ConQuest DICOM server version 1.4.1 (released 03/03/2003). This server was developed within the E.U. ConQuest project as a small image archiver. It was used to connect ConQuest imaging applications to the hospital's equipment to receive images conforming to the DICOM standard (C-STORE). The DICOM server is an adapted version of the University of California at Davis DICOM software (Personal PACS). The user interface has been developed at the Radiotherapy Department of the Netherlands Cancer Institute (NKI). In addition, the original Davis code has been extended significantly by the ConQuest . The server talks DICOM on the front end and stores image data in files in archive directories. The image files are stored either in chapter 10 DICOM format and batch converted to PNG format for web use. Conversion to PNG will losslessly create a file with fixed brightness and contrast from default values embedded in the DICOM file. This lossless compression produces a final image that is 1/10 the size of the original image, and the decreased bandwidth allows much faster transfer of images to the consulting physician at his terminal.

As the physicians evaluating the scans can be using any of a number of screens within the facilities and at home, it was imperative that a method be available to quickly and easily determine that the monitor in use is correctly calibrated. The proposed solution, described by Tobin et al., and advocated by the American College of Radiology, is the use of a standard image containing lines and grey scales produced by the Society of Motion Picture and Television Engineers (SMPTE) [3], as shown in Figure 3. The SMPTE image has been described in detail in the literature [3, 4]. Other test patterns have also been proposed [3,4]. Thus a physician who can detect the brightness and contrast differences, spatial resolution and aliasing, and continuous gray scale subtleties should reliably read a CT image digitally delivered by the community hospital's radiology department.

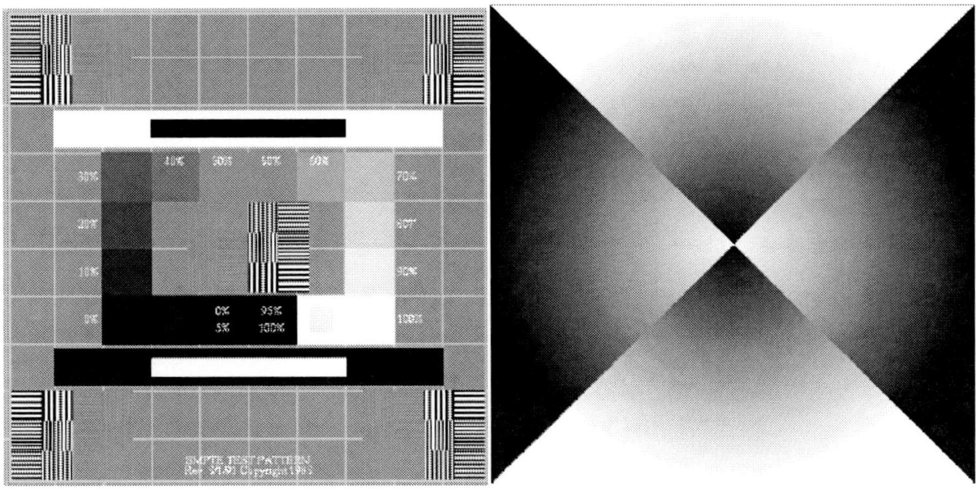

Figure 3. The gray scale is shown at left depicts as a series of squares in the center of the image that range from black (0%) to white (100%) in a semi-rectangle. The 0% and 100% squares each contain smaller squares within them that represent signal level steps of 5% and 95%, respectively. You should be able to visually differentiate the inner square from the larger square that contains it. In each corner of the image as well as in the very center, inspect the 6 squares filled with varying widths of alternating black/white horizontal and vertical lines. You should be able to differentiate all the lines, from fat to narrow (6 pixels, 4 pixels, and 2 pixels) and both horizontally and vertically. In the gray scale image at right, No concentric ring-like features should be present. If such features are present, the images from BrighamRad displayed on the workstation will be displayed at less than optimal quality.

To confirm the accuracy of nonradiologist readings by physicians involved with REACH, charts of all patients evaluated with the REACH system at 2 sites within a span of 6 months were reviewed on site. The REACH consultant's CT scan interpretation via the live system was compared to the final printed radiologist's report in the medical record. There was 100% correlation between the readings. This was true both for patients treated with tPA as well as for patients not treated, regardless of the reason, including abnormal CT scan findings. Of note is the fact that two patients had their CT scan interpreted by the primary care physician in the rural ED as normal, although these patients actually had intracranial bleeds which were detected by the REACH consultant using the system. These were confirmed in the final radiologist report.

## Client Side Software

It is possible to build useful functionality into even relatively thin clients. By utilizing a custom developed ActiveX control, the newer versions of the REACH client provide an intuitive window and leveling interface. Additionally, these REACH clients provide consulting physicians with a method to identify and calculate lesion volume, bringing the robust tools available at complex imaging workstations to remote clients, demonstrating how thin clients can easily accommodate evolving user requirements.

One goal of remote client development is to provide remote users with a familiar experience relative to that which they would encounter locally. This involves integrating familiar functionality into the remote client, such as window and leveling, as well as maximizing the speed and responsiveness of the system. Due to network infrastructure limitations mentioned earlier, the latter can provide a daunting challenge, but these potential challenges can be surmounted with adequate software design.

Speed and responsiveness are often constrained by limited network bandwidth in telestroke applications. Transmission of real time video and image studies place significant demands on the available bandwidth. Fortunately, these challenges are not unique and have been encountered since the inception of distributed network applications. Telestroke systems can take advantage of techniques that have been developed to limit the bandwidth consumed by both video and still images. Compression and buffering are two methods that can be employed to increase the perceived speed and responsiveness of the remote system.

Compression involves eliminating redundant information during transmission at the cost of processing overhead at the server and client side. Both the video stream and still images from imaging studies can be compressed for transmission. Numerous image and video formats support compression, but the choice of image and video format must support the requirements of the telestroke system.

Image compression schemes can be roughly divided into lossless and lossy compression. In lossless compression schemes the information that encodes an image is reorganized such that it takes up less space, but every single element of data is still present in the image when it is decompressed. In lossy compression, some information is discarded and irretrievably lost in the compression process. The art of lossy compression involves selectively discarding only visually imperceptible information. Unfortunately, additional spurious information (artifacts) may also be inserted into the image during this process. Because medical imaging places additional demands on image compression technology that are not often encountered in consumer applications, the loss of information as well as the introduction of artifacts renders lossy compression inadequate in many medical imaging applications. However, the results of lossy compression are perfectly adequate in distributed network applications that utilize video. In fact, real time video streaming would not be feasible without the superior compression ratios available through lossy compression.

At the telestroke application implementation level, image compression occurs after the imaging study is stored in the PACS system. Image data must be extracted from the storage modality (usually DICOM compliant) and converted to a compressed image before it is transmitted to the remote client. Once again software development time and expense can be minimized by utilizing available software components to convert the images to well supported formats. There are some drawbacks in using image formats developed for consumer use. Most consumer formats support a maximum of 8 bits per color channel. As a result, data is lost when medical images containing 16 bits per channel are converted to these formats. Newer revisions of two image standards do provide support for 16 bits per channel. The Portable Network Graphics (PNG) format, and Joint Photographic Experts Group 2000 (JPEG2000) standard both support 16 bits per channel, as a well as numerous other valuable features such as gamma correction, alpha channel transparency, and various modes of lossless compression. Both standards are royalty and license free, but the 16 bit features are not yet widely supported at the client level. Most client computers require proprietary software to take full advantage of the capabilities of these image formats, but widespread support of the extended PNG as well as JPEG2000 features will become available within two years based on the adoption pace of previous standards. Furthermore, the DICOM compression committee (working group 4) has adopted JPEG2000 for integration into future DICOM standards.

While standardized support for 16 bit images may be forthcoming, current application require proprietary software development to accommodate the additional information encoded in a 16bit image. The REACH system accomplishes this by transmitting the entire unprocessed DICOM image to the client and extracting the 16 bit image information. This data is then encapsulated in a system specific format for manipulation and display.

Buffering is another method frequently used to improve performance when transmitting large amounts of information, such as real time video and medical image, over distributed networks. Typically, network bandwidth is not utilized consistently. Periods of high demand are punctuated by times of low network utilization. Buffering techniques take advantage of this characteristic by using periods of low network utilization to pro actively retrieve and store information. Sophisticated mathematical techniques may be employed to predict what information will be required by the user next. This information is then retrieved using reserve network bandwidth.

The REACH system employs a simple but effective buffering method. Physicians typically evaluate a single section, and then move to an adjacent section. The REACH client uses any available residual bandwidth to predictively retrieve adjacent CT slices, moving progressively away from the current section. This "window" containing the current and adjacent slices is updated as the physician moves through the study ensuring that the next image is immediately available when requested, while minimizing memory requirement on the client end.

## Server Side Software

Rapid deployment of web applications became essential to business survival during the internet boom at the turn of the century. To quickly tie all these disparate components together, the heart of the REACH system was devised with custom built server side scripting software, which dynamically generates custom HTML on the server end, and is delivered to the client browser as they surf through the site. This has been implemented to generate realtime patient information HTML pages to the physician. This scripting technology is complimented with a database backend, allowing for generation of tremendously dynamic content. The contents of a page can come from anywhere - databases, plain text files, searches, calculations, CT images - and be dynamically inserted before it is sent to the user.

Another benefit of developing the application as a server side scripted application is the ability to modify the application without interrupting service to the end users, and deploying upgrades centrally without having to be onsite. The current REACH system is developed with Internet Information Server (IIS) 3.0, but other options available are with Sun Java and PHP, an open source scripting language.

## Evaluation Results

The REACH system is currently rolled out in 8 rural hospitals in east Georgia, USA, as of May 2005. It has been used to evaluate 177 patients from March 2003 to April 2005, and 28 have received tPA, all without developing intracranial hemorrhage complications. This has been summarized in table 1. NIHSS scores ranged from 0 to 30 with a mean of 14.3 (sd=8.7, median 11.5). The mean onset to door time was 70.9 minutes (sd=70.8, median 50), the mean door to consult time was 45.1 minutes (sd=39.8, median 34), and the mean door to NIHSS completion was 62.9 minutes (sd=50.8, median 51). The mean onset to needle time was 135.33 minutes (sd=51.45, median 134.5). Rapid improvement defined as a drop of 4 or more points at 24 hours occurred in 12 of 28 patients. The in-hospital mortality rate was 2/24 or 8%. About one quarter of the REACH tPA-treated patients were treated within 90 minutes of the onset of symptoms and over half were treated within 2 hours. This compares favorably to urban systems of stroke care where 28% of the tPA-treated patients were treated under 2 hours. Just as importantly, over 54 patients that were evaluated in rural areas were not urgently transported to our tertiary care center when they were remotely diagnosed with symptoms that were rapidly improving or too mild. This allowed savings to the health care system that, though not directly tangible, were nonetheless real.

**Table 1. Tally of REACH patients evaluated between March 2003 and April 2005**

| | |
|---|---|
| Total tPA treatments | 28 |
| Too Mild (NIHSS < 4) | 27 |
| Rapidly Improving | 26 |
| Beyond Time Window | 25 |
| Intracranial Hemorrhage | 22 |
| Seizures | 9 |
| Uncontrolled Hypertension | 1 |
| Bleeding Contraindication | 0 |
| Prolonged INR | 4 |
| Poor Medical Condition | 0 |
| Other contraindication (infarct, edema) | 1 |
| Conversion Reactions | 4 |
| Other | 24 |
| Evaluation not completed | 6 |
| Total | 177 |

Another important aspect of the imaging capabilities provided by the REACH system was the ability to rapidly assist the local ED in other diagnoses that was urgent and emergent. When the CT image presented by the rural hospital staff to the neurologist consultant as a normal finding in Figure 4, the consulting physicians were able to assist the rural staff in confirming the diagnosis of intracerebral or subarachnoid hemorrhage, with subsequent rapid transfer to tertiary care center, a diagnosis that could possibly have been dangerously prolonged.

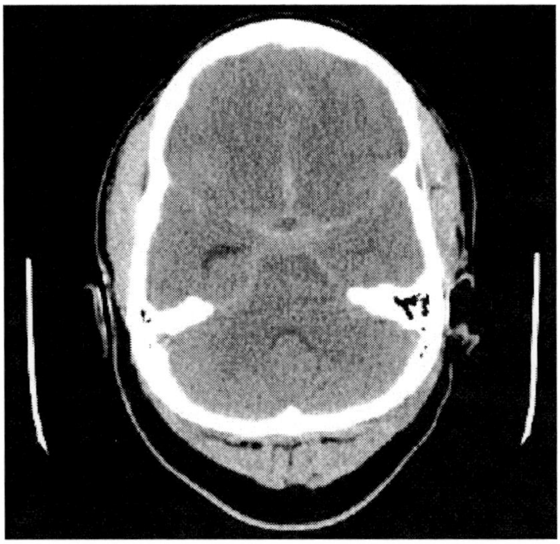

Figure 4. CT image of patient presenting 40 minutes after passing out while washing her car. A diagnosis of subarachnoid hemorrhage was made with the assistance of telestroke imaging.

These data show that the REACH telestroke system can assist rural facilities in safely delivering tPA by non-neurologists, provided that there is some baseline training and consultation assistance. Education, increased awareness, and commitment to some form of stroke pathway are essential to expeditiously evaluate and screen acute stroke patients for proper treatment options.

Furthermore the imaging data collected is useful in providing epidemiological data for further study. With other data jointly recorded through the telemedicine system at the time the scan is obtained, such as baseline NIHSS, estimated time of onset, estimated onset to ER door time, door to CT, as well as demographic data such as age, gender, race, later studies can be performed to determine whether further correlations exist between hemorrhagic incidence in particular populations, or outcomes in infarct reduction or hemorrhage volume in particular subpopulations. The volume of data collected is overwhelming and the various ways in which it can be analyzed and studied has not yet been fully appreciated.

## C. Take-Home-Message

There is a large opportunity for telestroke and telestroke imaging to fill the needs of areas that face delays in neurologic care, such as in smaller health community and dense urban areas. This can be accomplished by utilizing low cost modular off-the-shelf components that will allow rapid upgrades in implementing the latest cutting edge techniques to deliver imaging.

One field that is rapidly advancing and which will provide ubiquitous imaging-on-demand throughout a medical facility, large or small, is the advent of wireless Internet technology. This technology will ultimately place much of the needed real-time data, including the latest patient imaging, into the physicians' hands. It will certainly streamline bedside consults and allow for remote consults to become much more commonplace. By utilizing modular off-the-shelf wireless components, telestroke programs that wish to deliver images to handheld and remote devices will be able to keep up with the ever improving mediums. For instance 802.11b was the initial standard developed to provide data transmission at 11Mbps in the 2.4Ghz range. Shortly thereafter 802.11g was recently finalized and provides 54Mbps in the 2.4Ghz range. A third standard, 802.11a, will allow data transfer at 54Mbps in the 5Ghz range, allowing for less interference from other sources in the 2.4Ghz range such as cordless phones and microwaves.

As the electronics industry manages to pack more processing power into smaller and smaller form factors, the economies of scale will allow widespread availability of handhelds and tabletPCs in the health care field that will be wirelessly connected to the Internet, and constant access to patient data. Telestroke imaging will also benefit from the ability of smaller and more powerful handheld devices to display and manipulate the images wireless delivered. If powerful enough, these images can be manipulated in real time, and even streaming video can be included in the evaluation. Finally all this information collected from the patient can be digitally stored, processed, and analyzed, as well as used as teaching tools and learning material.

The future of telestroke imaging lies in the digital realm. It is a large field, tying broad arenas such as digital image processing, database servers, wireless communication, telecommunications infrastructure, and thin clients together to deliver vast but pertinent information to the evaluating physician regardless of temporal and spatial location.

## References

[1] *Digital Imaging and Communications in Medicine* (DICOM). Published by the National Electrical Manufacturers Association. Copyright 2003.

[2] K.E.B. Hickman, *The SSL Protocol*, December 1995.

[3] http://www.rsasecurity.com/rsalabs/node.asp?id=2293. Accessed April 2005.

[4] Reiner BI, Siegel EL, Flagle C, et al. Effect of filmless imaging on the utilization of radiologic services. *Radiology* 2000;215:163–7.

[5] Reiner BI, Siegel EL, Hooper FJ, et al. Radiologists' productivity in the interpretation of CT scans: A comparison of PACS with conventional film. *AJR Am. J. Roentgenol.* 2001;176:861–4.

[6] Weatherburn G, Bryan S, Cousins C. A comparison of the time required by radiologists for the preparation of clinico-radiological meetings when films and PACS are used. *Eur. Radiol.* 2000;10:1006–9.

[7] Wagner SC, Morrison WB, Carrino JA, et al. Picture archiving and communication system: Effect on reporting of incidental findings. *Radiology* 2002;225:500–5.

[8] Lev MH, Farkas J, Gemmete JJ, et al. Acute stroke: Improved nonenhanced CT detection-benefits of soft-copy interpretation by using variable window width and center level settings. *Radiology* 1999; 213: 150 - 155.

[9] Dayhoff RE, et al., Integrating Medical Images into Hospital Information Systems. *J. Dig. Imag.*1991; 4:87-93.

[10] Fener EF, Hanlon WB. A Functional Model for PACS Beyond Radiology. *S/CAR 92 Proc. Symp. Foundation 1992*, Baltimore, MD, pp. 289-295.

[11] American Heart Association, Heart and Stroke Statistical Update. Dallas, TX, 2001.

[12] CDC Atlas of Stroke Mortality: http://www.cdc.gov/cvh/maps/strokeatlas/index.htm

[13] McNamara R, Position Statement on the user of Intravenous Thrombolytic Therapy in the Treatment of Stroke. http://www.aaem.org/positionstatements/thrombolytictherapy .shtml

[14] Use of intravenous tPA for the management of acute stroke in the emergency department. *Position Statement Ann. Emerg. Med.* 2002;40:551.

[15] Adams JG, Chisholm CD on behalf of the SAEM Board of Directors. The Society for Academic Emergency Medicine Position on Optimizing Care of the Stroke Patient. *Acad. Emerg. Med.* 2003 10: 805.

[16] Canadian Association of Emergency Physicians Committee on Thrombolytic Therapy for Acute Ischemic Stroke. Thrombolytic Therapy for Acute Ischemic Stroke. http://www.caep.ca/004.cjem-jcmu/004-00.cjem/vol-3.2001/v31-008.htm

[17] Rosenbloom M, Jaffe W, Adams J. Patient care efficiency and medical error reduction using PDA based medical information. *Acad. Emergency Medicine*. 8: 587-588.

[18] Robinson R, Burk M. Identification of drug-drug interactions with personal digital assistant-based software. *American Journal of Medicine*. 2004; 116.

[19] Goldberg R, Kuhn G, Andrew L, et al. Coping with medical mistakes and errors in judgement. *Ann. Emergency Medicine* 2002;39:3.

[20] Bodenheimer T, Grumbach K. Electronic Technology. A spark to revitalize primary care? *JAMA*. 2003;290.

[21] Martin S. MD's computer, PDA use on the upswing. *CMAJ* 2002; 167: 794.

[22] Martin S. More than half of MDs under age 35 now using PDAs. *CMAJ* 2003;169. 952.

[23] Khan A, Geria KR, Frank J, Davidson S. Utilization of PDAs by Emergengy medicine and Pediatric residents. *Acad. Emergency Medicine*. 2004; 11:498.

[24] Scott PA, Temovsky CJ, Lawrence K, et al. Analysis of Canadian Population with Potential Geographic Access to Intravenous Thrombolysis for Acute Ischemic Stroke. *Stroke* 1998; 29: 2304.

[25] Marler JR, Tilley BC, Brott TG, et al. Early Stroke Treatment Associated with Better Outcome. *Neurology* 2000;55:1649-1655

[26] http://www.rsasecurity.com/rsalabs/faq/3-6-3.html

[27] http://www.cs.rice.edu/~astubble/wep_attack.pdf

[28] Brott T, Adams HP, Olinger CP, et al. Measurements of acute cerebral infarction: a clinical examination scale. *Stroke* 1989;20:864–870.

[29] Brott T, Adams HP, Olinger CP, et al. Measurements of acute cerebral infarction: a clinical examination scale. *Stroke*. 1989;20:864–870.

[30] Wityk R, Pessin MS, Kaplan RF, et al. Serial assessment of acute stroke using the NIH Stroke Scale. *Stroke*. 1994;25:362–365.

[31] Shafqat S, Kvedar JC, Guanci MM, et al. Role of telemedicine in acute stroke: feasibility and reliability of remote administration of the NIH stroke scale. *Stroke*. 1999; 30: 2141-2145.

[32] Wang S, Lee SB, Pardue C, et al. Remote Evaluation of Acute Ischemic Stroke: Reliability of National Institutes of Health Stroke Scale via Telestroke. *Stroke* 2003 34: e188 - e191.

[33] Tobin M. Evaluation of Teleradiology Image Quality Using a SMPTE Test Pattern. http://www.mikety.net/Articles/MD.SMPTE/SMPTE.html (Accessed 4/2003).

[34] Society of Motion Pictures and Television Engineers (SMPTE). Specifications for Medical Diagnostic Imaging Test Pattern for Television Monitors and Hard-copy Recording Cameras. Recommended Practice RP 133-1986. *SMPTE Journal* 1986; 95: 693-695.

[35] Gray JE, Lisk KG, Haddick DH, et al. Test Pattern for Video Displays and Hard-copy Cameras. *Radiology* 1985; 154: 519-527.

[36] Gray JE. Use of the SMPTE Test Pattern in Picture Archiving and Communication Systems. *Journal of Digital Imaging* 1992; 5(1): 54-58.

[37] Halpern EJ, Esser PD. An Improved Phantom for Quality Control of Laser Scanner Digitizers in Picture Archival and Communications Systems. *Journal of Digital Imaging* 1991; 4: 241-247.

[38] Esser PD, Halpern EJ, Amis ES. Quality Assurance of Picture Archiving Communication Systems with Laser Film Digitizers. *Journal of Digital Imaging* 1991; 4: 248-250.

[39] Grotta JC, et al., Intravenous tissue-type plasminogen activator therapy for ischemic stroke: Houston experience 1996 to 2000. *Arch. Neurol.*, 2001. 58:2009-13.

In: State-of-the-Art Imaging in Stroke, Volume 2
Editor: Bernhard Schaller, pp. 285-326
ISBN 978-1-60021-499-8


*Chapter X*

# Brain Functional Imaging for Evaluation of Brain Function and Neuronal Plasticity

***P. M. Rossini, G. Dal Forno*, F. Vernieri* and C. Altamura****
Clinical Neurology, University Campus Bio-Medico, Rome, Italy
*AFaR-Department of Neuroscience, Ospedale Isola Tiberina, Rome, Italy
IRCCS Centro S. Giovanni di Dio-Fatebenefratelli, Brescia, Italy

## A. Introduction

It has been traditionally taught that adult brain has no significant ability for self-repair or reorganization following injuries that cause neuronal death. On the other hand, it is common in clinical practice to see slow but consistent recovery over a period of weeks and months following lesions of apparently stabilised neurological deficits, such as stroke. Degrees of spontaneous recovery range widely, even in light of very similar acute lesions and clinical pictures.

Several explanations, not mutually exclusive and often overlapping, have been given for the recovery of lost function. For example, in stroke syndromes, reabsorption of perilesional edema, interindividual variability of perfusion patterns and arterial collaterals have been proven to play a major role. However spontaneous recovery following an ischemic neural damage may persist beyond the time needed for structural changes secondary to the brain infarct. This observation suggests that other mechanism beside cerebral reperfusion or resolving of inflammatory processes may contribute to recover some cerebral functions.

Additional and more general mechanisms for human CNS functional recovery though, that despite extensive animal research had been elusive and had not explained the molecular basis of plasticity, are now being understood and described thanks to new techniques for their functional study in vivo. Multiple representations of the same function in the cortex (e.g. motor control), presence and amount of alternative neural routes (e.g. *ipsilateral* corticospinal fibers), unmasking of functionally silent connections, as well as changes in synaptic efficacy and remodelling, are all important contributors to the *plasticity* of the human CNS.

A better understanding of the mechanisms underlying recovery (or deterioration) of function after a CNS lesion, as well as those leading to maladaptive or unfavorable outcomes, would be essential for directing specific and effective rehabilitative strategies as well as avoiding potentially harmful interventions.

In this chapter we review those anatomical and physiological aspects of the nervous system that likely play a major role in post-lesional functional improvement, with special emphasis on the sensorimotor system. In addition methods that allow for in-vivo evaluation of plastic phenomena will be reviewed.

# B. Experimental Knowledge

## Mechanisms of Plasticity of the Central Nervous System

In the last few decades, experimental research has shown that mature CNS does have a degree of reorganization following exercise and even the capability for self repair following injury, although the definite clinical demonstration of the actual linkage between functional recovery and plastic reorganization is still missing.

The term *"plasticity"* describes the capacity for pliancy and malleability. When applied to a dynamic and biologic system, such as brain function and behavior, the concept of plasticity usually includes the *potential for change* as well as all the mechanisms of self-repair and/or of reorganization of neural connections. Plastic phenomena are probably at the basis of learning as well as of damage repair in fact cortical maps can be modified by sensory input, experience and learning. Indeed, cortical representation areas probably undergo continuous transient changes during routine life experiences, in response to repeated stimuli as well as to sensory deprivation, movement patterns, and cognitive tasks. For example, transient enlargement of cortical representation areas over a few days has been demonstrated in response to the repeated performance of a skilled movement pattern, such as the learning of a piano exercise [1]. Such changes are likely to become stable, depending on the duration of the "exposure" to a stimulus or motor pattern, as exemplified by the permanent and asymmetric enlargement of the cortical representation area of the left fingers in string players or of the lips in trumpet players [2, 3].

The physiology at the basis of the rapid "plastic" changes of the CNS, probably include a number of cellular and anatomical phenomena. The true anatomical distribution of a neural network is indeed much larger than the area of its usual functional influence, as exemplified by the multiple representations of each muscle and joint area in the motor cortex (see below).

Modifications of the synaptic efficacy within neuronal networks have been favoured by many as underlying learning and memory, as well as some of the cortical plasticity related to acquisition and recovery of sensorimotor function.

The functional status and distribution of a network probably depends on the balance between excitation and inhibition, with some areas being kept silent, or 'masked', by a mechanism of active tonic inhibition mediated through GABAergic input. This active inhibition can be altered or removed, causing a rapid change in size or distribution of the functional network, a process called "unmasking" [4].

Other relatively fast processes that most likely play a pivotal role in the functional strengthening or weakening of existing synapses are long term potentiation (LTP) and long term inhibition or depression (LTI or LTD), respectively [5]. LTP and LTI are neurophysiological mechanisms, by which information is stored in the CNS. LTI is probably based upon Na+ or Ca2+ channels at least for short-term changes, while LTP-like mechanisms include glutamate dependent NMDA receptor activation for long-term changes, a process that can be antagonized by GABA-inhibition [6]. Ever since it was discovered in the hippocampus, LTP has been regarded as the prototypic mechanism of modified synaptic efficacy. LTP can occur with different mechanisms, such as modification of the input to a postsynaptic cell, the concomitant synchronous input to the synapse from another cell, or postsynaptic depolarization. Therefore, converging inputs from various sources, including cortico-cortical and subcortical-cortical connections, could interact and lead to the reshaping of cortical input-output somatotopy [7].

The release of neurotrasmitters from diffuse projection systems, such as noradrenalin synthesized by the locus coeruleus cells, dopamine by the lateral tegmentum and serotonin by the raphe nuclei, are all also likely to modulate synaptic efficacy [8]. The role of Nitric Oxide, as a potential modulator of cortical plasticity is also under investigation [9].

A fourth process likely to play a role in CNS plasticity, although conceivably over a longer time frame, is neuronal sprouting and formation of new synaptic connections. These changes at a cellular level are probably strongly influenced by local neurotransmitter and neurotrophic factors release, and synaptic protein synthesis. In particular dendrites and dendritic spines, the main site for synaptic connections, undergo continuous remodeling [10], a process most likely modulated also by interaction with neighboring astrocytes. The elements that govern local neurotrophic factor release probably include a number of physiological as well as pathological stimuli. For example, it is well documented that ischemia is a strong inducer of gene expression in the brain [11] and a number of growth factors can reduce infarct size in experimental models [12]. On the other hand, in experimental stroke, placement in an enriched environment, with the possibility of performing various activities as well as interactions, results in better recovery, as compared to standard laboratory environments [13]. These findings may be related to direct stimulation of trophic factor release through environmental stimulation, a mechanism probably operating also in normal non-pathologic situations, such as experience-based or use-dependent plasticity.

In addition to cellular and synaptic mechanisms, the CNS functional anatomy seems to be organized, even through a certain degree of relative redundancy, so that damage can be at least in part functionally compensated. Furthermore, all damaging and restorative mechanisms are strongly influenced by the remote effects of the loss of excitatory/inhibitory modulation from a damaged area onto adjacent or distant brain centers connected via cortico-cortical and transcallosal projections, a phenomenon called diaschisis. For instance cortico-cortical inputs to the primary motor cortex (MI) are dominated by those from the supplementary motor area, premotor cortex and primary sensory cortices 1, 2 and 3, where spatiotemporal maps allow the integration of the proprioceptive, tactile and visual cues necessary for manual actions [14]. Voluntary motor activity in humans requires sensory feedback from the moving part [15]. After a stroke, for example, patients with poor improvement of hand motor control show severe metabolic depression in the thalamus [16]. Together with the output for movement, simultaneous discharges to primary somatosensory cortex (SI) are fired by MI, probably providing the "efferent copy" of the motor program which the sensory feedback should be matched with [17].

An appropriate sensory feedback from the paretic hand, therefore, seems fundamental for long-term motor recovery and neuronal reorganization beyond the limits of the usual sensorimotor areas.

In healthy humans the organization of the sensorimotor areas is rather symmetrical between the two hemispheres, and this has been demonstrated with different methods of functional brain imaging, particularly for hand control. When a hemispheric lesion occurs, adjacent or distant, but functionally connected neuronal aggregates, can progressively take over for the lost neurons [18) and this reorganization, is expected to modify interhemispheric symmetry in terms of absolute surfaces, number of "recruited" neurons, and spatial coordinates. Symmetry can thus be used as an important parameter to study brain lesions.

The motor system seems to be the most obvious one to study as a model for basic plasticity phenomena because it controls readily evident human behaviours, yet it is also complex enough to be representative of many other functional systems. We will, therefore, review more in detail the neurophysiology of sensorimotor function, particularly for hand and arm control.

## Technologies for Non-Invasive Functional Brain Imaging

Different imaging techniques are nowadays available for investigating brain function, mapping areas of activation during a cognitive or motor task or in response of a sensory stimulus. Some measure regional blood flow and metabolic changes linked with function-related variations in neuronal firing level, whereas other techniques analyze the electromagnetic properties of brain neurons (Table 1.)

PET is a relatively invasive technique involving inhalation or injection of radioactive substances. This technique produces quantitative maps of brain activity using tracer kinetic modeling of the radioactive compound. For instance, regional cerebral blood flow (rCBF), a marker of synaptic activity in the structurally intact brain (so-called `neurovascular coupling`), can be measured using various radioisotopes. While the subject lies in the scanner, radiation detectors, positioned all around the head, detect the anatomical location within the subject's brain where the encounter of a positron and a natural electron, reciprocally annihilating, produces gamma radiations. The source of these radiations can in turn be mapped showing the position of the radioisotope in space, that is where the blood is preferentially flowing while the subject performs a particular `activation` task [19]. The anatomic location of the activation can be determined by mapping the signal changes into a standardized co-ordinate system and superimposed onto a standardized three-dimensional MR image of the human brain [20]. Although initially possible only across a group of subjects, recent advances in PET technology have made possible to detect significant activations in individual subjects and to map these changes on their own MRI's, resulting in substantial improvement in spatial resolution and anatomical registration.

**Table 1. Core principles of various functional imaging techniques**

| Technique | Core Principle |
|---|---|
| Positron Emission Tomography<br>Near InfraRed Spectroscopy<br>Functional Magnetic Resonance } | Regional blood flow and metabolic changes |
| High Density ElectroEncephaloGraphy<br>MagnetoEncephaloGraphy<br>Transcranial Magnetic Stimulation<br>MRI detection of weak magnetic field } | Electromagnetic properties of neuronal firing |

Temporal resolution of PET is poor, as each measurement of rCBF takes around 90 seconds and cannot be repeated for at least 6 minutes. On the other hand, spatial resolution can be at the 5–10 mm level. Because of dosimetry, only a limited number of scans can be obtained in a single session in a given subject. A major advantages of PET is that radioisotopes can be incorporated into specific ligands to the receptors one wants to study. This technique is however rather expensive, invasive and complex in execution, requiring a cyclotrone to produce in loco the short decaying radioisotopes needed. Though PET had an 'historical' role in producing the first cerebral mapping in vivo outside the neuro-surgery room, because of its invasiveness and poor temporal resolution its utilization has become less relevant since the introduction of fMRI.

Functional MRI derives its signal from changes in deoxyhemoglobin concentrations in response to cerebral activity, without the need to inject or inhale exogenous substances. The fundamental signal detected by fMRI derives from hydrogen atoms, abundantly represented in water molecules of the brain. When subjected to a magnetic field, these atoms absorb energy with a characteristic radiofrequency and, after a short period, this energy is re-emitted at the same radiofrequency with a gradual return to a steady state. The MRI scanner measures the sum of the re-emitted radiofrequency energy which decays over time in dependence of presence of inhomogeneities in the magnetic field. Greater inhomogeity induces decreased image intensity, because each hydrogen atom is exposed to a slightly different magnetic field strength and their radio-frequency emissions annul one another. Oxyhemoglobin is weakly diamagnetic and interferes very little with the magnetic field, while deoxyhemoglobin is a paramagnetic molecule and its variations in concentration can be detected generating fMRI activation with an inverse correlation. The detected signal is called "blood oxygen-level dependent (BOLD) signal" [21] and it was first described by Ogawa [22] in rat brain studied with strong magnetic fields (7 and 8.4 T). Since then, several experimental study have analyzed the origin of its signal to clarify the complex cascade that, from neural activation, finally generates the decrement of deoxyhemoglobin concentration detected by MRI. Though these phenomena are only partially understood, it is generally accepted, however, that fMRI activation is based on neuro-vascular coupling, i.e. the vascular response to a neural activation to supply glucose and oxygen.. Neuronal activation secondary to a task increases the need for energetic molecules and within two seconds an initial consumption of oxygen and a transitory increase of deoxyhemoglobin concentrationis observed. This transient phenomenon is believed to cause the initial deflection of fMRI time course below baseline, defined as "initial dip". Even though several studies seem to confirm this hypothesis, the real meaning of the "initial dip" is still uncertain. However, this phenomenon has stirred interest because it may reflect a rapid increase of the cerebral metabolic rate of oxygen (CMRO) before the cerebral blood flow (CBF) increase, and this phenomenon may be more localized to the area of increased metabolism, while the following CBF increase may instead cover a wider area.

Two seconds after enhancement of the neural firing rate, a local increase of CBF is observed, with a subsequent oversupply of oxygen. The CBF increases much more than $CMRO_2$ producing a reduction of the oxygen extraction fraction (OEF) and the total deoxyhemoglobin present in an image voxel is detected by the MRI scanner as the positive component of the time course, generating ultimately the BOLD signal [21]. Nevertheless, BOLD signal is probably due to a complex interplay including OEF, $CMRO_2$, blood oxygen saturation and blood volume in addition to the CBF. In fact, the relative changes in CBF and $CMRO_2$ determine the level of oxygenation of the blood, while the CBV determines the total amount of blood (and thus the total deoxyhemoglobin present in each voxel). For instance, a post-stimulus undershoot of the BOLD signal is common and may last for 30 seconds or more [23], while the CBF response typically shows either a shorter and weaker post-stimulus undershoot or no undershoot at all [24]. The post-stimulus undershoot is probably generated because the CBV is slower to recover than the CBF and CMRO. Then, if the oxygen extraction fraction returns to baseline at the end of the stimulus, but the venous blood volume remains elevated, total deoxyhemoglobin will be higher than baseline, reducing the BOLD signal [25]. The undershoot in the BOLD signal can also be explained as a reduction of the neuronal activity after stimulation [26], leading to a matching undershoot in CBF. Therefore, among the causes of the post-stimulus undershoot could be a mismatch in the CBF and CBV post-stimulus recovery, a CBF undershoot following reduction of neuronal activity, or a combination of both.

Other physiological factors may modulate BOLD signal intensity, such as vascular geometry, haematocrit and basal oxygenation levels. Baseline CBF has also been observed to have a strong effect on the BOLD magnitude response to the same stimulus. For example, if baseline CBF is increased by breathing $CO_2$, the BOLD response to the same task is reduced substantially. Interestingly, however, the CBF change appears to remain the same despite baseline changes [27]. Similar results have been found with injection of acetazolamide, a carbonic anhydrase inhibitor. Carbonic anhydrase catalyzes the conversion of $CO_2$ to bicarbonate ions, which increases the capacity of the blood for removing CO. Inhibiting this enzyme may lead to increased $CO_2$ concentration in the brain, so the mechanism of action for increasing CBF may be the same as for $CO_2$ itself. This observation is of paramount interest when fMRI is used to analyze cerebral activation in patients affected by cerebrovascular disease, as discussed below.

Even if s the BOLD effect is primarily due to changes in local deoxyhemoglobin content, two additional sources of signal change must be considered: the intravascular and the extravascular signals. Both compartments are in fact affected by the magnetic field gradients created by the presence of deoxyhemoglobin, which cause the MR signal to decay faster when deoxyhemoglobin increases. Although the amount of extravascular signal is much greater than the intravascular signal, the sensitivity of the latter to blood oxygenation is much higher. The result is that the intravascular contribution likely accounts for half or more of the signal change observed at 1.5 T-field intensity. As mentioned before, the total deoxyhemoglobin content could change either by changing the oxygen extraction fraction or by changing the volume of the venous blood, so the role of volume changes must be considered [28]. Finally, diffusion effects can also be important for the smallest vessels.

Although the hemodynamic process responsible for the BOLD signal has been thoroughly investigated, the nature of the bio-chemical signal that couples neural activity to vascular response is yet to be fully clarified. In fact, it is widely accepted that a CBF increase follows directly synaptic activity enhancement and a number of studies using a variety of different techniques have shown data suggesting a linear relationship between neural activity and subsequent hemodynamic response [29]. A particular attention must be paid to those utilizing intra-cortical electrodes and intense magnetic fields in animal models. Very recently, the correlation between firing rate and BOLD was also confirmed with MRI/MRS (magnetic resonance spectroscopy) studies in rats, whereby a linear relationship between $CMRO_2$, glutamatergic neurotransmitter flux, and neural activity has been demonstrated [30].

On the other hand, blood flow increases proportionally to glucose consumption which is in turn linked to synaptic activation. Empirical studies suggest that cortical cells firing activity contributes minimally to cerebral metabolic demand. For this reason if firing frequency duplicates, the effect on regional metabolism should be modest if compared to the changes measured by functional imaging techniques. On the other hand, the major cause of cortical consumption of oxygen and glucose is the re-equilibration of ionic concentrations trough the $Na^+/K^+$ ATPase pump [31] and the recycling of neurotransmitters following synaptic activity. The intracellular/extracellular sodium gradient is in fact far from equilibrium, and pumping sodium against this gradient causes thermodynamically very high energy consumption. For this reason, the most costly aspect of neural activity is likely to be the excitatory synaptic activity whith glutamate dependent sodium channels opening. In a recent animal experiment, blocking voltage-dependent $Na^+$ channels substantially reduced the CBF response [32], supporting once more the idea that the dominant energy consuming process in the brain is the recovery from excitatory activity. Finally, there is evidence suggesting that inhibitory activity does not elicit a measurable BOLD response [33].

It has been hypothesized that fMRI signal is generated by non-oxidative metabolism of glucose. This theory would explain, on one hand, the proportionality between blood flow and glucose consumption, and on the other hand, the uncoupling between blood flow and oxygen consumption. In particular, astrocytes play a crucial role in neurotransmitters recycling, burning up energy to remove glutamate from the extra-cellular space and transform it in glutamine. The glutamate released by excitatory synapses, stimulates a concomitant glucose up-take from the blood by astrocytes surrounding synapses and intra-parenchimal capillaries. To recycle the neurotransmitters, astrocytes take the glycolysis pathway utilizing glucose and producing lactate. According to this hypothesis, blood flow changes are thus necessary to supply the glucose requested by astrocytes, independently from blood oxygenation. The alternative theory proposes that blood flow increase is necessary to supply the oxygen requested by neuronal metabolism. In accordance with this hypothesis, the apparent uncoupling between blood flow and oxygen consumption is the consequence of oxygen transportation. In fact, an excessive increase in blood flow is requested to support a slight change of oxygen metabolism, since its extraction (through passive diffusion) is less efficient for high flow levels. This second hypothesis is founded on two considerations. First, oxygen consumption is proportional to neural firing, although in a different level than blood flow. Second, estimation of the metabolic costs of cerebral activity shows that energy is mainly consumed by neurons, proportionally to their firing rate, while only a small percentage of energy is utilized by astrocytes. In fact, neurons obtain energy from the oxidative metabolism of lactate, while astrocytes do only from non-oxidative glycolysis. Finally, astrocytes might transiently derive their energy supply directly from glycogen during intense neural activity, so to avoid augmentation of glucose transportation. In summary three signals could be at the basis of neuro-vascular coupling, causing the hemodynamic response: lactate produced by astrocyte metabolism (implying a strong relation between synaptic activity and BOLD contrast), a diffusible molecule generated by neuronal spiking (such as nitric oxide), or an intrinsic stimulus of arterioles secondary to transient oxygen decrease (causing the initial dip). However, the vaso-dilation underlying the increased blood flow has also been hypothesized to be associated with passive dilation of venules and veins because of their balloon-like elasticity. [34].

In the last few years, a new fMRI technique called arterial spin labeling (ASL), has been introduced, that allows measuring both the BOLD signal and CBF simultaneously.

With ASL, magnetization of the arterial blood is inverted and, after a suitable delay to allow tagged blood to enter the desired image plane, an image is acquired. The experiment is then repeated without tagging the arterial blood and another image is acquired as a control. The image difference, "control minus tag", is then a direct reflection of how much arterial blood was delivered to each voxel and so providing a CBF map. With dual echo acquisition, with subsequent acquisitions alternating between tag and control, the data can be processed to yield essentially independent measurements of the local CBF and BOLD time series. Although currently such technique is not widely available, it seems to offer the best prospects for providing data that will allow quantitative analysis of the BOLD effect and a more accurate interpretation of its signal when utilized in stroke patient. With the use of this technique Uludag˘ and collaborators [35], evaluated cerebral activation and deactivation to visual stimulus in healthy subjects with a task characterized by eye open and closing . On the basis or their findings, they propose a mechanistic model of *feed-forward neurovascular coupling*. According to this model, neural activity produces and/or releases vasoactive agents that increase or decrease CBF, so that the change in CBF directly reflects the change in neural activity, independent of the resting level CBF. This way, the change in CBF for a given stimulus would not depend on baseline CBF, but on baseline neural activity. In the $CO_2$ experiments mentioned before, baseline neural activity presumably remained constant, despite the alteration of baseline CBF, so the increment of CBF with activation remained the same. In this study, neural activity was presumed to be reduced with eyes closed, and the corresponding reduction in CBF was interpreted as a result of neurovascular coupling. On the other hand, the larger increment of CBF change should then reflects the larger change in neural activity between resting and activated states. The authors suggest also that this feed-forward neurovascular coupling model could be used to investigate the mechanisms of action of other exogenous agents that alter CBF, such as caffeine or alcohol, to test whether these drugs alter baseline CBF through direct effects on vessels or secondary to neuronal changes.

Anothe issue, only lately clarified, is which current determines the hemodynamic response among those induced by neuronal activity,. Recent reports suggest that the evolution of the BOLD signal is more closely related to the so-called local field potential (LFP) variation than to spiking activity changes of single or multiple neurons (MUA: multiple-unit spiking activity). LFPs, represent slow waveforms, that include synaptic potentials, after-potentials of somato-dendritic spikes, and voltage-gated membrane oscillations reflecting the input of a given cortical area as well as its local intracortical processing, including the activity of excitatory and inhibitory interneurons. The LFP may be interpreted as the result of the cooperative activity in neural populations. In summary, combined physiological and fMRI experiments suggest that the BOLD signal mainly reflects the incoming specific or association inputs into an area and the processing of this input information by the local cortical circuitry [36]. Kim and collaborators recently [37] confirmed this finding, in a study combining fMRI analysis and microelectrode registration of neural activation in response to a visual stimulus in cortical area 18 of the cat. The authors observed also an approximated linear coupling between BOLD and neuronal activity if a large enough activity area is considered. Together with previous studies by other groups [29, 38], these results suggest that the functional ''activation'' area identified in the published BOLD studies with relatively large voxel sizes of about 3–5 $mm^2$ may accurately reflect the underlying neuronal activity. However the data of this study indicate that in cat area 18, only less than 50% of the variance in neuronal modulation, during stimulation with simple moving gratings, can effectively be accounted for, if voxel sizes of 2.6-2.6 $mm^2$ or less are used. Voxels of sub-millimeter scale, therefore, should be interpreted with great caution. and sub-millimeter resolution fMRI imaging would seem to call for the mapping of MR signal with sources other than the T2*-based BOLD contrast.

Although the BOLD signal change is very small, this is offset by the acquisition of repeated time-series, so the technique has sufficient sensitivity to detect activations from individual subjects. The acquisition frames of fMRI depend on the specific collection sequence used, but it can be less than 100ms for a single scan, allowing to perform multi-slice imaging of the whole brain within a short time period. Temporal resolution of fMRI is dictated by the hemodynamic response timing of the neurovascular coupling phenomenon, which is about 12 seconds. It is nevertheless possible to detect differences in peak activation time between brain regions in the order of two seconds, thanks to the previously mentioned initial dip detection. The signal reaches its plateau after 6–12 sec and returns to baseline, although a prolonged post-stimulus undershoot is often evident [23, 34]. This post-stimulus undershoot has been suggested to be secondary to passive dilation of venules and veins as mentioned above. Conversely, spatial resolution of fMRI is currently the highest among functional imaging techniques, up to less than 1 mm provided a sufficient signal-to-noise ratio.

Both PET and fMRI can provide a detailed relationship between function and anatomy and comprehensively map the distributed network subtending a given motor act. There are, however, intrinsic limitations in either techniques. In particular, the length of the examined epochs necessary to compute a statistically significant activation (seconds to minutes) make it difficult to discriminate the temporal sequence of a phenomenon and to differentiate neuronal firing decrease from increase (exciting vs inhibiting net effects). In the case of movement paradigms, the activation directly linked to motor programming and execution cannot be distinguished from the sensory feedback from the moving parts, and the chronological relationship (hierarchy) between activated areas cannot be studied [39].

On the other hand, the other functional techniques which base their signal on the direct analysis of magneto-electrical properties of neural firing, have a better temporal resolution despite an inferior spatial resolution. Other human brain mapping technologies based on metabolic signals have begun to contribute to our understanding of brain plasticity. Near-infrared spectroscopy (NIRS) is an emerging technology that non-invasively measures brain activation by monitoring changes in the absorption of near-infrared light by hemoglobin-containing species in cerebral blood. The functioning principle of this technique is schematized in Figure 1. Changes in concentration of hemoglobin are directly proportional to the variation of regional blood volume and with this technique, small changes in light intensity are almost proportional to the variations of total hemoglobin concentration. NIRS, providing a real-time assessment of fluctuations in cerebral hemoglobin, has been used to estimate the CBV [40]. Moreover, NIRS, through the measurement of oxyhemoglobin (oxy-Hb) and deoxyhemoglobin (deoxy-Hb) concentrations, allows the determination of oxygen saturation of the blood in vivo, in a simple and noninvasive way. NIRS can be designed to be relatively insensitive to head motion, and by using compact instrumentation it can be applied in stroke patients at bedside or in rehabilitation facilities. In addition, this technology is less expensive than PET or fMRI. Moreover, there is evidence indicating that it may be possible to detect optical signals directly related to neuronal activation [41]. The physiological basis of these event-related optical signals (EROS) is not well understood, but it may include cell swelling or membrane polarization associated with neuronal activity, resulting in local light-scattering changes. Thus, optical imaging may provide insights into both the electrophysiological (fast) and hemodynamic (slow) processes underlying other brain imaging signals [42].

The temporal resolution of NIRS is similar to that of fMRI (approximately 1 s), though the sampling rate is typically several orders of magnitude greater, thereby allowing a more accurate detection of the hemodynamic response evolution. Disadvantages of NIRS, as compared to PET and fMRI, are its relatively poor spatial resolution (approximately 3 cm) and depth penetration (approximately 1 cm beneath the deep margin of the skull); however, in a multimodal imaging experimental setting this technique could allow a more complete analysis of metabolic changing secondary to cerebral activation.

Transcranial brain stimulation (TMS) [10], is a safe, and non-invasive technique increasingly used in investigations of brain plasticity. In contrast to the other technique that record brain activity, TMS also interacts with the pattern of cortical activation. In fact, TMS, through a brief and intense magnetic field, created by a circulating electric current within a coil applied directly to the scalp, permits the mapping of underlying cortical representation areas [43].

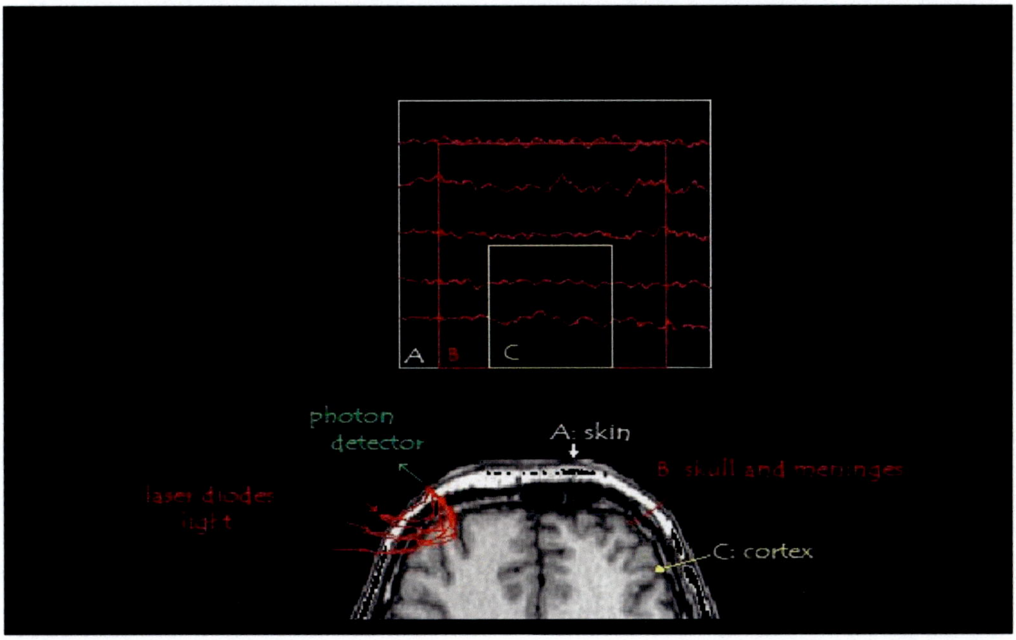


Figure 1. The image explain the functioning principle of NIRS technique. Near infrared light (NIR 700-900 nm) is emitted by laser diodes, variably distant one from the other, and it goes through skin, skull, CSF and meninges (A-B) to finally reach the cortex (C). Haemoglobin contained in the cerebral vessels partially absorbs the NIR light, which is subsequently backscattered from the brain and recorded by a photon detector. The light attenuation change in compartment C is measured to determine fluctuations in cerebral haemoglobin and thus to estimate CBV variation.

This magnetic field penetrates human tissue painlessly, and if the current amplitude, duration and direction are appropriate, it induces electric currents that can depolarize neurons or their axons. One obvious limit of TMS is, however, that the technique allows only cerebral mapping of the motor cortex, differently from other methods mentioned above.

When applied over the scalp regions corresponding to the motor strip, the magnetic stimulus triggers cortico-spinal pathway directly or through cortico-cortical connections. The effect of the magnetic stimulation may be registered with epidural electrodes or generally, less invasively, in the connected “target” muscles where a transient electromyographic response (Motor Evoked Potentials = MEPs) is detected. Thanks to this technique, the excitability threshold and propagation properties of cortico-spinal fibers responsible for target muscle activation can be examined. The development of coil stimulators of various shapes, sizes, and orientation allows for preferential excitation of discrete brain regions [17].

In particular, the circular coil positioned on the vertex of the scalp stimulates within a distance of centimeters from its edge, a relatively non focal stimulation. Activation occurs maximally in an circular area of the same size under the coil. This coil may be useful to measure amplitude, latency and morphology of MEPS, but it does not allow a precise somatotopic mapping of motor cortex or selective electrical stimulation. Conversely, an eight-shaped coil permits to map cerebral organization and reorganization with focal stimulation in consecutive positions of the scalp distant 1 centimeter one from the other. The current induced under the midregion is in fact, twice that under each of the edges [44].

Upper extremity muscles representation areas usually line up in a proximal to distal and medial to lateral location along the central sulcus [45]. The area of a TMS map is a function of both the area of the underlying corticospinal map and the distance from the coil to the corticospinal neurons that can be activated. The higher is the intensity of the TMS stimulus, the larger is the area of the MEP map, and the higher is the excitability of cortical neurons, the greater the ease to stimulate them at a given distance from the coil.

Intensity and latency of motor responses can be also be traced on bi-dimensional maps drawn from the vertex and other anatomical landmarks. It is not only cortical excitability that must be defined: the area of MEP maps also depends on the excitability of spinal mechanisms. The magnetic field train activates a portion of the corticospinal projections that produces an action potential in spinal motoneurons. If these neurons are far from their threshold, they will not discharge and no MEP will be recorded. In this case, the stimulation point on the scalp will be outside the area of the MEP map. Conversely, if spinal excitability is high, the same excitatory post-synaptic potential (EPSP) will discharge the motoneuron and produce a MEP. The cortical point will be then classified as inside the cortical map. An alternative strategy to evaluate MEP excitability is to map the motor thresholds for a specific movement at particular scalp locations [46]. Cortical motor threshold is defined as the minimum intensity that produces a MEP in the target muscle on 50% of trials [47, 48]. This is a complex measure since, although the initial cortical elements activated are likely to be large-diameter myelinated axons, as mentioned before, MEPs are evoked only after a sequence of synaptic relays in both cortex and spinal cord. Thus, although the threshold of the cortical axons is likely to be relatively dependent of the level of synaptic activity in the cortex, the MEP threshold will also depend on the excitability of synaptic relays. The evoked movement will be related to the first recruited muscle at the point of stimulation. Relatively discrete and reproducible movements can be evoked in distal hand muscles, but only rarely in more proximal muscles because of their higher threshold. TMS mapping studies can also be carried out using other types of measures. For instance, the duration of the cortical silent period or the TMS-induced delay in voluntary movement can be used to map the inhibitory effects of TMS.

The analysis of electromyographic response of ten different muscles of the upper limb at the same time demonstrated activation cluster and muscles aggregation also during focal stimulation [49]. This observation suggests the presence of a motor network along the pre-central part of M1. Changes in cortical maps that are use-dependent or consequent to a lesion, usually demonstrate two main characteristics. The first is the enlargement or restriction of the excitable area, without changes in the amplitude-weighted center of the motor output maps, or center of gravity (CoG), possibly due to the recruitment or inhibition of a fringe of adjacent neurons. The second is the migration of the excitable area outside the usual boundaries, possibly due to a lesion affecting the brain district where lays the "hot spot" (the point of maximum response of the target muscle) (Figure 2). Such a "migration" may be apparent, and due to the activation of a secondary hot spot previously hidden by the predominant one, or it may be in fact real, due to the progressive activation of new synaptic connections.

Whether mapping studies focused on excitability or on location, one of the main findings has been that both features can be influenced by the level of sensory feedback. For example, removing feedback in healthy subjects by temporary anesthesia can increase excitability of corticospinal projections to muscles proximal to the block [50].

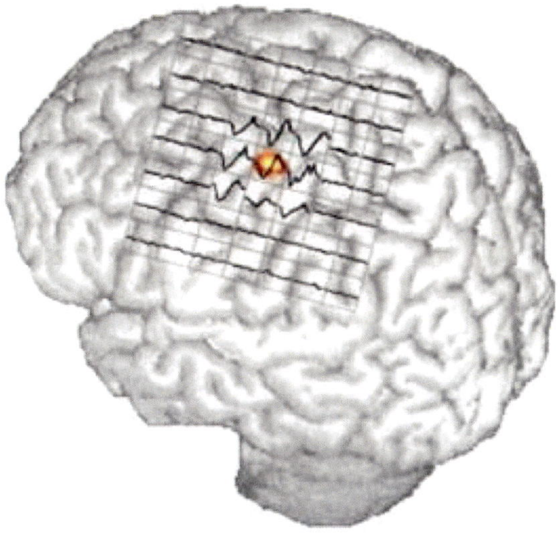

Figure 2. The figure shows the superimposition on a brain model, of the grid of stimulation sites and MEPs recorded from the abductor digiti minimi muscle of a healthy volunteer. The coloured area represents the hot-spot (red) corresponding with the center of gravity (yellow).

This effect is however transient, it occurs during the period of anaesthesia, and it returns to normal shortly after the block. Nevertheless, other types of sensory alteration can cause also longer lasting changes. It was observed [51] that stimulation of peripheral sensory afferents for several minutes can lead to changes in MEP maps that last 30–60 min after the end of sensory stimulation. Besides, paired stimulation of peripheral afferents and TMS of sensorimotor cortex can also lead to similar long lasting changes in corticospinal excitability.

At present, beside the possibility to map the motor cortex, TMS is used in two additional ways to investigate neuronal plasticity. First, single and paired pulse TMS techniques is a powerful tool for studying mechanisms of intracortical inhibition and excitation [52], differently from blood flow based neuroimaging methods, such as PET and fMRI, where in the activated brain regions, excitatory or inhibitory neuronal activities cannot be distinguished. . Second, in addition to recruiting positive phenomena, TMS can be used to interfere with normal neuronal activity during perception, motor execution, or higher-level cognitive processes to explore the functional relevance of cortical reorganization. This disruptive effect of TMS on cortical function is often referred to as a “virtual lesion”. It occurs because the stimulus transiently synchronizes the activity of a large proportion of neurons under the coil inducing a long lasting generalized IPSP (inhibitory post-synaptic potential) that reduces cortical activity for the next 50–200 ms depending on stimulus intensity.

Moreover, repetitive TMS (rTMS) can produce changes in excitability of cortical circuits that outlast the period of stimulation, opening the possibility of intervening directly with the mechanisms of cortical plasticity in the intact human cortex. Nevertheless, in this case, specific safety issues need to be taken into account. If rTMS is applied at high frequency and intensity to the cortex, it may even induce epileptic seizures. However, the risks can be minimized by careful selection of subjects, stimulus threshold and strict adherence to safety guidelines [53]. On the contrary, when rTMS is applied at low frequency, it mainly inhibits cortical excitability in the healthy. These properties are currently under evaluation to test the theoretical therapeutic effect of this technique. In particular, low frequency rTMS is currently employed in the research context as a therapeutic tool for drug-resistant epilepsy. On the other hand, high frequency rTMS has been successfully used to treat mood disorders, and very recently, potential beneficial effect have been theorized on the plastic phenomena following ischemic strokes. However, clinical application of this technique as a therapeutic tool has yet to be approved.

Advanced EEG methods permit to eliminate the contribution of volume currents, to obtain reference free recordings and to disentangle locoregional rhythmic or transient neuronal activities produced by both tangentially and radially oriented generators from discrete brain regions underlying the exploring electrode [54]. However, EEG data are measurements of potential differences on the scalp, thus EEG signals are produced by ohmic flow of current in the head, that are highly sensitive to the conductivity of the brain, skull, and extracranial tissue. Consequently, the main pitfall of this technique is the so-called "inverse problem" that is to localize regions of neural activation from the analysis of the obtained electric dipole.

Nevertheless, a promising computational EEG approach comes from the analysis of the coherence of the EEG rhythms (theta, alpha, and beta) simultaneously generated in different cortical areas. Coherence analysis studies non-invasively and with a high temporal resolution, the connectivity of different brain regions, and how this connectivity changes in relation to task activation. Coherence EEG, as well as the study of the coherence between EEG and EMG signals during voluntary motor activity, are very promising methods that might permit a more in depth study of neuronal plastic changes secondary to either physiological brain function or to disease states [55].

Recently, high-spatial density EEG (using more than 64 sensors) has been successfully used to improve the spatial resolution of this technique. This new interesting method [56] has been applied for multimodal integration with fMRI. Besides the detection of cerebral activation, this approach allows the analysis of cerebral connectivity (i.e. *functional binding* among different brain regions) with a good spatial resolution. As cerebral connectivity could play a fundamental role in cerebral reorganization, its analysis is of great relevance in revealing plastic phenomena following ischemic damage. In fact, it could clarify the time sequence and the connection among the different cerebral structures detected as 'activated' by the fMRI.

Magnetoencephalography (MEG) is a non-invasive functional imaging technique, which detects magnetic fields induced by neural firing. In fact, it does not require inhalation or injection of radio-labeled molecules or contrast agent and patients are not subjected to magnetic fields, permitting also repeated measures. MEG can identify spatially the synchronous firing of neurons from restricted cortical areas, in relation to either spontaneous cerebral activity or in response to external stimuli, and allows the analysis of neuronal activation with temporal resolutions of a millisecond or less. Differently from EEG, the MEG signal is not influenced by extra-cerebral tissue layers overlying brain. It allows to localize and measure the weak magnetic field induced by intracellular currents in a shallow brain region exactly below the recording sensor, without any contributions from volume currents. Neuronal action potentials and post-synaptic potentials (particularly those of pyramidal cells) may be simplified as current dipoles generating a magnetic field in accordance to the "right hand thumb rule". Signal detected from MEG derives essentially from post-synaptic potential because of the possible temporal summation of these currents and a lower extinction velocity. MEG is able to detect at the scalp magnetic fields induced by dipole intensity currents of 10 nA x m, so that approximately one million synapses activated simultaneously can generate an evoked response. Since there are approximately $10^5$ pyramidal cells per $mm^2$ of cerebral cortex, and thousands of synapses for each neuron, hypothetically the simultaneous activation of few synapses of each neuron within an area of a square millimeter should be sufficient to induce a detectable signal on the scalp. In practice, though, larger areas actually need to activate simultaneously to annul electromagnetic fields generated by currents flowing in opposite directions. Magnetic fields induced by living creatures are much lower than magnetic signals from non-biological sources in urban areas, for this reason quite important measures must be taken to obtain a magnetically shielded recording environment. In humans, the highest magnetic field is generated by the cardiac muscle (40-50pT), whereas in the vigilant brain it is physiologically represented by rhythmic spontaneous activity (alpha rhythm). Fields evoked by sensory stimulation have even weaker intensity (around 10-100 fT). For this reason, background activity may limit the signal-to-noise ratio but it is interrelated among different sensors and it can be theoretically discriminated from signal source. The peculiarity of the bio-magnetic technique is to detect extremely weak signals in the presence of a background noise at least 100 times superior. This is possible thanks to superconducting devices called SQUIDs (Superconductiong Quantum Interference Devices) which must be kept at a temperature of -269 °C with a liquid helium cryostat. The sensors are able to detect only perpendicular components of the magnetic field, thus the signal detected records preferentially the tangential component of current dipoles generated in the depth of gyri. Magnometers can record a magnetic field derived by intracellular currents or by a combination of both intra- and extra- cellular currents, depending on its orientation with respect to the scalp. If the axis of the magnometer is perpendicular, in order to detect only the radial component of an extra-cranial field, the signal detected is related only to intra-cellular currents. On the other hand, if the axis is rotated and also the tangential component of the field is measured, the recording derives from both currents. The aim of the MEG examination is to map the distribution on the scalp of the magnetic field generated by neural firing and use the obtained maps to calculate the most plausible distribution of current sources. The fundamental problem in source localization is to estimate the neural current distribution which has generated the detected field ("the inverse problem"). In fact the distribution of the current in a conductor cannot be deduced univocally based on the magnetic field induced. To get around this problem researchers model the magnetic response on one of the possible current dipoles (the Equivalent Current Dipole: ECD). It is possible, this way, to map the sensory homunculus through the analysis of the magnetic response (somato-sensory evoked field,SEF) induced by stimulation in different sites (Figure 3).

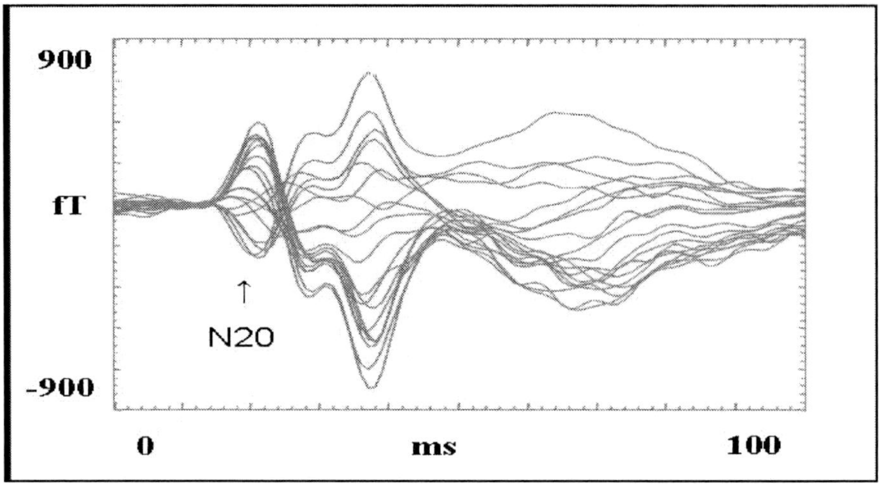


Figure 3. MEG time-course signal registered from parietal-frontal channels after electrical stimulation at the contra-lateral median nerve. The arrow indicates the first detectable response (N20), 20ms after the stimulus, which reflects SI activation.

This model arises logically from the physiological observation that the main neuronal sources of MEG consist of palisades of cortical pyramidal cells, with elongated apical dendrites oriented perpendicularly to the cortical surface. This dipole would express, in statistical terms, where the center of gravity of the active layers lies at that particular time, with variable intensity, position and direction. The values of these parameters are chosen at every instant in time in order to minimize the discrepancy between the theoretical field generated by the dipole and the one measured by the sensor. The parameter that evaluates this difference permits to recognize if the model is inadequate to explain the magnetic distribution measured and to determine the confidence interval for the estimated localization (goodness of fit). From a more theoretical point, it can be argued that detection of a single dipole solution of the inverse magnetic source reconstruction problem does not prove the existence of such a dipole, even when the so-called ''goodness of fit'' is 100%.

Integration of MEG data with anatomical images generated by magnetic resonance imaging is defined as "magnetic source imaging (MSI)". Superimposition of MEG activation to anatomical images is made possible by common reference points (nasion, and pre-auricolar point bilaterally) digitalized to generate a system of coordinates. Simple placement of vitamin E capsules detectable MRI, on the subject's head anatomical landmarks, allows the anatomical superimposition of MEG maps onto radiological images. MRI planes are set parallel to the above-defined localization coordinate system to achieve a highly precise superimposition [57]. This approach has gain great advantage to cerebral mapping with MEG and has been successfully utilized for epilepsy neurosurgery, granting a spatial resolution of about 5 mm.

In summary, MEG follows the spatial and temporal evolution of a dipolar generator source, which is modeled as a current dipole, able to explain 90% or more of the magnetic field distribution over the scalp. It has a very high time resolution, in the order of one millisecond or less. Due to its physical properties, MEG allows a precise 3D-localisation of the firing neuronal pool whenever it produces a dipolar field distribution at the scalp level

[58]. Besides the spatial properties, the strength of ECDs (roughly reflecting the number of neurons firing synchronously), and their orientation can also be measured, while response (SEF) morphology provides indirect information on the underlying neural circuitry. Decrease or increase of dipole strength can be due to restriction or enlargement of the responsive area studied, possibly because of recruitment of fringes of neurons surrounding those usually firing in response to the incoming stimulus. These variations can be secondary to dynamic phenomena, such as use-dependent modulation of synaptic efficacy, changes of excitatory/inhibitory input from adjacent or remote lesioned brain areas (diaschisis), or changes in the amount of sensory information.

MEG and EEG differ fundamentally from fMRI and PET, in both the physiological processes that are measured and the properties of the inverse problem that are solved to produce functional images. Neuronal activation can be detected indirectly with both fMRI and PET through imaging of localized contrast changes resulting from the hemodynamic effects of this activation. Aside from the potential problem that neuronal activation and hemodynamic changes may not always be co-located, these methods are limited in temporal resolution by hemodynamic time constants. In contrast, MEG and EEG signals are the direct extra-cranial manifestations of neuronal activation and can record changes in the millisecond scale at which they occur. Consequently, it may be possible with MEG or EEG not only to detect networks of neuronal assemblies, but also to determine causality within these networks. The other major difference between MEG or EEG and fMRI or PET is in the form of the inverse problems. In fact, both fMRI and PET involve reconstruction of images from a large number of independent samples so that stable images can always be computed at the expense of some mild loss in resolution, thus in this case the inverse problem is not relevant.

In contrast, the MEG or EEG inverse problem involves estimation of brain activation from at most a few hundred spatial samples so that highly restrictive assumptions are required to compute a stable inverse. This presents significant challenges both in the selection of a model that reflects these assumptions and also in the interpretation of the resulting inverse solutions.

To finally resolve the spatial or temporal resolution limits of the mentioned techniques, the challenge that today's researchers are facing is to detect directly the magnetic field generated by neuronal currents. The well-understood sensitivity of MRI to magnetic field variations was first utilized about a decade ago to map electric current density in homogenous and heterogeneous media. Detection of the neuronal currents resulting from brain activity is much more difficult, since these currents are approximately three orders of magnitude smaller, much more transient, and perhaps localized to a smaller region in space. These ionic currents induce subtle and transient magnetic flux density changes, depending on their temporal and spatial coherence. The parallel component of these fields alters the magnetic phase of surrounding water protons and thus influences the phase and/or magnitude of the MRI signal in dependence of the size and geometry of the synchronous current sources.

Evoked or spontaneous magnetic fields (EMF or SMF) measured on the scalp (around 2–4 cm away from the current source) by MEG are on the order of $10^{-12}$ (spontaneous) to $10^{-13}$ (evoked) Tesla. Details about neuronal currents spatial scales are not well known. As mentioned before, It is assumed that at least 50,000 or more cortical neurons, occupying an area of few squared mm must coherently act to produce magnetic fields detectable by MEG.

This spatial scale is approximately that of a typical MRI voxel. The magnetic field peak values and durations depend on stimulus type. Calculations suggest that current sources causing EMFs, assuming an approximate MRI scale of 1–2 mm, could create local peaks of current changes generating a magnetic field in the order of $10^{-9}$ to $10^{-10}$ T, lasting for less than 100 msec. On these basis, researchers are trying to define a new MRI-based methodology for detection of weak and transient changes in magnetic field secondary to neural firing, and other physiologically relevant transient fields in the order of $10^{-10}$ T and lasting for a few dozens of msec [59, 60].

This new methodology would bring great advantage to cerebral mapping, allowing detecting, with excellent spatial and temporal resolution, neural activation and consequently the temporal and spatial evolution of neural circuitry at the basis of both cerebral physiological function and plastic reorganization following different types of damage. However, the complete development and the subsequent diffusion of this method, will likely take some time to actually take place. In the meanwhile, researchers should optimize the use of the currently available imaging techniques. Spatial and temporal resolutions of the various techniques are summarized in table 2.

**Table 2. Comparison of the temporal and spatial resolutions of various functional imaging techniques**

| Technique | Spatial resolution | Temporal resolution |
|---|---|---|
| High density Elettroencephalography | 2-3 cm | Milliseconds |
| Magnetoencephalography | 5mm | Milliseconds |
| Transcranial magnetic stimulation | 1 cm | - |
| Positron emission topography | 5-10 mm | 90 sec |
| Functional magnetic resonance | 1 mm | 2 sec |
| Near infrared spectroscopy | 3cm | ~ 1sec |
| MRI detection of weak magnetic field | 1-2 mm | Milliseconds |

# C. Clinical Knowledge

## Mapping Cerebral Plasticity

Somatotopy is one of the most relevant aspects of motor and sensory cortical representations. Hughlings Jackson hypothesized the idea of cortical areas systematically organized to control movement of different parts of the body, for the first time, in the 1870. He had taken his inspiration by the observation of epileptic patients experiencing motor focal seizures. In the same period, Fritsch and Hitzig, stimulated electrically cortices of dog brains, providing a direct proof of somatotopic organized cortices. This idea was finally conformed by the well-known Penfield's *Homunculus* and Woolsey's *Simiunculus* [61]. Furthermore, subsequent experimental studies by means of intra-cortical stimulations clarified that each body part has multiple cortical representations, sometimes overlapping. A main representation in one particular spot of the pre-central gyrus seems to exist, though at the same time other neuronal clusters inside the gyrus, yet in a smaller amount and in a different combinations with other body-districts, are present. Another relevant characteristic of cortical somatotopy is the symmetrical representation between the two hemispheres. In fact, despite a small inter-subject variability of the cortical representation, a strong symmetry is present between the two hemispheres of the same subjects. These observations represent the basis for the functional mapping of cerebral reorganisation following learning or neural damage, which may alter this inter-hemispheric symmetry. Nowadays, all the above-mentioned techniques of non-invasive imaging had permitted an accurate mapping of brain functions and in particular, the somatotopic representations in healthy controls.

Talairach and Tournoux, in the 1988, elaborated a coordinate system to allow a precise localization of different functional areas as a guide for stereotactic neurosurgery of sub-cortical structures. This system today permit to normalize the data obtained from a single case and using the proportional system, the normalization applies to all brains. This normalization permits statistical studies, since the measurements can be reduced to a common scale. The Talairach space was modeled on the anatomical data of a single subject (the cadaver of a 60-year-old woman). The coordinate system is based on the line which crosses the inter-hemispheric fissure between the superior edge of the anterior commissure (AC) and the inferior edge of the posterior commissure (PC). This line is called the AC-PC line (or Y axis), and has a relationship with sub-cortical gray structures, dividing the thalamus from the subthalamic region. The two other reference lines of the system are defined with respect to the AC-PC line: the coronal AC line (VAC or Z axis), and the PC line (VPC). The VAC is a line laying in the coronal plane, traversing the superior margin of the anterior commissure and perpendicular to the AC-PC line. The origin of both Y and Z axes is given by their intersection. The VPC (or X axis) is perpendicular both to the AC-PC and the VAC line, and shares the same origin. This way, every single spot of human brain is defined by three values (X, Y, Z) that measure its distance, expressed in millimeters, with respect to the axis origin in the anterior, superior and right direction. The Talairach coordinate system, in the attempt to standardize anatomical areas with high inter-subject variability, presents several limits. First of all, it expresses the distance of a point from the axis origin with absolute numeric values, not proportionally to the real volumes of the brain under analysis. To avoid this problem, it is necessary to "normalize" anatomical brain images to make them fit the "standard" brain proportions. This way, an incorrect positioning of the fundamental axis causes considerable errors in the coordinate calculation. However, the main limit of the Talairach and Tournoux system is encountered in the conversion from stereotactic coordinates to the correspondent Brodmann areas. As a consequence, correspondence among the stereotactic space, cyto-architecture and anatomical structures (sulci and gyri) must be considered as probabilistic. For this reason, to match functional activation with a specific anatomical region, beside the evaluation of its stereotactic coordinates, is often necessary to consider positions with respect to cerebral structures easily detectable in the static brain imaging, considered as landmarks. For instance, the hand area is located in correspondence of an inverted $\Omega$ or a horizontal $\varepsilon$ shaped knob on the superior part of the pre- and postcentral gyrus.

The hand region is the brain area most thoroughly investigated, because of this clear anatomical landmark and its relevant function. For instance, complete hand recovery represents one of the major goals of rehabilitation in stroke patients; therefore plasticity mapping studies usually focus their analysis on both sensory and motor cortex of the hand region. In fact both motor activity and sensory feedback are fundamental for a complete recovery.

Several cerebral mapping studies of functional imaging evaluated stereotactic coordinates for primary sensory hand area with different kind of stimuli and agreed to indicate the following values:

- X = - 43 (variable values from -43 to – 47)
- Y = - 28
- Z = + 52

The primary sensory hand area is localized on the anatomic region corresponding to primary motor area, in the post-central gyrus, however with respect to the motor Ω, it is more widely extended. Stereotactic coordinates of primary motor hand area were obtained with a finger tapping task:

- X = - 35 (variable values from - 34 to - 38)
- Y = - 26
- Z = + 55 (variable values from 53 to 57).

Value variability is probably due to inter-subject anatomical differences, to the occasional inclusion of motor/ sensory activation areas correspondent to the fingers or the palm and to the above mentioned limits of this coordinate system. Moreover, sensory coordinates were evaluated with various kinds of stimuli that may activate different sub-areas of SI.

A more recent alternative to Talairach and Tournoux space is the Montreal Neurological Institute (MNI) space. This standardized space, differently from the Talairach system, is the combination of several MRI scans on right-handed normal controls. The MNI system is slightly larger, taller from AC to top by 5mm and deeper from AC to bottom by 10mm than the Talairach proportional grid system. It is currently employed by Statistical Parameter Mapping (SPM), the National fMRI Database, and the International Consortium for Brain Mapping. On the other hands, the Talairach system is used by other widespread processing tools, such as the Brain Voyager.

However, in an fMRI study Sanes and collaborators did not find a precise somatotopy of fingers and wrist, but a spatial overlapping, with a highly distributed circuitry in the hand region of MI, where different muscles and/or movements are widely mixed. On the other hand, more recent studies individuated a somatotopic gradient at least for simple movement of the fingers, though observing a significant overlap also in this case. Nevertheless, the time resolution of fMRI technique does not allow designing the potential hierarchy within the neural circuit controlling a specific muscle or movement. In spite of this observation, considering that M1, SMA and other motor related structures in the brain must develop neural signals (for reach and grasp movements) that control more than 50 muscles with 27 degrees of freedom (for the fingers, wrist and elbow), the exclusion of a highly integrative function for brain motor structures seems unlikely. Thus, understanding how M1, and other supraspinal motor related regions are organized must go beyond simple straightforward concepts of somatotopy and include the demonstrated complex features of anatomic and functional organization. The existence of multiple yet discrete efferent micro- and macrozones from primary motor cortex, is now accepted as the essential organisational principle of this area. Animal studies demonstrate that the MI is organized so that a particular movement can be elicited through stimulation of different MI regions, often several millimeters apart and separated by non-responsive districts [62]. In addition, bi-directional projections interconnect motor cortex areas for different muscle districts.

Any movement, therefore, differently from what traditionally believed according to the labelled-line hypothesis, seems to be controlled not by single groups, but by a whole network of neurons, distributed throughout the MI cortex. In this model, the motor output from overlapping cortical territories converges onto single muscles. Similarly, the output from any given cortical site diverges onto multiple muscles, while horizontal intracortical projections interconnect subregions within MI. This pattern explains the considerable overlap in cortical representation of the entire musculature in area 4, particularly for hand muscles.

The multiple representations of each muscle and contiguous joints, the overlap of outputs to different motoneurons, as well as the large cortical representation of hand and fingers, are probably the anatomical substrate for the extraordinary repertoire of possible movement strategies as well as the coordination of action initiated by many muscles at different joints. In other cortical maps, such as SI, the connections are quite precise and each finger, for example, is mapped in a very ordered somatotopic arrangement. Functionally, in fact, strict coordination of different muscle fields is essential, and, for instance, the stability of the proximal arm and girdle are necessary for the successful execution of finger movements. Moreover, while movements occur in a three-dimensional space with several degrees of freedom, the body surface may be envisioned as a two-dimensional sheet, reproduced as a surface in a point-to-point fashion in SI. Multiple representations underlying different motor functions of separate body parts, along with distributed and cooperating neural networks may, therefore, overlap spatially and temporally, offering flexibility in motor learning as well as progressively substitute a related dysfunctional area more easily than highly specialized and unique groups of cells would, being thus fundamental for functional (or maladaptive, see below) plasticity. In fact, cerebral plasticity secondary to different stimuli, such as exercise or sensory deprivation, determines a functional instability of cortical motor circuitry, continually modifying regional body representation [63].

Sensory perception and its role in motor control involve large brain areas including primary somatosensory, visual, and motor cortices, as well as secondary sensory and motor areas. Basal ganglia and thalamic relays significantly contribute to motor planning, sensory perception and sensorimotor integration. Supplementary motor and premotor cortices play a pivotal role in motor preparation and execution which, on their own, are carried out via corticospinal fibers from primary motor cortex, under the parallel control of other descending systems, while cerebellar relays constantly monitor motor output and execution. Functional connections between SI and motor cortex are also fundamental for motor control. In fact, in addition to direct input to MI from the thalamus, the somatosensory cortex is also a major source of input to the motor cortex, and is the only type of primary sensory cortex with direct access to MI.

Experimental evidence for a separate functional organization within different areas of SI is available. Input form deep receptors is projected to areas 3a and 2, after a relay in the anterodorsal shell of the VPL thalamic nucleus, while the cutaneous input, relayed from the central core of VPL, is projected selectively to cortical areas 3b (more densely) and 1. In the primate, the representation of the glabrous skin of each digit in area 3b, occupies about 1-2 square mm. Digit 1 is more laterally represented, while digit 5 is the most medial one. Cells from areas 1 and 2 analyze more complex, 'associative' features of a stimulus, such as velocity or presence of edges, which cross over different districts of the receptor surface of area 3b. Area 3b, on the other hand, extracts quantitative data relative to a stimulus in a given skin locus. Internal connections between the SI areas are extensive: area 3b projects mainly to areas 1 and 2, while area 1 is also reciprocally connected with areas 2 and 3b.

Kurth and collaborators [64] stimulating electrically different body-districts and detecting the consequent fMRI activation, demonstrated a fine spatial discrimination, besides the somatotopic representation of SI. In fact, in the hand area, are present multiple discrete representation for the fingers that are extended in a medio-lateral direction from the thumb to the little finger. Subsequent studies [65] observed different degrees of discrimination in different areas, with the highest somatotopic discrimination in the 3b area, followed by 3a and 1 and then the 2 area.

Differently from SI, SII area is relatively poorly known as about its precise spatial extension as well as its structural and functional organization. This area is located in the upper arm of the lateral sulcus. The topography of SII has been recently clarified by fMRI [66] and MEG/fMRI studies [67], which by applying sensory stimuli in different body-districts, mapped the elicited cerebral response observing, also in this case a somatotopic representation. The secondary sensory area of the hand has been specifically studied by Ruben and colleague with fMRI [68]. By stimulating with painless electric discharges the little finger, the index finger and the thumb, they observed a finger somatotopic organization in the parietal operculum both controlaterally and ipsilaterally. Though with minor spatial discrimination for each finger and greater overlapping with respect to SI, fingers were represented approximately in the middle of the lateral sulcus, while the thumb was observed medially, next to the bottom of lateral sulcus and the posterior pole of the insula. The presence of a bilateral signal is probably secondary to inputs reaching SII both ipsi- and controlaterally, but since only about 30% of SII neurons, have bilateral receptive field, the ipsilateral activation is weaker.

The extensive knowledge of sensory-motor somatotopy and the presence of anatomical reference points permit narrowing the analysis on the functional region of interest (ROI) during mapping of brain activations. A ROI based approach in fact allows direct, unbiased measurement of activity in an anatomical region, assuming that functional divisions follow anatomical divisions. Moreover it improves the ability to identify topographic changes (for example in sensory-motor mapping -central sulcus- or social perception mapping -superior temporal sulcus-) and complements voxel-based analyses.

## Experience-Dependent Plasticity Tracked via Functional Imaging

Numerous examples of neural plasticity can be found in physiologic conditions, such as skilled or repeated training, as well as in instances of permanent or transient deafferentation of cerebral cortical areas.

In the auditory system plasticity is an inherent phenomenon, which can be demonstrated behaviorally throughout life in processes subtending the identification of new voices or the learning of new languages. Both adults and children can learn to distinguish speech sounds that they could not hear before training. The firing patterns of single auditory neurons, as well as auditory cortex function, are altered as a consequence of training and learning new behaviors [69]. The mismatched negativity (MMN) evoked potential is a powerful tool to demonstrate functional plasticity in the auditory cortex. The MMN is a cortical response probably originating in non-primary auditory areas, normally obtained when an acoustic change is introduced in a repetitive sequence of acoustic stimuli, and it is largely attention-independent and sensitive even to barely perceivable changes. Krause et al [70] have shown that in normal adults the MMN can be greatly incremented after only a few hours of specific listening discrimination training, directed at the recognition of slightly different acoustic stimuli. These neurophysiologic changes, attesting to cortical plastic phenomena occurring in response to training, were long lasting and specific to the training. Simple repeated exposure to varying stimuli, in fact, tends instead to cause a decrement in MMN over time.

The auditory cortical plasticity effects of training have been demonstrated also in children with learning disabilities and dyslexia. Dyslexic children often show poor phonemic awareness, a dysfunction most likely at the basis of their poor word recognition skills. Intensive remedial training and tone-speech discrimination exercises can induce behaviorally measurable improvement in performance. The brain plasticity changes subtending such phenomena have recently been studied with Magnetic Source Imaging (MSI), a neuroimaging method that provides real-time spatiotemporal maps of brain activation, by measuring electrical currents generated by cortical neurons during a task. Simos et al. [71], have shown a long lasting bihemispheric change in the patterns of cortical activation in children with dyslexia before and after intensive remedial training. Dyslexic children, when compared to controls, had an abnormal baseline cortical activation pattern in response to a pseudoword reading task, showing poor left posterior superior temporal gyrus activation and aberrant increased activation on the corresponding right cortical areas. After intensive remedial training resulting in behavioral improvement of reading skills, the dyslexic children showed a measurable "normalization" of the cortical activation pattern on MSI, similar to the pattern seen in controls.

Cortical plasticity effects of training have also been studied in musicians. MEG studies of auditory stimulation with noise-burst or tones have shown that the electromagnetic signal generator sources for noise-burst were separated and located posteriorly from those for tones, in musicians with an "absolute pitch", but not in non-musicians. These results have been ascribed to presence of distinct neural networks in the auditory cortex of musicians, which may result from plastic reorganization of the cortex because of training. In skilled musicians, also, the cortical representation areas are enlarged to a degree correlated with age at which musical training had begun, with no differences between musicians with an absolute or relative pitch [72], suggesting rather extensive and important plastic cortical rearrangement during the early years of life. The auditory system matures poorly in the absence of appropriate acoustic stimulation and even unilateral sensorineural hearing loss, despite the mostly bilateral cortical projections from the peripheral auditory system, may modify information processing in central auditory pathways. On the other hand, the auditory system retains a great degree of plasticity despite prolonged periods of deafness, proven by the successful restoring of cortical stimulation obtained through cochlear implantation, both in children and in adults. In otosclerotic patients studied before and after corrective surgery, a significant recovery of air conducted auditory function has been demonstrated. Moreover, the usual tonotopic organization of the auditory cortex during pure tone stimulation, which was missing in presurgical recordings, was reacquired after surgery together with a significant improvement of acoustic function.

Interestingly, enhanced visual function in deaf individuals has been in part demonstrated, suggesting compensatory enhancement of an intact sensory modality when another function is deficient, similarly to the case of greater tactile or auditory skills in blind subjects. Studies using Event Related Potentials (ERP) have demonstrated that in deaf subjects, the parietal regions are strongly activated by moving visual stimuli, a phenomenon that occurs only to a small degree in normal hearing individuals [73]. This suggests reorganization of cortical areas normally not involved in visual processing and/or an extension of visual cortical fields outside their normal boundaries. In congenitally deaf individuals the functional enhancement of the visual sensory modality seems to relate particularly to peripheral fields where stimuli cause larger evoked potentials and faster reaction times in deaf compared to normal hearing subjects. A recent fMRI study of visual attention to peripheral field stimuli has shown significantly greater activation of the motion sensitive cortical areas in congenitally deaf individuals compared to controls [74].

Similarly to conditions of auditory cortical deafferentation, combined Event Related Potentials and PET studies in blind humans have indicated significant activation of visual cortical areas in response to auditory stimuli and during haptic mental rotation tasks, as well as while reading the Braille alphabet or performing other tactile discrimination tasks, activities not associated with any cortical activation in individuals with normal vision. Studies with TMS have shown an enlargement in the motor hand area representation in Braille readers, and more so in congenitally blind individuals [75].

Recruitment of visual cortex for somatosensory processing occurs in blind subjects but not in those with normal vision. This cross-modal plasticity may contribute to sensory compensation in subjects with early onset blindness and may account in part for the superior tactile perceptual abilities of blind subjects. Repetitive TMS causes a temporary disruption of cortical function, and when applied to the visual cortex of subjects with early onset blindness during identification paradigms of Braille or embossed Roman letters, it induces errors in both tasks, distorting tactile perceptions. This has no effect on tactile performance in non-visually impaired individuals, while it is known to disrupt their visual performance.

The degree of reorganization occurring in late onset blindness is less well characterized. In fact, the previously mentioned repetitive TMS-induced dysfunction of Braille reading in congenitally and early-onset blind persons, does not occur in late onset blind individuals. Likewise, PET technology has shown that congenitally blind subjects demonstrate task-specific PET activation of extrastriate visual areas and parietal association areas during Braille reading, while subjects with post-pubertal visual loss show additional activation in the primary visual cortex alone [76]. Animal models using blind-raised monkeys have demonstrated crossmodal activation in extrastriate areas with somatosensory stimulation, but no response in primary visual cortex. The differential activation between late-onset and congenitally blind subjects suggests the possibility of reciprocal activation by visual imagery in subjects who have experienced vision early in life.

TMS studies of cortical motor output maps in blind workers have shown rapid and reversible modulation in relation to activity with a larger motor output for the first dorsal interosseous muscle (FDI) of the Braille reading hand. This appeared greater immediately after their working shift compared to after 2 days of rest. Similar changes were not evident in other muscles (ADM) not involved in the Braille reading process.

The role for TMS in studying plastic changes of the human motor system in the acquisition of new fine motor skills is further evidenced by recent work by Liepert et al. In this study, a brief training session of synchronous movements of the ipsilateral thumb and foot induced a transient shift of the center of gravity (CoG) of the hand muscle examined (APB), of about 7 mm medially, towards the foot area. The changes observed, which disappeared approximately 1 hour following the experiment, were ascribed to cortical modulation interactions between hand and foot representation areas in motor cortex. Cortical modulation phenomena may be in part the basis for commonplace performance improvements in speed and accuracy occurring following practice of complex motor tasks. Similarly, the cortical motor areas targeting the contra-lateral long finger flexor and extensor muscles in subjects learning a one-handed, five-finger piano exercise, were shown to increase in size and the activation threshold to decrease after only 5-days of training.

Focal TMS of the motor cortex evokes isolated movements of the thumb, in the same direction of a thumb movement exercise practiced for several minutes prior to stimulation. Substantially smaller effects, instead, follow direct stimulation of corticofugal axons with transcranial electrical stimulation, thus pointing to the cortex as the site of plasticity. Training, therefore, established a rapid and transient change in the cortical network encoding the kinematic details (direction of movement) of the practiced movement.

Experience-dependent reorganization of the adult MI may underlie the acquisition and long-term retention of motor skills. Functional MRI studies have shown that after 4 weeks of training of a specific motor sequence, the extent of cortex activated by the task is enlarged in trained subjects compared to subjects who had not practiced the same sequence previously, and that these changes persisted for several months [77].

Use-dependent aberrant plastic reorganization of the brain, may represent the substrate for some neurological deficits or dysfunctions. Focal dystonia, for example, tends to occur with repetitive synchronous movements of the fingers, a movement pattern that is part of many human activities, for example instrument playing in musicians. MEG recordings have shown that the mean distances of ECDs in the SI area corresponding to the fingers is smaller for the affected hand of dystonic musicians, compared both to the non-affected hand in the same subjects, or to the hands of non-musician controls, suggesting fusion of motor output.

Mental imagery of movements - not evoking a contraction - may increase the capability of acquiring new motor skills. Such a technique has been successfully applied as a training procedure, in order to improve the actual performance without receiving any feedback about the results and TMS represents an excellent tool to demonstrate motor output changes taking place during the ideation of movement. Several Authors have described facilitatory effects of motor imagery, as evidenced by a decrease in the excitability threshold, induced by "thinking about" a movement [17, 78-80]. Non-motor mental activity and alerting stimuli "per se" have been shown to potentiate the amplitude of MEPs in the target muscles, in strict time relationship with a desynchronization of the background EEG activity of the stimulated brain areas [81]. Movement imagery can thus direct a specific facilitation on the prime-mover muscle involved in a mentally simulated movement. This process is specifically and asymmetrically affected when the motor cortex, contralateral to the affected limbs, is stimulated with focal TMS, in early unilateral Parkinson's disease patients [82], suggesting a crucial role of motor imagery in normal movement initiation and execution. Better understanding of motor imagery mechanisms in both physiologic and pathologic conditions, is likely to lead to more effective rehabilitative approaches.

This extended analysis of cerebral mapping in healthy subject is at the base of a full comprehension of the plastic reorganization following an ischemic damage. Functional imaging, in fact, permits to study also the changes of neural circuitry following a cerebro-vascular event.

## D. Mapping Cerebral Plasticity after Stroke: What is the Best Strategy?

To date, all functional imaging techniques in spite their increasing technology, still present limits in spatial or temporal resolution and explore cerebral function from different points of view. Moreover, when evaluating brain plasticity in older subjects and in patients affected by cerebrovascular disease, the analysis may encounter further difficulties. This is the case of the techniques based on metabolic aspect of cerebral activation. Changes in cerebrovascular ultrastructure during aging result largely from arteriosclerotic changes, which probably decrease the elasticity and compliance of affected vessels. Aging is also associated with a decrease in resting cerebral blood flow, cerebral metabolic rate of O2 consumption and vascular reactivity. In fact, the latency of the midpoint of the trailing edge of the BOLD response tends to increase with age. Therefore, in order to avoid the potential confounds resulting from this effect, it may be appropriate to use the latency of the leading edge or the peak intensity of the BOLD signal, rather than its trailing edge or the area under the signal, as the salient variable in event-related studies that compare groups of different ages [83]. There is evidence that the BOLD signal shows a decreased signal-to-noise ratio in older subjects, also because of a greater level of noise (mainly because of head motion). In individuals with cerebrovascular disease, neurovascular coupling has also been found to be altered in an increasing number of reports. These findings have implications for fMRI studies that aim to compare neural activity between aging or diseased populations and young or healthy subjects. It might be necessary to screen subjects carefully for cerebrovascular abnormalities [84]. Previous reports hypothesized that anatomical stenosis or occlusion of the carotid artery are the direct cause of an impaired neurovascular coupling because of a post-stenotic compensatory dilation that might reduce the dynamic range of vascular dilatation. Following a single case observation of negative BOLD signal ipsilaterally to carotid artery occlusion [85], the same research team analyzed BOLD activation in a group of patients with carotid stenosis [86] and a previous cerebrovascular event. In this study, patients underwent fMRI evaluation during a motor task and during inhalation of air enriched with $CO_2$ to evaluate vasomotor reactivity (VMR) (Figure 4). They observed reduced or negative BOLD signals in the affected compared to the unaffected hemisphere in patients with alteration of VMR. On this basis the authors conclude that extra- or intracranial artery disease influences CVRC and consequently the BOLD signal. A more recent study [87] demonstrated the absence of the BOLD signal in the affected and sometimes in the unaffected hemispheres of stroke patients in presence of detectable neural activation recorded with MEG (Figure 5). These patients had received an electrical stimulation at the wrist. In order to clarify the origin of this uncoupling, the authors investigated the possible role of the lesion site, white matter hyper-intensities observed in magnetic resonance, current medication, risk factors, anatomy of the neck vessels, and cerebral vasomotor reactivity as measured by transcranial Doppler during $CO_2$ inhalation. Neither neuronal activation properties, nor any of the considered factors (in particular presence of carotid stenosis or occlusion) were related to the lack of fMRI activation, with the exception of altered vasomotor reactivity, which was on the contrary strongly related. One interpretation suggested by the authors is that, despite the efficient release of particles mediating the cerebrovascular reaction (K+, H+, Adenosine, Nitric Oxide etc.) [88], the hemodynamic response was scanty because of a vascular tree already maximally dilated. In this case normal function can nevertheless be maintained until energy substrates are sufficient. This was the first report of an absent fMRI activation in spite a detectable neuronal response; in previous studies, however, stroke patients had been asked to perform a different task, namely finger tapping. These different results could be secondary to motor preparation and execution (i.e. the amount in attention and motor programming) strategies adopted for the paretic hand. It is, in fact, a common observation that mental and physical activities – even when outwardly normal – can be abnormally fatiguing for stroke patients.

Similarly, Binkofski and Seitz reported [89] a transient absence of BOLD activation despite clinical improvement of hand function and integrity of the motor cortical output system as verified by preserved MEPs. These observations are of predominant relevance when evaluating cerebral plasticity in stroke patients. In a recent study, Stefanovic and collaborators characterized the hemodynamic and metabolic down-regulation accompanying neuronal inhibition. They employed pulsed arterial spin labeling (PASL) to quantify CBF and BOLD signals at the same time and a motor task paradigm previously shown to produce robust ipsilateral neuronal inhibition. In all subjects, BOLD, CBF and $CMRO_2$ signals increased in the contralateral and decreased in the ipsilateral primary motor (M1) cortex, thereby establishing that the sustained negative BOLD response is probably a marker of neuronal deactivation. On the other hand, ipsilateral activation of the unaffected hemisphere of stroke patients is often observed during a motor task and it is hypothesized to correlate with poor functional recovery [90]. However, on the basis of the above considerations, it could be difficult to discriminate whether the finding of an absent ipsilateral BOLD signal actually represents the lack of neural activation or the effect of VMR impairment.

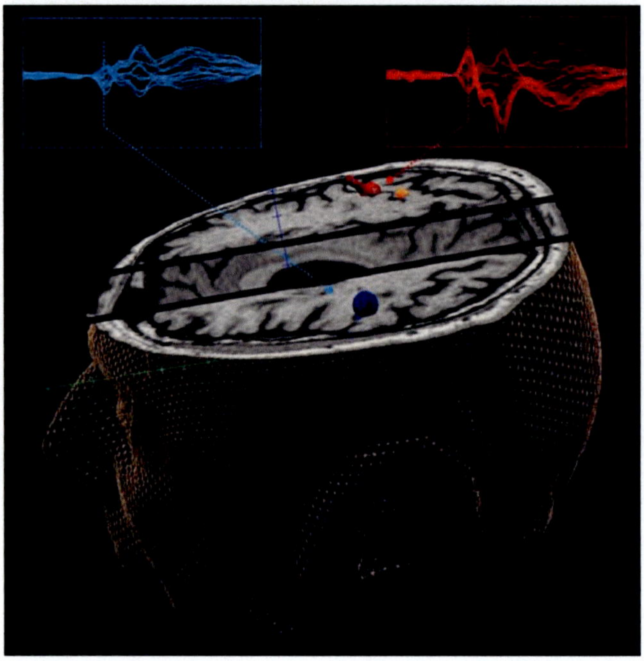

Figure 4. Example of neuro-vascular uncoupling. Red and light blue vectors indicate bilateral SI activation detected by MEG in a patient affected by an ischemic stroke of the left hemisphere. Differently, fMRI BOLD signal in the same subject is undetectable in the affected hemisphere. Top: Parieto-frontal channels.

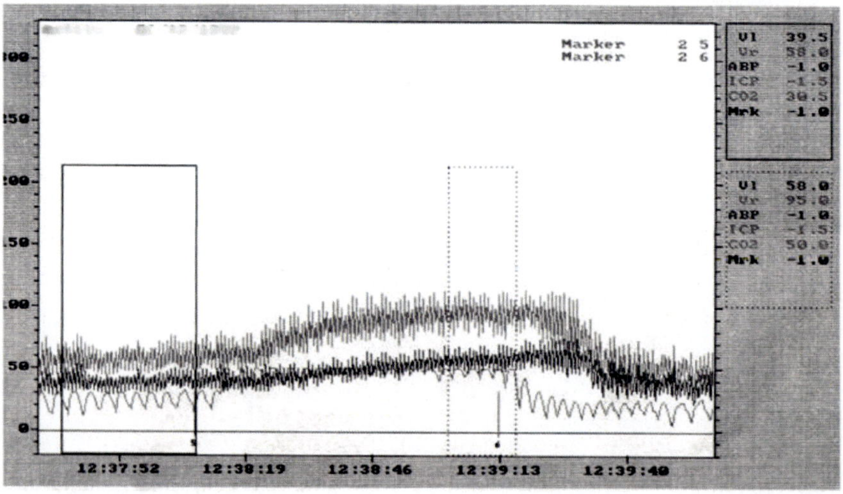


Figure 5. Example of altered vasomotor reactivity in a stroke patient affected by right hemiparesis. After a vasodilatatory stimulus, the mean blood flow velocity (MFV) of the right middle cerebral artery increases within the physiological range. The left MFV, on the contrary, does not significantly increase.

Similarly, if a negative BOLD signal is detected when examining stroke patients, it is debatable whether to attribute it to neuronal deactivation or to activation in presence of VMR malfunction.

At the same time, to clarify the mismatch previously observed between neuronal activation and BOLD signal, Seiyama and collaborators [91] co-recorded fMRI and near infrared optical imaging (NIOI) signals. The authors showed circulatory conditions generating positive, negative, and silent BOLD signals during brain activation, by expressing fMRI signals as a function of Hb species concentration obtained with NIOI. In fact, NIOI, although it was used only to measure the cortical function, revealed to be a useful tool for detecting BOLD-fMRI silent and negative brain activation and estimating its circulatory conditions.

Moreover, Seyama and colleague, based on their results, hypothesized that fMRI signals obtained with a 1.5-T MRI system reflect changes in the magnetic susceptibility of the tissue containing mainly venules and large veins but not capillaries, with a relative dispersion of the signal. Deoxyhemoglobin changes initially occur at the area of increased neuronal activity and subsequently propagate down the venous vasculature, including large draining veins that are distant from the site of elevated neuronal activity. Dilution by blood draining from "inactive" areas should ultimately diminish this nonspecific draining-vein effect and thus limit its spatial extent. An fMRI signal measured with a much higher magnetic-field system (4 T MRI) should present an amplified relative contribution of the capillaries, since it becomes greater with increased magnetic field strength with respect to the relative contribution of venules [92]. However, higher magnetic fields are not yet allowed, neither available for current clinical assessment. Moreover, these last observations suggest that a higher magnetic field could not be useful to detect cerebral activation in stroke patients. In fact, 4 and 7 T fMRI would derive the signal prevalently by the micro-vascular response, which is more greatly affected in these patients.

Advances in technology, or in the design or analysis of experimental paradigms, should make it easier to distinguish changes in neurovascular coupling from changes in neural activity. However the combination of functional imaging with other techniques, as previously reported with MEG or TMS, might also be very helpful in this regard. These techniques, in fact, offer different information of the alteration secondary to an ischemic event taking into account neuronal firing properties and the related hemodynamic and metabolic phenomena as two sides of the same coin. If fMRI offers a more accurate spatial resolution, MEG and TMS have grater advantage in the analysis of the temporal sequence of cerebral activation and/or morphology and other properties of neuronal activation (i.e. excitability) [93, 94]. In summary, until new technologies are available, a multimodality integration approach will be the only option to analyze properly neural activity and to map cerebral plasticity, particularly in stroke patients.

Another aspect that must be considered when evaluating cerebral plasticity in stroke patients is the choice of an appropriate task. Finger tapping is the most frequently used paradigm in these studies, as the motor recovery represent the essential goal of rehabilitation and it may reflects movement execution as implemented in everyday life. One pitfall of this paradigm is that the task performance can not really be controlled for effort in paretic limbs even when movement parameters are carefully matched. In this respect, electric stimulation is a more sensitive experimental paradigm, not only because its physical parameters are measurable and its neuronal recruitment is more selective, but also because it recruits approximately the same amount of neurons in each hemisphere. This type of stimulation, therefore, allows standardization of the procedure across different subjects, across sessions, and during a follow-up. Moreover, abnormalities of brain responses to sensory stimuli are still of paramount interest in testing hand control, since sensory feedback plays a pivotal role in motor control [95, 96]. According to these observations, when evaluating stroke patients, a more accurate experimental paradigm should include both motor task and sensory stimulation. Moreover, with this paradigm neural reorganization following cerebrovascular accidents may be investigated more precisely, expanding the analysis the sensory-motor circuit.

A future challenge is to find prognostic markers among all parameters analyzed by the above-mentioned techniques and to understand the plasticity phenomena that permit functional recovery. If these goals are accomplished, functional imaging techniques will be able to play also an important role in clinical practice and in rehabilitation strategies.

## Monohemispheric Lesions and Stroke

All the above mentioned techniques have been performed in different experimental settings in the attempt to clarify the plastic mechanisms allowing functional recovery. Although a full comprehension of these phenomena is far to be achieved, significant progress was made in the last decade. Taking advantage of the different features of functional imaging techniques, various aspects of brain reorganization have been evaluated. In fact, numerous factors can influence degree and mode of plasticity after a stroke, such as site and extent of the lesion, diaschisis, and pre-stroke organization of the motor areas, in particular the amount of ipsilateral uncrossed corticospinal fibers [97].

When damage to a functional system is partial, a within-system recovery is possible, whereas after complete destruction, substitution by functionally related systems remains the only alternative. Experimental and clinical studies have shown that approximately 1/5 of the pyramidal fibers is sufficient to ensure restitution of fractionated hand finger movement. In this case, this within-pyramidal system reorganization is probably one of the best mechanisms for functional recovery of the motor control of hand and upper limb. However, complete lesion of the pyramidal neurons of a brain region is often observed. In this case, rather than a complete substitution of function, the main mechanism underlying recovery of motor abilities involves enhanced activity in preexisting networks.

Both longitudinal and cross-sectional PET and fMRI studies have documented abnormal activation patterns during sensory stimulation or movement of a paretic hand even after full clinical recovery. In particular, an unusual involvement of ipsi-lesional non-motor and contra-lesional motor areas has been observed producing asymmetrical activation.

However, because of the considerable logistic complexity, these studies were conducted in only a limited number of patients and only few longitudinal studies have been published to date.

Enhanced bilateral activation of motor pathways has been reported, both in cortical and subcortical infarct, together with recruitment of sensory and secondary motor structures normally not involved in the task, as well as displacement of primary motor peak activation toward the face area. Additionally, interesting findings have been a strong peri-infarct activation [98], and ipsilesional premotor cortex activation [99]. The overactivation of the ipsilesional motor cortex was observed also after sub-cortical stroke and might reflect an excessive recruitment of this cortical field in an attempt to perform the task despite corticospinal tract damage. Thus, recovery would be optimal when M1 is not only preserved structurally, as after subcortical - as opposed to cortical - strokes, but is also capable of enhanced workload, ie, it is not completely disconnected. In this case, the unmasking of previously silent synapses, as well as enhanced input from neighboring PM and SMA, would implement this overrecruitment of the affected-side M1.

The posterior shift and inferior extension of M1 activation observed both in cortical and subcortical strokes might represent unmasking/disinhibition of synaptic connections within the cortico-spinal tract system [100]. Analysis of this asymmetry is facilitated by the anatomical reference points and the system coordinates mentioned above, that allow comparing data across different subjects or techniques.

Functional reorganization of the motor output following a hemispheric stroke has been consistently observed also via TMS and MEG. Recordings of Somatosensory Evoked Fields (SEFs) over the controlateral parietal regions, were performed 9 or more weeks after a first-ever monohemispheric stroke, via separate electrical stimulation of median nerve, thumb and little finger of both hands. Only the initial part of the SEFs, which contains the most stable, repeatable and attention independent waves (N20m, P30m), were analyzed. The Equivalent Current Dipole (ECD) characteristics (spatial co-ordinates and strength) were calculated at 1msec intervals in the 15-50 msec post-stimulus epoch. The "hand extension" area was also calculated as the distance in millimeters between the centers of the ECDs activated by fifth and the first finger stimulation. A MEG-brain MRI common reference system was defined on the basis of anatomical landmarks. All the SEF parameters, including interhemispheric differences, had been previously tested in a group of healthy subjects and the abnormality threshold defined. Excessive interhemispheric signal strength asymmetry was found for at least one stimulated district in 63% of patients with recordable SEFs from the AH, and nearly 80% of ECD pairs from homologous districts exceeded the normative range. When latency delays were accompanied by ECD spatial displacements, these always affected the N20 component generator sources. With the integration of MEG data with MRI anatomical information, it was shown that all identified ECDs were localized outside the area of the anatomical lesion. The classical "homunculus" somatotopy, seen in the healthy hemisphere, was maintained even for the 'migrated' sensory hand areas (thumb more lateral, little finger more medial and median nerve in between). A significant enlargement of the hand area was seen in the AH, with a medial shift of the little finger, and a tendency of both finger representations to shift anteriorly. Abnormal parameters were infrequently encountered in UH. Greater interhemispheric asymmetry, reflective of cortical reorganization, correlated with worse clinical recovery, in agreement with longitudinal functional imaging studies of post-stroke aphasia showing that better recovery was associated with return of left hemisphere perilesional activity, while persistent activation of homologous areas in the non-dominant hemisphere probably represent maladaptive plasticity [97].

In stroke patients MEPs recorded in a relaxed muscle state are often absent with TMS of the affected hemisphere. However, with this technique excessive asymmetry of the hand muscle motor maps between the Affected and the Unaffected Hemispheres (AH *vs* UH) has also been observed. Such asymmetries are due to "map migration", usually on the medio-lateral axis. Often an antero-posterior shift of several millimeters of the CoG has also been reported. This is particularly frequent and stable over time, in patients in the chronic stages, while it can be seen as a transient dynamic phenomenon in first few months after a stroke. TMS studies performed in the acute (4-72 hours), subacute (one week) and chronic stages (6 months) after a stroke showed increased excitability thresholds and prolonged MEPs latencies (when present) acutely, in the AH, while responses from the UH remained normal in each recording session. Interhemispheric differences between AH and UH were significant for all the parameters studied. The responses from the AH changed significantly during follow-up, with most parameters showing a partial recovery: latencies of MEPs decreased and amplitudes increased, though they were still altered at the 6th month, but also the clinical improvement was still ongoing. Interhemispheric differences between AH and UH were the most altered neurophysiological parameters, particularly for excitability thresholds. MEP amplitudes, acutely, had a positive correlation with clinical picture and with long term outcome, the higher the MEP amplitude, the better the outcome. No correlation was found between side (right vs left) or type of the lesion (cortical vs subcortical) and neurophysiologic parameters.

Hemispheric motor output was also studied at two different times after a stroke (T1= 8 weeks; T2= 16-18 weeks). Excitability thresholds were significantly higher and the MEP amplitudes smaller in the AH despite a stronger TMS employed. The area of cortical output to the target muscle was asymmetrically restricted, compared to controls and with the patients' UH. The percentage of altered parameters was significantly higher in T1 and in those suffering from subcortical lesions, possibly due to the large number of densely packed fibers affected by a subcortical lesion and to a less efficient short-term "plastic" reorganization. Anomalous "hot spot" sites were observed more frequently in the cortical group. In T2, the parameters of "subcortical" patients' were improved to the same level of the "cortical" group. A significant enlargement of the AH hand motor cortical area was found in 67% of cases in T2 compared with T1, together with clinical improvement. [49]. When followed up in post-stroke epochs, various MEPs parameters improved; the steepest parts of the recovery slopes being concentrated in the 40 to 80 days post-stroke. Similarly, recent reports documented for the first time rapid plastic changes in the cortices of rats, during the hyperacute stage after a lesion (up to 6 hours from the ischemic event). In particular, neuronal hyperexcitabily was observed, associated with rapid expansion of receptive fields following peripheral electrical stimuli in the peri-lesional area of the somato-sensory cortex [93].

Beside inter-hemispheric activation asymmetries, in terms of both site and excitability, were reported other finding describing brain plasticity. In fact both cerebral hemispheres ipsi- and contralateral to a stroke, may play an important role in functional recovery in the acute and subacute stages. The remote effects of the lesioned area, or "diaschisis", suggest that acute neuronal failure in the ischemic area induce modulatory effects on cortical excitability of unaffected districts of the same hemisphere, via cortico-cortical connections, and of the contralateral UH via transcallosal fibres. Transient hyperexcitability of the UH contralateral to a neocortical infarction has been documented in animal models [101]. The relationship between clinical recovery and early cortical excitability to TMS after a stroke has been studied, as a possible prognostic tool. MEPs from upper limb muscles have always been obtained in patients who fully recover finger control. The study of intracortical inhibition (ICI) and facilitation early after a stroke sheds light on some plasticity mechanisms. A TMS study of large MCA infarctions, with single and paired pulse TMS of the UH, showed a decrease of ICI, 2 weeks after the stroke. This finding corresponds to results obtained in animal studies. In rats the ICI was associated with GABA (A) receptors downregulation and glutamatergic activity enhancement. Since ICI changes are supposed to be modulated by GABAergic activity the decreased ICI in the UH of patients with large infarctions may indeed reflect GABA activity downregulation. This effect could be due either to damage of transcallosal fibers and loss of the physiological interhemispheric inhibitory modulation, or to enhanced use of the unaffected arm in daily activities, since ICI is modified in a task- and use-dependent manner. A disinhibition in the UH is also supported by the finding of enlarged MEP amplitudes when stimulating this hemisphere after a stroke.

A loss of ICI was observed instead in the AH, in stroke patients with either small motor deficits at onset or rapid spontaneous motor recovery, while ICI in the UH was not different from age-matched controls. This result corresponds to animal studies describing loss of GABAergic inhibition immediately surrounding a cortical lesion. On this basis, it has been suggested that the rapid clinical improvement of some patients might be induced by motor cortical disinhibition, secondary to the remote effects of structurally intact areas (′diaschisis′) and/or to the pre-existing organization of the motor areas (i.e. the amount of ipsilateral uncrossed corticospinal fibers).

A recent report [94] described a dissimilar result in a population of postacute stroke patients with mild to moderate motor impairment. In this study analysis of the ICI/ICF with paired TMS of the UH and AH showed significant interhemi-spheric asymmetries of the early inhibitory part of the recovery curves, resulting from enhanced intracortical excitability of the AH (defective AH ICI) and a normal intracortical inhibition of the UH (effective UH ICI). The author speculated that the significant inter-hemispheric asymmetry of inhibition caused by a defective AH ICI, associated with an effective UH ICI, could be considered a good neurophysiological marker of cortical plasticity as a mechanism for poststroke functional recovery.

Nevertheless, the role of ipsilateral cortico-spinal connections is still controversial, particularly their contribution to motor recovery after a unilateral lesion. In several studies ipsilateral MEPs (iMEPs) could be elicited by TMS either over the UH of stroke patients or over the AH. The iMEPs were usually obtained stimulating anteriorly and medially to the primary motor cortex, suggesting activation of corticospinal pathways from premotor areas. Outcome was variable, some authors finding a correlation between iMEPs and motor recovery, while for others the opposite was true.

Interhemispheric differences have also been evaluated with fMRI. Data were analyzed using a Laterality Index (LI), ranging from +1 to –1, as an indicator of shift of the motor network activation towards the UH, . In clinically stabilized, chronic strokes LI is more broadly distributed compared to controls, due to prominent contralesional activation, while in controls there is preservation of the normal interhemispheric balance. Interestingly one study [90] has observed a positive correlation between LI changes over time and concomitant finger motion recovery, documenting that the greater the activation shift towards the UH (> LI value), the worse the recovery. This finding suggests that contra-lesional SM1 activation seems less efficient than ipsilesional activation for adult stroke recovery. An alternative hypothesis to explain these contralesional activations stems from the finding in healthy subjects of ipsilateral SM1 activation during complex as well as non-dominant hand motor tasks, suggesting some sort of bi-hemispheric cooperation. After a stroke affecting the CST, execution of a simple motor task might involve the recruitment of this bilateral network, normally engaged only with more complex tasks.

Interhemispheric differences are of interest also in MEG studies. For instance, for the "hand area", in particular, parameters were abnormal in 20 % and 13 % of subcortical and cortical lesions, respectively, due to enlargement of the "hand area" size (39 ±7 mm in subcortical strokes, 27 mm in cortical lesions, vs. 16 ±5 mm in healthy controls). The area enlargement did not significantly correlate with the clinical outcome.

One way to specifically examine intervention induced plastic reorganization is to study patients in the very chronic stages of their illness when the probability of spontaneous recovery is negligible, or to study the short-term effects of interventions (e.g., within a single day), where changes observed after a single therapeutic session are likely due to the intervention itself rather than to spontaneous improvements. Some studies have looked at the intervention-induced effects on motor reorganization of constraint-induced movement therapy (CIMT). With TMS, repeated baseline measurements have shown highly reproducible results in strokes occurred more than 6 months prior. Prior to CIMT, the patients had higher motor thresholds and smaller motor output maps in the AH. After therapy, motor output maps in the AH had increased by approximately 40% while those in the UH had decreased, though not significantly. Thus, the AH cortical map had become larger than that in the UH. Both changes presumably reflect use-dependent mechanisms that are increased by the use of the paretic hand during training and decreased use of the non-affected hand. Such neurophysiological changes were paralleled by significant clinical improvement of motor function. Motor thresholds had remained identical after CIMT, and since they are determined in the *center* of the cortical representation area, it was concluded that enlargements of the motor output maps were due to excitability increase at the *borders* of the representation area, possibly through GABA-dependent modulation of horizontal intracortical inhibitory circuits. After CIMT, the Center of gravity (CoG) of the motor output maps, had shifted significantly in the AH mainly in the medio-lateral axis, presumably indicating recruitment of additional adjacent brain areas. Similar results have also been reported in monkey studies [102]. In the subsequent 6 months after CIMT the motor output map sizes equalized (<area in AH, >area in UH), while motor performance remained unchanged. These changes were interpreted as indicators of improved connectivity between neuronal populations, allowing a reduction of cortical excitability while maintaining performance. In contrast, a MEG study found a large shift of movement-related cortical potentials in the UH 3 months after CIMT. CIMT and manipulation of monoamine neuromodulators have been shown, in randomized controlled trials, to enhance motor recovery via stimulation of use-dependent connections. The facilitatory effects of different interventions studied with TMS showed that contraction of the target muscle exceeded all other facilitatory techniques such as preinnervation of more proximal or contralateral homologous muscles, or passive cutaneous stimulation. These results confirm that increased or repetitive use has facilitatory effects and improves motor performance.

Functional MRI studies have reported that specific rehabilitative procedures, either passive or active, are able to induce significant changes in brain activation. In patients with recent subcortical strokes, 3 weeks of intensive rehabilitation –as compared to standard stimulation- resulted in enhanced activation of ipsilesional sensorimotor primary cortices. Similarly, in a group of patients with cortical or subcortical chronic stroke, predominant activation of contralesional MI cortex during active motor tasks before training, evolved in a preferential ipsilesional MI activation with intense training of the paretic arm, and resulted in a significant clinical improvement [103].

# E. Aspect to the Future

Altogether, findings from PET, fMRI, TMS and MEG studies suggest that reorganization of the motor output from a lesioned hemisphere can still taking place several months after a stroke (Table 3). The time course and degree of motor recovery in humans could largely depend on the degree of damage to the previously described distributed motor network, since different motor areas operate in a parallel rather than in a hierarchical fashion and parallel descending pathways might be able to compensate functionally for each other.

**Table 3. Summarizes the post-stroke plastic phenomena observed with different functional imaging techniques. The prognostic value of such phenomena is also analyzed. Most phenomena observed in the acute phase following an ischemic event seem to have a maladaptive significance and tend to return to normality when clinical recovery takes place. It is still unclear whether the observed plastic changes are epi-phenomena or the cause of a poor recovery**

| Post-stroke plastic phenomena | | |
|---|---|---|
| • Inter-hemispheric activation asymmetry | Extension of the affected side activation<br>Displacement of the affected side activation | As clinical recovery takes place, the activation balance between the AH and UH shifts and the amount of overactivated areas on both sides decreases |
| • Bilateral activation of SM1 for movement of the affected hand | | |
| • Increased activity in primary and secondary motor areas in the affected hemisphere | | |
| • Acutely increased excitability thresholds and prolonged MEPs latencies (when present) in the AH measured with TMS | | During follow-up responses from the AH changed significantly showing a partial recovery: in the AH latencies of MEPs decreased and amplitudes increased |
| • Transient hyperexcitability of the UH/AH (controvertial results) with alteration of ICI, measured by TMS | | Negative or Positive prognostic factor? |

The post-stroke interval of some studies was long enough to suggest that the observed modifications were due to corticospinal tract reorganization, rather than recovery from perilesional edema and 'early' cortical hypoexcitability. Recovery of sensory deficits can also play a significant role, since the modulation of the tonic sensory flow from the skin enveloping the target muscle significantly affects the amount of its cortical representation. Future research will hopefully lead to new technologies allowing cerebral mapping with a high temporal and spatial resolution. In the meanwhile multimodal integrated techniques could provide enough information for a complete analysis of post-stroke plastic change. When these plastic phenomena will be totally clarified, new therapeutic strategies could be attempted to avoid maladaptive processes and promote favorable ones. Moreover, new prognostic factors would be available for the clinical practice, maybe even in the iper-acute phase. Nevertheless, functional imaging could gain a central role to guide neuro-rehabilitation programs.

## F. Take-Home-Message

Since the introduction of functional imaging techniques, research has made notable progress in the study of brain plasticity. It was traditionally taught that adult brain has no significant ability for reorganization following injuries or training, but cerebral functional imaging demonstrated that it is possible and relevant for clinical recovery. This consideration is particularly important when applied to ischemic brain injuries, which today are the most common cause of chronic disability. Unfortunately, the techniques currently available do not permit a complete analysis of neuronal activation properties since none of them presents high degree of temporal and spatial resolution. Moreover, recent reports evidenced that methods based on metabolic vascular response (e.g. fMRI) may be defective even in detecting neuronal activation when performed in stroke patients. In fact, an impaired cerebro-vascular reactivity does not allow a proper vascular response, impeding the blood oxygen over-supply, detected by these techniques, to take place [87]. In the next future, functional methods will be able to detect the weak magnetic fields induced by neuronal currents with a higher spatial resolution, eliminating these shortcomings. Despite this, integrated approaches have already permitted a thorough investigation of post-stroke plastic reorganization. Different phenomena were described in the acute and chronic phase of an ischemic event, with variable relation to clinical recovery. However, it is yet to be clarified whether these changes are just epi-phenomena or causes of the functional improvement, or if they even represent forms of maladaptive reorganization. When post-stroke plastic changes will be completely understood and interpreted, new drugs will be tried to avoid the sequelae of ischemia and to aid recovery. Moreover, functional imaging techniques will play an important role in guiding rehabilitation programs. Though this prospective seems far in the future, technology progresses faster and faster, thus, in the next decades research will hopefully accomplish important goals in the cure of stroke.

# References


[1] Pascual-Leone A, Nguyet D, Cohen LG, et al. Modulation of muscle responses evoked by transcranial magnetic stimulation during the acquisition of new fine motor skills. *J. Neurophysiol.* 74:1037-1045, 1995.

[2] Elbert T, Pantev C, Weinbruck C, et al: Increased cortical representation of the fingers of the left hand in string players. *Science* 270:305-307, 1995.

[3] Schulz M, Ross B, Pantev C.Evidence for training-induced crossmodal reorganization of cortical functions in trumpet players. *Neuroreport* 14:157-61, 2003.

[4] Jacobs KM, Donoghue JP: Reshaping the cortical motor map by unmasking latent intracortical connections. *Science* 251:944-947, 1991.

[5] Sakamoto T, Porter LL, Asanuma H: Long-lasting potentiation of synaptic potentials in the motor cortex produced by stimulation of the sensory cortex in the cat: a basis of motor learning. *Brain Res.* 413:360-364, 1987

[6] Hess G, Jacobs KM, Donoghue JP: N-Methyl-D-aspartate receptor mediated components of fiels otentials evoked in horizontal pathways of rat motor cortex. *Neuroscience* 61:225-235, 1994.

[7] Crair MC, Malenka RC: A critical period for long-term potentiation at thalamocortical synapses. *Nature* 375:325-328, 1995.

[8] Le Doux J: *The emotional brain; the mysterious underpinnings of emotional life*. New York: Touchstone Press, 1996.

[9] Kara P, Friedlander MJ:Dynamic modulation of cerebral cortex synaptic function by nitric oxide. *Prog. Brain Res.* 118:183-98, 1998.

[10] Fisher M, Kaech S, Knutti D, et al.: Rapid actin-based plasticity in dendritic spines. *Neuron*. 20:847-854, 1999.

[11] Akins PT, Liu PK, Hsu CY: Immediate early gene expression in response to cerebral ischemia. Friend or foe? *Stroke* 27:1682-1687, 1996.

[12] Kawamata T, Dietrich WD, Schallert T, et al: Intracisternal basic fibroblast growth factor enhanced functional recovery and upregulates the expression of a molecular marker of neuronal sprouting following focal cerebral infarction. *Proc. Nat. Acad. Sci. USA* 94:8179-8184, 1997.

[13] Johansson BB, Ohlsson A-L: Environment, social interaction, and physical activity as determinants of functional outcome after cerebral infarction in the rat. *Exp. Neurol.* 139:322-327, 1996.

[14] Rossini PM, Pauri F: Neuromagnetic integrated methods tracking human brain mechanisms of sensorimotor areas 'plastic' reorganisation. *Brain Res. Rev.* 33:131-54, 2000.

[15] Pantano P, Formisano R, Ricci M, et al: Motor recovery after stroke. Morphological and functional brain alterations. *Brain*. 119:1849-1857, 1996.

[16] Binkofski F, Seitz RJ, Arnold S, et al.: Thalamic metabolism and corticospinal tract integrity determine motor recovery in stroke. *Ann. Neurol.* 39:460-470, 1996.

[17] Rossi S, Pasqualetti P, Tecchio F, et al.: Corticospinal excitability modulation during mental simulation of wrist movements in human subjects. *Neurosci Lett.* 243:147-151, 1998.

[18] Weder B, Knorr U, Herzog H, et al: Tactile exploration of shape afetr subcortical ischaemic infarction studied with PET. *Brain* 117:593–605, 1994.

[19] Newberg A, Alavi A, Reivich M: Dtermination of regional cerebral function with FDG-PET imaging in neuropsychiatric disorders. *Semin. Nucl. Med.* 32:13-34, 2002.

[20] Watson JDG, Myers R, Frackowiak RSJ et al: Area V5 of the human brain: evidence form a combined study using positron emission tomography and magnetic resonance imaging. *Cereb. Cortex* 3:79-94, 1993.

[21] Arthurs O, Boniface S: How well do we understand the neural origins of the fMRI BOLD signal? *Trends Neurosci.* 25:27-31, 2002.

[22] Ogawa S, Lee TM, Kay AR, et al. Brain magnetic resonance imaging with contrast dependent on blood oxygenation. *Proc. Natl. Acad. Sci. USA* 87:9868–9872, 1990.

[23] Frahm J, Kruger G, Merboldt KD, Kleinschmidt A) Dynamic uncoupling and recoupling of perfusion and oxidative metabolism during focal brain activation in man. *Magn. Reson Med.* 35:143–148, 1996.

[24] Obata T, Liu TT, Miller KL, et al. Discrepancies between BOLD and flow dynamics in primary and supplementary motor areas: application of the balloon model to the interpretation of BOLD transients. *Neuroimage*.21:144-53,2004.

[25] Buxton RB, Uludag K, Dubowitz DJ, Liu TT. Modeling the hemodynamic response to brain activation. *Neuroimage*.;23 Suppl 1:S220-33, 2004.

[26] Logothetis N. The Underpinnings of the BOLD Functional Magnetic Resonance Imaging Signal. *J. Neurosci.,* 23:3963–3971, 2003.

[27] Li TQ, Kastrup A, Moseley ME, et al. Changes in baseline cerebral blood flow in humans do not influence regional cerebral blood flow response to photic stimulation. J Magn Reson Imaging. 5:757-62, 2000.

[28] Boxerman JL, Bandettini PA, Kwong KK, et al. The intravascular contribution to fMRI signal change: Monte Carlo modeling and diffusion-weighted studies in vivo. Magn. *Reson. Med.* 34:4–10, 1995.

[29] Rees G, Friston K, Koch C. A direct quantitative relationship between the functional properties of human and macaque V5. *Nat. Neurosci.* 3:716–723, 2000.

[30] Smith AJ, Blumenfeld H, Behar KL. et al Cerebral energetics and spiking frequency: the neurophysiological basis of fMRI. *Proc. Natl. Acad. Sci. USA* 99:10765 10770, 2002.

[31] Ames A. CNS energy metabolism as related to function. *Brain Res. Brain Res. Rev.*,34(1-2):42-68, 2000.

[32] Kida I, Hyder F, Behar KL. Inhibition of voltage-dependent sodium channels suppresses the functional magnetic resonance imaging response to forepaw somatosensory activation in the rodent. *J. Cereb. Blood Flow Metab.* 21:585-91, 2001.

[33] Waldvogel D, van Gelderen P, Muellbacher W, et al. The relative metabolic demand of inhibition and excitation. *Nature*.;406:995-8, 2000.

[34] Buxton RB, Frank LR, Wong EC, et al. A general kinetic model for quantitative perfusion imaging with arterial spin labeling. *Magn. Reson. Med* 40:383-96, 1998.

[35] Uludag K, Dubowitz DJ, Yoder EJ, et al. Coupling of cerebral blood flow and oxygen consumption during physiological activation and deactivation measured with fMRI. *Neuroimage* 23:148-55, 2004.

[36] Logothetis NK. MR imaging in the non-human primate: studies of functional and of dynamics connectiviy. *Curr. Opin. Neurobiol.* 13:630-42, 2003.

[37] Kim DS, Ronen I, Olman C, et al. Spatial relationship between neuronal activity and BOLD functional MRI. *Neuroimage*; 21:876-85, 2004.

[38] Heeger, D.J., Huk, A.C., Geisler, W.S., et al.. Spikes versus BOLD: what does neuroimaging tell us about neuronal activity? *Nat. Neurosci;* 3: 631– 633, 2000.

[39] Frostig RD, Lieke EE, Ts'o DY, et al. Cortical functional architecture and local coupling between neuronal activity and the microcirculation revealed by in vivo high-resolution optical imaging of intrinsic signals. *Proc. Natl. Acad. Sci.* 87:6082-6086, 1990.

[40] Vernieri F, Tibuzzi F, Pasqualetti P, et al. Transcranial Doppler and near-infrared spectroscopy can evaluate the hemodynamic effect of carotid artery occlusion. *Stroke.*;35:64-70, 2004.

[41] Gratton G, Fabiani M, Corballis PM, et al. Fast and localized eventrelated optical signals (EROS) in the human occipital cortex: comparisons with the visual evoked potential and fMRI. *Neuroimage,* 6:168-180, 1997.

[42] Dale AM and Halgren E: Spatiotemporal mapping of brain activity by integration of multiple imaging modalities. *Curr. Opin. Neurobiol.*, 11:202–208, 2001.

[43] Barker AT, Jalinous R, Freeston IL: Non invasive stimulation of human motor cortex. *Lancet* 1:1106-1107, 1985.

[44] Barker AT. The history and basic principles of magnetic nerve stimulation. *Electroencephalogr. Clin. Neurophysiol. Suppl.* 1999;51:3-21.

[45] Wassermann EM, McShane LM, Hallett M, Cohen LG: Noninvasive mapping of muscle representations in human motor cortex. Electroencephalogr *Clin. Neurophysiol.* 85:1-8, 1992.

[46] Classen J, Liepert J, Wise SP, Hallett M, et al: Rapid plasticity of human cortical movement representation induced by practice. *J. Neurophysiol.* 79:1117-1123, 1998.

[47] Rossini PM, Barker AT, Berardelli A, et al: Non-invasive electrical and magnetic stimulation of the brain, spinal cord and roots: basic principles and procedures for routine clinical application. Report of an IFCN committee. *Electroencephalogr. Clin. Neurophysiol.* 91:79-92 1994.

[48] Rothwell JC. Paired-pulse investigations of short-latency intracortical facilitation using TMS in humans. *Electroencephalogr. Clin. Neurophysiol. Suppl.*;51:113-9, 1999.

[49] Rossini PM, Caltagirone C, Castriota-Scandberg A, et al: Hand motor Cortical area reorganization in stroke: a study with fMRI, MEG and TMS maps. *NeuroReport* 9:2141-2146, 1998.

[50] Ridding MC, Rothwell JC. Afferent input and cortical organisation: a study with magnetic stimulation. *Exp. Brain Res.* 126:536-544, 1999.

[51] Ridding MC, McKay DR, Thompson PD, et al. Changes in corticomotor representations induced by prolonged peripheral nerve stimulation in humans. *Clin. Neurophysiol* 112:1461–1469, 2001.

[52] Shimizu T, Hosaki A, Hino T, et al: Motor cortical disinhibition in the unaffected hemisphere after unilateral cortical stroke. *Brain* 125:1896-907, 2002.

[53] Wassermann EM, Grafman J, Berry C, et al.: Use and safety of a new repetitive transcranial magnetic stimulator. *Electroencephalogr. Clin. Neurophysiol.*;101:412-7, 1996.
[54] Babiloni C, Babiloni F, Carducci F, et al: Human brain oscillatory activity phase-locked to painful electrical stimulations: a multi-channel EEG study. *Hum. Brain Mapp.* 15:112-23, 2002.
[55] Mima T, Toma K, Koshy B, et al: Coherence between cortical and muscular activities after a subcortical stroke. *Stroke* 32:2597-2601, 2001.
[56] Babiloni F, Cincotti F, Babiloni C et al: Estimation of the cortical functional connectivity with the multimodal integration of high-resolution EEG and fMRI data by directed transfer function. *Neuroimage*.;24:118-31, 2005.
[57] Rossini PM, Tecchio F, Pizzella V, et al: On the reorganization of sensory hand areas after mono-hemispheric lesion: a functional (MEG)/anatomical (MRI) integrative study. *Brain Res*. 782:153-166, 1998b.
[58] Williamson SJ, Kaufman L: Evolution of neuromagnetic topographic mapping. *Brain Topogr*. 3:113-127, 1996.
[59] Bodurka J, and Bandettini PA. Toward direct mapping of neuronal activity: MRI detection of ultraweak, transient magnetic field changes. Magn Reson Med, 47:1052-8. 2002
[60] Xiong J, Fox PT, and Gao J-H: Directly mapping magnetic field effects of neuronal activity by magnetic resonance imaging. *Hum. Brain Mapp.* 20:41– 49, 2003.
[61] Penfield W and Rasmussen T. The Cerebral Cortex of Man. New York: MacMillan, 1950.
[62] Penfield W and Boldrey E: Somatic motor and sensory representation in cerebral cortex of man as studied by electrical stimulation. *Brain* 60:389-443, 1937.
[63] Sanes JN and Donoghue JP. Plasticity and primary motor cortex. *Annu. Rev. Neurosci.* 23: 393–415, 2000.
[64] Kurth R, Villringer K, Curio G, et al: fMRI shows multiple somatotopic digit representations in human primary somatosensory cortex. *Neuroreport* 11:1487-1491, 2000.
[65] Iwamura Y Hierarchical somatosensory processing Current Opin in Neurobiol 8:522-528, 1998
[66] Disbrow E, Roberts T, Krubitzer L: Somatotopic organization of cortical fields in the lateral sulcus of Homo Sapiens: evidence for SII e PV. *J. Comp. Neurol.* 418: 1-21, 2000.
[67] Del Gratta C, Della Penna S, Ferretti A, et al: Topographic organization of the human primary and secondary somatosensory cortices: comparison of fMRI and MEG findings. *NeuroImage;* 17, 1373–1383., 2002.
[68] Ruben J, Schwiemann J, Deuchert M, et al. Somatotopic organization of human secondary somatosensory cortex. *Cereb. Cortex*; 11: 463-473, 2001.
[69] Recanzone GH, Schreiner CE, Merzenich MM: Plasticity in the frequency representation of primary auditory cortex following discrimination training in adult owl monkeys. *J. Neurosci.* 13:87-103, 1993.

[70] Krause N, McGee T, Carrell TD, et al: Central auditory system plasticity associated with speech discrimination training. *J. Cogn. Neurosci.* 7:25-32, 1995.

[71] Simos PG, Fletcher JM, Bergman E, et al: Dyslexia-specific brain activation profile becomes normal following successful remedial training. *Neurology* 58:1203-1213, 2002.

[72] Pantev C, Oostenveld R, Engelien A, et al: Increased auditory cortical representation in musicians. *Nature* 392:811-814, 1998.

[73] Neville HJ, Mills DL, Lawson DS: Fractionating language: different neural subsystems with different sensitive periods. *Cereb. Cortex* 2:244-58, 1992.

[74] Bavelier D, Tomann A, Hutton C, et al: Visual attention to the periphery is enhanced in congenitally deaf individuals. *J. Neurosci.* 20:1-6.2000.

[75] Pascual-Leone A, Torres F: Plasticity of the sensorimotor cortex representation of the reading finger in Braille readers. *Brain.* 116:39-52,1993.

[76] Cohen LG, Weeks RA, Sadato N, et al: Period of susceptibility for cross-modal plasticity in the blind. *Ann. Neurol.* 45:451-60, 1999.

[77] Karni A, Meyer G, Jezzard P, et al.: Functional MRI evidence for adult motor cortex plasticity during motor skill learning. *Nature*; 377:155-8, 1995.

[78] Abbruzzese G, Trompetto C, Schieppati M: The excitability of the human motor cortex increases during execution and mental imagination of sequential but not repetitive finger movements. *Exp. Brain Res*; 111:465-72, 1996.

[79] Rossini PM, Rossi S: Clinical application of motor evoked potentials. *Electroencep. Clin. Neurophysiol;* 106:180-194, 1998.

[80] Izumi SI, Findley TW, Ikai T, et al: Facilitatory effect of thinking about movement on motor evoked potentials to transcranial magnetic stimulation of the brain. *Am. J. Phys. Med. Rehab.*; 74: 207–213, 1995.

[81] Rossini PM, Desiato MT, Lavaroni F, et al: Brain excitability and electroencephalographic activation: non-invasive evaluation in healthy humans via transcranial magnetic stimulation. *Brain Res.*; 567:111-9, 1991.

[82] Filippi MM, Olivieri M, Pasqualetti P, et al: Effects of motor imagery on motor cortical output topography in Parkinson's disease. *Neurology;* 57:55-61, 2001.

[83] Richter W, Richter M. The shape of the fMRI BOLD response in children and adults changes systematically with age. *Neuroimage;* 20:1122-31, 2003.

[84] D'Esposito M, Deouell LY, Gazzaley A. Alterations in the BOLD fMRI signal with ageing and disease: a challenge for neuroimaging. *Nat. Rev. Neurosci*; 4:863-72, 2003.

[85] Rother J, Knab R, Hamzei F, et al.: Negative dip in BOLD fMRI is caused by blood flow--oxygen consumption uncoupling in humans. *Neuroimage*; 15:98-102, 2002.

[86] Hamzei F, Knab R, Weiller C, et al. The influence of extra- and intracranial artery disease on the BOLD signal in FMRI. *Neuroimage.* 20:1393-9, 2003.

[87] Rossini PM, Altamura C, Ferretti A, et al.. Does cerebrovascular disease affect the coupling between neuronal activity and local haemodynamics? *Brain*;127:99-110, 2004.

[88] Villringer A, Dirnagl U. Coupling of brain activity and cerebral blood flow: basis of functional neuroimaging. *Cerebrovasc. Brain Metab. Rev.*; 7:240-76, 1995.

[89] Binkofski F, Seitz RJ. Modulation of the BOLD-response in early recovery from sensorimotor stroke. *Neurology.* 12;63:1223-9, 2004.

[90] Calautti C, Baron JC: Functional neuroimaging studies of motor recovery after stroke in adults: a review. *Stroke.*;34:1553-66, 2003.

[91] Seiyama A, Seki J, Tanabe HC, et al. Circulatory basis of fMRI signals: relationship between changes in the hemodynamic parameters and BOLD signal intensity. *Neuroimage* ;21:1204-14, 2004.

[92] Ogawa S, Lee TM, Barrere B. The sensitivity of magnetic resonance image signals of a rat brain to changes in the cerebral venous blood oxygenation. *Magn. Reson. Med.* 2:205-10, 1993.

[93] Fujioka H, Kaneko H, Suzuki SS, et al.: Hyperexcitability-associated rapid plasticity after a focal cerebral ischemia. *Stroke*;35:346-8, 2004.

[94] Cicinelli P, Pasqualetti P, Zaccagnini M, et al. Interhemispheric asymmetries of motor cortex excitability in the postacute stroke stage: a paired-pulse transcranial magnetic stimulation study. *Stroke.*;34:2653-8, 2003.

[95] Rossini PM, Tecchio F, Pizzella V, et al. Interhemispheric differences of sensory hand areas after monohemispheric stroke: MEG/MRI integrative study. *Neuroimage*; 14:474-85, 2001.

[96] Rossini PM, Calautti C, Pauri F, et al.: Post-stroke plastic reorganisation in the adult brain. L*ancet Neurol.;*2:493-502, 2003.

[97] Cramer SC, Nelles G, Benson RR, et al: A functional MRI study of subjects recovered from hemiparetic stroke. *Stroke* 28:2518-27, 1997.

[98] Seitz RJ, Hoflich P, Binkofski F, et al.: Role of the premotor cortex in recovery from middle cerebral artery infarction. *Arch. Neurol.* 55:1081-1088, 1998.

[99] Pineiro R, Pendelbury S, Johansen-Berg H, et al.: Functional MRI detects posterior shifts in primary sensorimotor cortex activation after stroke: evidence of local adaptive reorganization? *Stroke* 32:1134-1139, 2001.

[100] Buchkremer-Ratzmann I, August M, Hagemann G, et al.: Electrophysiological transcortical diaschisis after cortical photothrombosis in rat brain. *Stroke* 27:1105-1111, 1996.

[101] Nudo RJ, Milliken GW: Reorganization of movement representations in primary motor cortex following focal ischemic infarcts in adult squirrel monkeys. *J. Neurophysiol.* 75:2144-2149, 1996.

[102] Carey JR, Kimberley TJ, Lewis SM, et al: Analysis of fMRI and finger tracking training in subjects with chronic stroke. *Brain* 125:773-88, 2002.

In: State-of-the-Art Imaging in Stroke, Volume 2
Editor: Bernhard Schaller, pp. 327-345
ISBN 978-1-60021-499-8


*Chapter XI*

# Functional Imaging of Motor Recovery after Stroke

***John W. Krakauer****
The Neurological Institute, Columbia University Medical Center
710 West 168th Street New York NY 10032

## Introduction

Stroke remains the leading cause of adult disability worldwide [1] despite significant advances in its prevention and acute treatment. Thus there is urgent need to better understand the neural mechanisms of stroke recovery in order to develop more scientific rehabilitation approaches and more effective pharmacological therapies. There has been an explosion over the past 15 years in the use of functional brain imaging to study how the mature brain reorganizes after stroke and other forms of brain injury. The purpose of this chapter is twofold: to provide a critical review of what has been learned so far about stroke recovery, specifically motor recovery, from functional imaging and to address methodological and theoretical limitations to the technique for elucidating mechanisms of brain recovery.

## Selection of Patients and Controls

Determining general principles for recovery from stroke is challenge because of the heterogeneity of the condition with regard to onset and etiology, patient age, lesion location, lesion size, and severity of the behavioral deficit [1]. All these factors, unless accounted for, may lead to changes in brain activation that confound interpretation of results as they pertain to recovery. The elderly recruit additional regions compared to the young even when they perform very simple motor tasks [2] and show differences in BOLD response [3]. It is

* Tel: 212 305 1710; Fax: 212 305 1658; email: jwk18@columbia.edu

therefore essential to use age-matched control subjects in functional imaging studies of stroke recovery to avoid misattributing aging-related changes to reorganization after stroke. Recovery from subcortical strokes can be slower that recovery from cortical strokes, which suggests that different restorative mechanisms may be operating in the two cases. In addition, there is evidence to suggest that cortical and subcortical strokes have differential effects on cortical excitability in the contralesional hemisphere [4]. Specifically, a unilateral cortical stroke can lead to decreased transcallosal inhibition of the unaffected hemisphere while this is not seen for subcortical strokes.

Thus, it is probably better to study these two patient populations separately. Imaging studies in healthy subjects show more ipsilateral activation when movements are performed with the non-dominant left hand than with the dominant right hand [5]. Thus mixing patients with strokes in the dominant versus non-dominant hemisphere may make interpretation difficult. fMRI is the functional imaging technique of choice for most studies of brain reorganization after stroke, a technique that depends on a coupling between local cerebral blood flow and neuronal metabolism. Stroke can affect both small and large cerebral vessels and so potentially alter or uncouple this relationship. Indeed, studies have shown that the response can be reduced or absent in the hemisphere ipsilateral to a large vessel stenosis [6, 7]. This complicates interpretation of functional imaging studies of recovery because an area that is contributing to behavior may nevertheless fail to show a response. Restricting hypotheses to areas that are not supplied by the stenosed vessel, ascertained by MRA or a perfusion study, might overcome this problem but the contribution of residual areas around the lesion might be missed.

## Defining Motor Recovery

In order to design a meaningful functional imaging experiment that addresses motor recovery after stroke, motor recovery needs to be properly defined i.e. how it is to be measured. This is crucial issue that is surprisingly underemphasized in studies of recovery although it should be apparent that the regions or patterns of brain activation identified will depend on the behavior in the scanner and/or the out-of-scanner behavioral measures used for modeling or correlating with activation changes. A common way to measure motor recovery is to use either an absolute or a change score using a clinical scale. It is possible, even likely, that neural correlates will differ for a change in performance versus an absolute level of performance. In a patient with only a mild deficit or full clinical recovery, a change measure will be small or zero whereas an absolute measure will be maximal. Conversely, a patient with a severe initial deficit with only partial recovery will score higher on a change measure compared to an absolute measure. A change scale is likely to be more informative in moderate to severely affected patients, whereas an outcome scale is likely to be better in studies of patients with only mild hemiparesis. Psychophysical studies indicate that there may be a categorical difference in the mechanism of impairment for patients with mild versus patients with severe paresis [8, 9]. This suggests these two groups should be studied separately in functional imaging experiments. A further problem is that the term hemiparesis encompasses both positive and negative signs that almost certainly have separable underlying mechanisms (see Krakauer 2005 for more detailed discussion [10]).

Clinical scales can either measure impairment or disability. Impairment is the neurophysiological consequence of a brain lesion whereas disability refers to the consequence of the impairment on activities of daily living (ADLs). An example of a motor impairment scale is the Fugl-Meyer (FM) assessment. This scale was specifically designed for patients with hemiparesis after stroke and sought to address the lack of a quantitative measure of stroke recovery at the level of impairment that could be used to assess the efficacy of a given rehabilitation technique [11]. The rationale behind using an impairment measure is that a disability measure is inadequate to capture the dynamic process of motor recovery and unable to distinguish between true recovery, or vicariation, of function and compensation. Compensation allows a patient to achieve an ADL using alternative strategy (e.g. the patient with a right hemiparesis who learns to use her left hand). In contrast, complete motor recovery implies that the patient is performing the task in the same way as age-matched controls. Thus a patient may be rated as fully recovered on a disability scale but only partially recovered on an impairment scale. A recovery measure needs to be sufficiently sensitive to detect impairment despite the presence of compensatory strategies. This is of particular importance in functional imaging studies because compensatory strategies are also likely to cause novel patterns of activation. For example, use of more proximal limb muscles to aid distal control might lead to contralesional activation, as proximal muscles have more bilateral cortical representation, but this novel activation would not indicate reorganization after stroke. Although positing full recovery on an impairment scale serves to highlight the categorical distinction between recovery and compensation, it remains an open question whether true full recovery ever really occurs. A more sensitive quantitative measure of movement may reveal a subtle abnormality not apparent with the FM score as the FM primarily assesses movements across isolated single joints with much less emphasis on the kinematics of multi-joint movements. Thus depending on the resolution of the measurement tool, performance between patients and controls may or may not differ. This issue profoundly effects interpretation of imaging results. Any difference seen in patients might be the result of the performance difference itself rather than reorganization *per se*. The issue of performance confounds will be addressed again in the context of particular experiments later in the chapter.

## What Hypotheses about Recovery Are Best Addressed by Functional Imaging?

The increased access to MR scanners in hospitals, the user-friendliness of imaging analysis software packages, and the sheer seductiveness of the images themselves has led to a susceptibility to lose sight of the assumptions underlying functional imaging in general, and issues of restoration of function in particular. Investigators should have explicit hypotheses that are optimally suited to testing with functional imaging. As in other areas of scientific investigation, fishing expeditions are not desirable.

Functional imaging is a correlative technique and at best can prove necessity to but not sufficiency of a brain area to behavior. Identification of a novel area of activation does not in itself tell the investigator what the area is doing computationally. An implicit computational assumption, common in the literature, is that if novel areas are involved in recovery then they must be contributing to motor execution. Alternatively, inferring the computational function based on what that area is known to do from other data, risks circularity. Ideally activation in the identified brain area should correlate with a behavioral measure rather than just rely on a simple contrast. Interpretation is also complicated by the possibility that activation is related to factors that are hard to define or measure such as attention, task difficulty or effort rather than execution of the behavior *per se*.

Recovery of function may occur through a number of distinct mechanisms. Utall [12] has provided a list of possible hypotheses regarding the mechanism of recovery of function (Table 1). A well-conducted imaging study should be able to identify or distinguish between these possible mechanisms. We will address these mechanisms again below when we cover cross-sectional and longitudinal study designs.

Hemiparesis, as clinically defined, can result from lesions in a variety of cortical and subcortical locations. Ideally, group analysis would be reserved for studies in which the patients are homogenous with respect to lesion location and other factors. Unfortunately, this is difficult in practice and so far the best that has been managed is to separate cortical and subcortical strokes and subacute and chronic hemiparesis. Group analysis on a heterogenous patient population implicitly assumes that general patterns of recovery-related activation can be identified despite individual differences in lesion location, stroke onset and severity of paresis. This is an empirical question but it could also be that each patient recovers in their own way and that it is the inter-individual variability that is informative rather than average activation across subjects. It is also conceivable to have inter-intervidual variability due to differential expression of a common recovery network. A multivariate approach would be required to demonstrate this.

## Measurement of Motor Behavior in and Outside the Scanner

The functional imaging environment limits motor behavior. Although proximal arm movements can be studied with PET, MR studies are restricted to distal movements of the wrist and fingers or flexion/extension at the elbow. The majority of studies of motor recovery after stroke have used fMRI and almost exclusively employed finger tasks. A limitation of finger movement studies is that they are hard to quantify, being limited to measures of pinch force and tapping rate. Precise quantification is important because, as mentioned above, performance differences can lead to activation differences that might confound interpretation, although it is unlikely that large activation differences are caused by small differences in motor execution. Kinematic trajectory data are rarely obtained and more complex visuomotor control is infrequently studied [13]. Another option is to make the within-scanner task simple but correlate activation changes with more complex measurements obtained at another time outside the scanner. This approach is predicated on the notion that there are general patterns of activation for a range of motor behaviors.

Patients with stroke present a number of additional challenges in the scanning environment compared to age-matched healthy controls. First, patients have reduced stamina and so tire easily. Scans that last more than an hour are likely to yield diminishing returns. Second, there is a higher incidence of mirror movements, involuntary synchronous movements of limbs on the opposite side to the voluntarily moving limb, in the unaffected hand of patients with hemiparesis compared with either hand in age-matched controls [14]. Clearly the presence of mirror movements makes any conclusion about the contribution of ipsilateral motor areas to recovery invalid. This problem was encountered in the original pioneering PET studies of motor recovery after stroke [15-17]. Potential solutions to the mirror-movement problem include EMG measurements from the ipsilateral hand either during the scan or, more conveniently, obtaining arm and leg EMG measurements during pre-scan training in the supine position outside the scanner. Of course, the latter approach assumes that patients will behave in a similar manner once in the scanner. Third, it has been shown that patients with stroke make more unwanted head movements in the scanner when they move either their hand or foot [18]. Head motion causes misregistration of voxel locations to anatomical locations, leading to false-positive activations when the head motion is task-correlated and false-negative results because random motion decreases signal to noise. Unfortunately, patients make more random and more task correlated movements compared to age-matched controls and thus limit who and what can be studied in the scanner.

# Cross-Sectional Studies

The following three criteria, taken from Rickard (2000) [19], have been suggested for the ideal cross-sectional fMRI study of plasticity: (i) There must be clear evidence of complete behavioral recovery of function in the patient; (ii) the computational steps executed by the patient and the controls in the service of the task should be equivalent or differences readily identifiable and quantifiable. (iii) There must be statistically significant activation in a novel area not seen in controls.

Each of these three criteria merit further comment. Evidence for complete behavioral recovery implies that convincing measurements of impairment were obtained in the patient in the subacute period after their stroke. This is important because a return to normal behavior in the subacute period could just be a return to pre-morbid patterns of activation after resolution of transient metabolic abnormalities or edema. Thus, any seemingly novel pattern of activation might reflect how subjects accomplished the task before injury. To claim that patients have made a true recovery requires that their movements are kinematically equivalent, e.g. move at the same average speed and achieve similar accuracy for the within-scanner task, to movements with their unaffected hand, or preferably, to movements made by age-matched controls. Showing a result that is statistically significant at the population level implies, despite heterogeneity in lesion location and severity of the initial deficit, that there are patterns of activation common to all patients who recover from hemiparesis and assumes that these play a role in recovery although it is possible that idiosyncratic individual and lesion-specific mechanisms are equally important.

The initial pioneering PET investigations of motor recovery after subcortical stroke essentially followed the reasoning of the three criteria outlined above. The first study was of 6 patients, two months or more out from first hemiplegic stroke and with good to complete recovery [15]. Patients were required to make sequential finger-to-thumb opposition movements, three every two seconds, with the rate set by a metronome. Patients served as their own controls by performing with their good hand as well as recovered hand. Group analysis showed that finger movement with the good hand primarily activated the contralateral primary sensorimotor cortex and ipsilateral cerebellum. In contrast, finger movements with the recovered hand activated both ipsi- and contra-lateral primary sensorimotor cortex and both cerebellar hemispheres. In addition, they also showed bilateral insula, premotor and inferior parietal activations. The authors concluded that ipsilateral motor pathways may contribute to motor recovery after stroke. However, this interpretation is complicated by a number of limitations, which indicate that the criteria outlined at the beginning of this section were not met by this study. First, no quantification of the extent of the initial paretic deficit is provided. Second, the authors state that testing of power at the wrist and hand showed no deficit but do not quantify their testing nor describe how it was done. Third, finger opposition is not a power task and so strength testing may not be apposite as it is a well-known clinical observation that patients with hemiparesis can recover power before finger individuation. Fourth, there was no detailed measurement of the finger-opposition task itself and so it is possible that there may have been subtle differences in performance, the authors themselves mention the possibility of mirror movements and overflow activity from axial muscles. Thus, the statistically significant additional activations seen with the 'recovered" hand may not represent recovery-related reorganization. The same group performed a follow-up study in 10 patients with recovery from striatocapsular infarction [16]. At least four of the patients made mirror movements. The results were very similar to the first study, with patients showing bilateral primary sensorimotor and cerebellar activation, along with bilateral insula and inferior parieatal activation. However, other than using age-matched controls instead of the unaffected hand, the same limitations stated above apply to this second study. The main concern is that mirror movements may have been responsible for the ipsilateral activations observed. The authors make the valid point that mirror movements themselves might be part of the recovery process but this does not answer the question whether the additional ipsilateral activations are necessary for movement of the recovered fingers rather than just the unaffected ones. This question was addressed by a third PET study perfomed by this group in which they compared activation in individual patients to a group of age-matched controls [17]. Notably, ipsilateral primary sensorimotor activation was only seen in those patients who made mirror movements. However, all patients showed increased ipsilateral premotor and contralateral cerebellar activation compared to controls, suggesting that ipsilateral activations may also relate to movements of the recovered hand. Overall, it is apparent that these three studies, although groundbreaking both in terms of question and approach, were confounded by mirror movements and potentially confounded by inadequate quantification of the initial deficit, of the degree of recovery and of the motor task in the scanner.

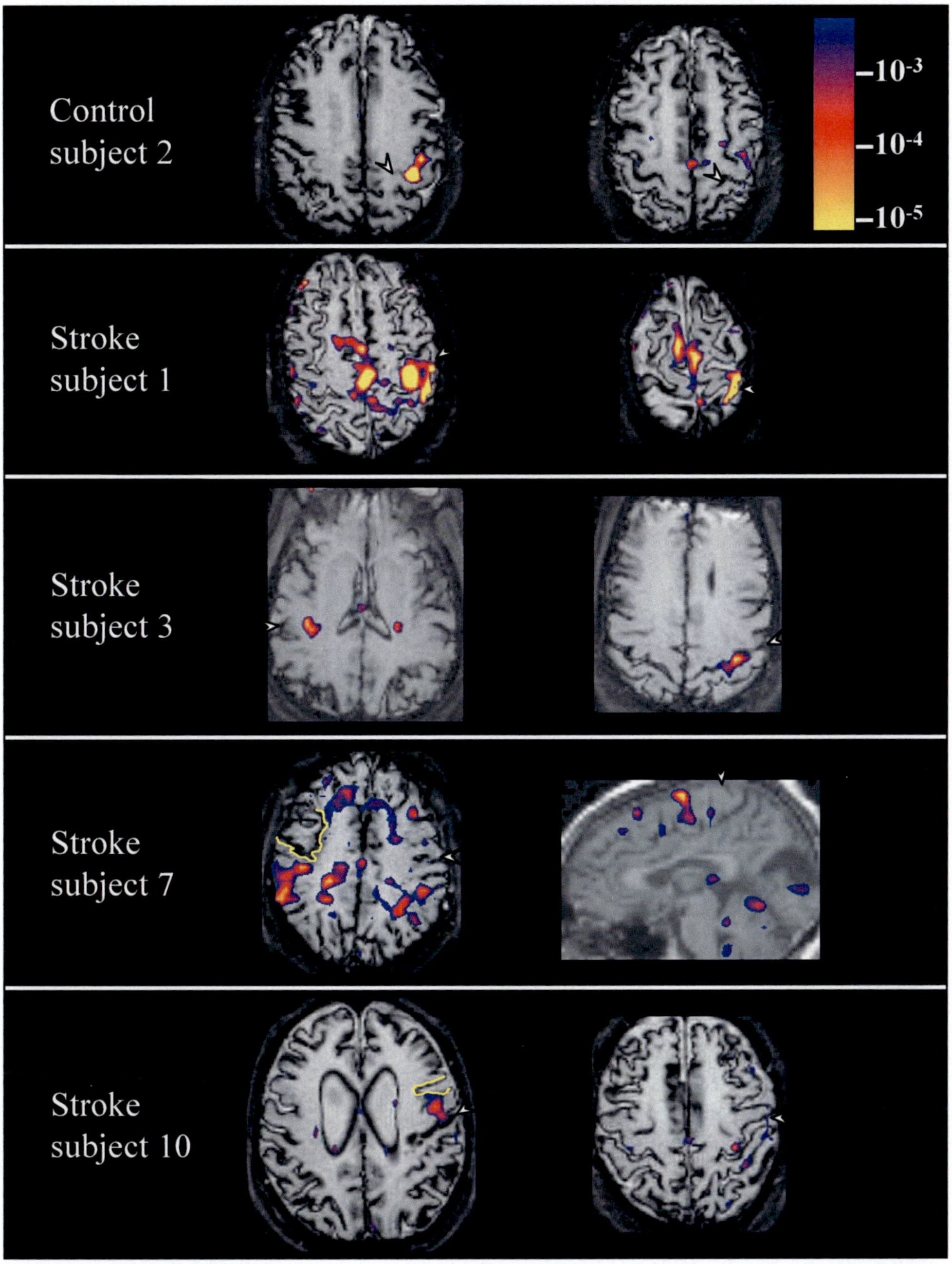


Figure 1. (Taken from Cramer et al. (1997), with permission). Axial fMRI activation images for a control subject and four patients recovered from hemiparesis, obtained by comparing rest with tapping of the right index finger. Increased activation in patients with stroke was identified by comparing the number of activated voxels within pre-chosen ROIs for each patient against a distribution generated from all control subjects' activations for the same task. Row 1. fMRI activation images for a control subject. The patients in rows 2 and 3 had left subcortical infarcts, located ventral to the images shown. In both patients there was significantly increased activation in the right (contralesional)sensorimotor cortex and in the SMA compared to controls. The patients in rows 4 and 5 had cortical infarcts (outlined in yellow). Two types of additional activation are apparent: increased activation in bilateral sensrimotor cortex and peri-infarct activation.

A similar rationale and approach to the aforementioned PET studies has been used in recent fMRI studies. In one such study [20], recovery was, like in the PET studies, defined on the basis of fairly crude strength criteria. The investigators used an index finger tapping rather than a finger-opposition task, applied a region-of-interest (ROI) analysis to compute a laterality index, and included patients with cortical strokes. Findings were very similar to the earlier PET studies with increased ipsilateral primary sensorimotor and premotor activation, and contralateral cerebellar activation, compared to controls (Figure 1). Importantly, only one patient was observed to make mirror movements in the scanner, suggesting that ipsilateral activation in primary sensorimotor cortex may not just be due to mirror movements but to recovery itself. These findings were confirmed in more recent prospective study [21], for which 8 patients were recruited with hemiparetic stroke from cortical or subcortical stroke within one month of the first motor measurement and who underwent 6 weeks of rehabilitation before undergoing functional imaging. The advantages of this study were that time after stroke was more uniform, motor performance was assessed before and after recovery, and EMG was obtained within the scanner to detect mirror movements. All the patients were deemed to have made excellent recoveries on the basis of grip force measurements and a functional battery called the Jebsen hand test. The main finding was that the patients, when they performed a 1 Hz finger opposition task, activated bilateral primary and premotor cortices even in the absence of EMG activity in the unaffected hand. In contrast, healthy subjects showed strictly contralateral activation of motor areas. Thus both PET and fMRI studies in patients with good clinical recovery indicate that additional contralesional brain regions are activated compared to controls despite similar motor performance and absent mirror movements.

As outlined above, studying patients with complete or near-complete recovery controls for performance confounds and thus allows comparison of activation patterns in patients and controls. However, this approach excludes the large number of patients who only make partial clinical recovery. To address this problem, cross-sectional studies have also been attempted in patients with only partial recovery or variable degrees of recovery.

One study used an event-related design and a near-isometric wrist extension task in 3 patients with chronic (> 6 months) hemiparesis and only partial clinical recovery [22]. The combination of a simple movement requirement and an event-related design, which permits elimination of poorly executed trials from image analysis, allows approximate matching of performance between patients and controls. Patients showed, as in studies of patients with excellent clinical recovery, increased activation in ipsilateral motor cortex despite the absence of detectable force production in the unaffected hand. A larger cross-sectional study recruited 20 patients with variable degrees of recovery after cortical and subcortical stroke [23]. One novel aspect to the study was to control for performance *within* the scanner but then correlate activation changes with performance variation on a composite *out-of-scanner* measure obtained on the same day as the fMRI. The within scanner task was a paced dynamic isometric handgrip task with a force requirement normalized to each patient's own maximum voluntary contraction. This was done in order to control for effort and relative performance. A second novel aspect to the study was to perform a principal components analysis on the whole data set of outcome measures to obtain a single representative outcome score, the first principal component, with which activation patterns across the patient group were correlated.

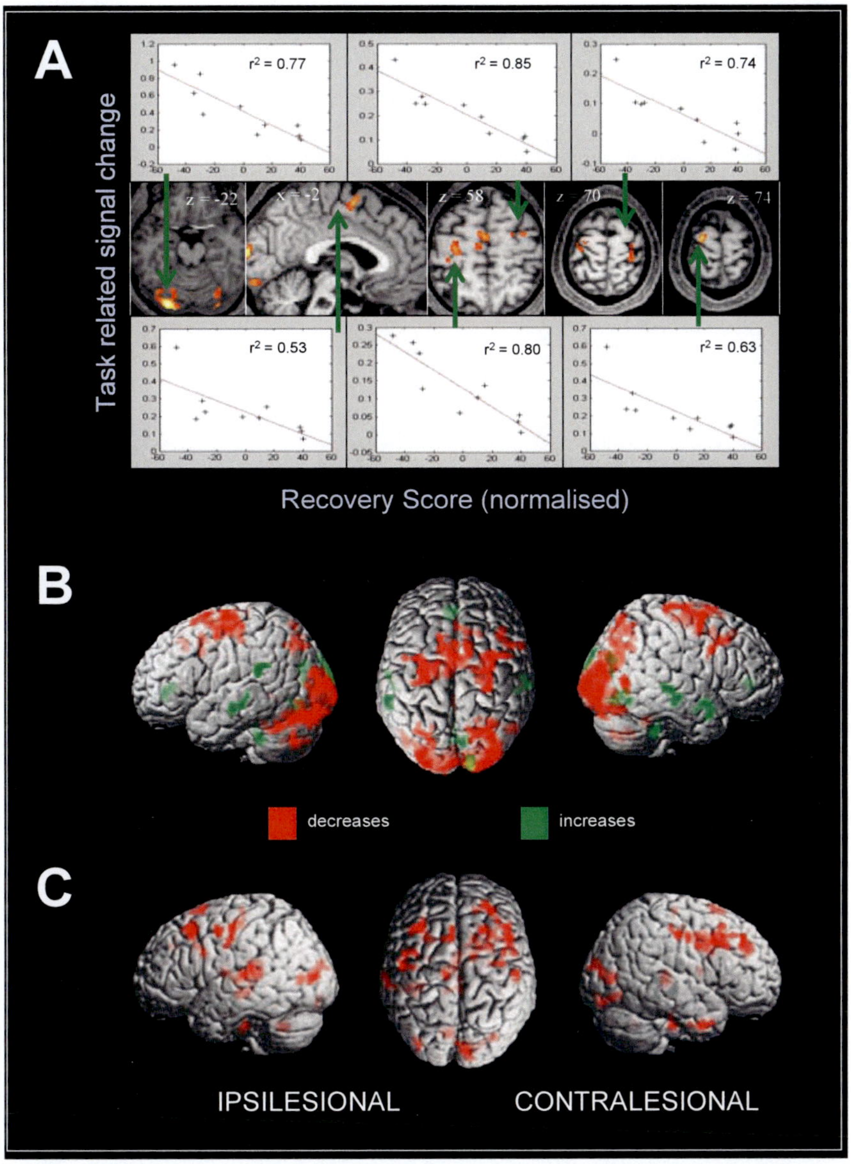


Figure 2. (Taken from Ward et al. (2003), with permission). A. Results of a single patient longitudinal analysis examining linear changes in task-related brain activations over sessions as a function of recovery. The patient had a left-pontine infarct resulting in right hemiparesis. Results are displayed on the patient's own normalized T1-weighted anatomical images (voxels significant at $p < 0.05$, corrected for multiple comparisons, with corresponding plots of size of effect against a normalized recovery score. The correlations coefficients were significant for all six of the selected brain regions. B. Results surface rendered, in three projections, on a canonical brain; red areas represent recovery-related decreases in task-related activation across sessions, and green areas represent task-related activation increases. C. Group 'recovery map' rendered on a canonical brain: brain regions in which linear reductions in task-related activation across sessions as a function of recovery were consistently detected for the whole group of patients. Random effects analysis, all clusters significant at $p < 0.05$, corrected for multiple comparisons). Images for patients with left-sided lesions were flipped about the mid-sagittal plane so that all patients were assumed to have a right-sided lesion. (left hemisphere is on the left, CL = contralesional; IL = ipsilesional).

There was no evidence for mirror movements by EMG when subjects performed the same isometric task outside the scanner. The main result of this study was that across the whole patient group and across stroke subtypes, there was a *negative* correlation between outcome and the degree of task-related activation in novel primary motor, premotor, parietal and cerebellar areas (Figure 2). There was no difference in task-related activation compared to the normal population in six patients with the best outcome. This study appears to contradict previous cross-sectional studies but can perhaps be reconciled with them by positing that in those studies, patients deemed fully-recovered would have been found to have a residual motor deficit with the more detailed outcome measure of the later study. A possible overall conclusion from the cross-sectional studies would be that activation of novel brain areas may represent functional reorganization but these areas are unable to mediate complete recovery. A problem with this interpretation, however, is that the additional activations could instead be due to the performance differences across patients rather than reorganization *per se*. An indirect answer to this issue of a performance confound came from an interesting cross-sectional study, which compared patients with chronic hemiparesis from cortical versus subcortical strokes [24]. The important finding was that despite comparable motor impairment, i.e. performance, in the cortical and subcortical groups, they showed significantly different patterns of brain activation when they moved the paretic limb. Specifically, whereas patients with subcortical stroke recruited canonical corticocerebellar regions along with ipsilateral post-central gyrus, patients with cortical stroke only showed activation around the stroke cavity, in mesial frontal areas and ipsilateral post-central gyrus. As performance did not differ across the two groups, these results suggest that novel patterns of brain activation represent post-stroke reorganization.

In general it is safer to infer that novel activation is related to restoration of function if there is a well-documented initial deficit followed by a recovered state at the time of imaging. This is especially true for studies of studies of higher cognitive functions, such as language, where a novel pattern of activation may reflect a pre-morbid pattern rather than reorganization. The functional anatomy of the motor system is more consistent across subjects, however, and makes it possible to ask the question whether the absence of a motor deficit in the presence of a lesion is because the brain has reorganized to maintain normal motor performance. This argument has had more traction with slow progressive disease than in stroke. For example, patients with multiple sclerosis without focal deficit or with only a single episode of optic neuritis show increased ipsilateral fMRI motor activation that correlates with lesion burden [25]. A conclusion from this result is that the additional ipsilateral activation maintains normal motor function despite the presence of lesions expected to cause a motor deficit. A similar result has been obtained recently in patients with critical carotid or middle cerebral artery stenosis or occlusion causing unilateral hemispheric hypoperfusion without infarction [26]. Patients showed increased motor activation in the normally perfused hemisphere despite the absence of any motor deficit on examination (Figure 3). An analogous result was obtained in a recent functional imaging study of movements of the ipsilesional arm in patients with right MCA infarction. The main finding was that although there were no observable behavioral differences in the left arm of patients and controls, patients showed significantly more bi-hemispheric activation [27]. Taken together, the results in the contralateral arm of patients with hemispheric hypoperfusion and in the ipsilesional arm of patients with unilateral stroke show that altered patterns of brain activation occur in the absence of an observable neurological deficit.

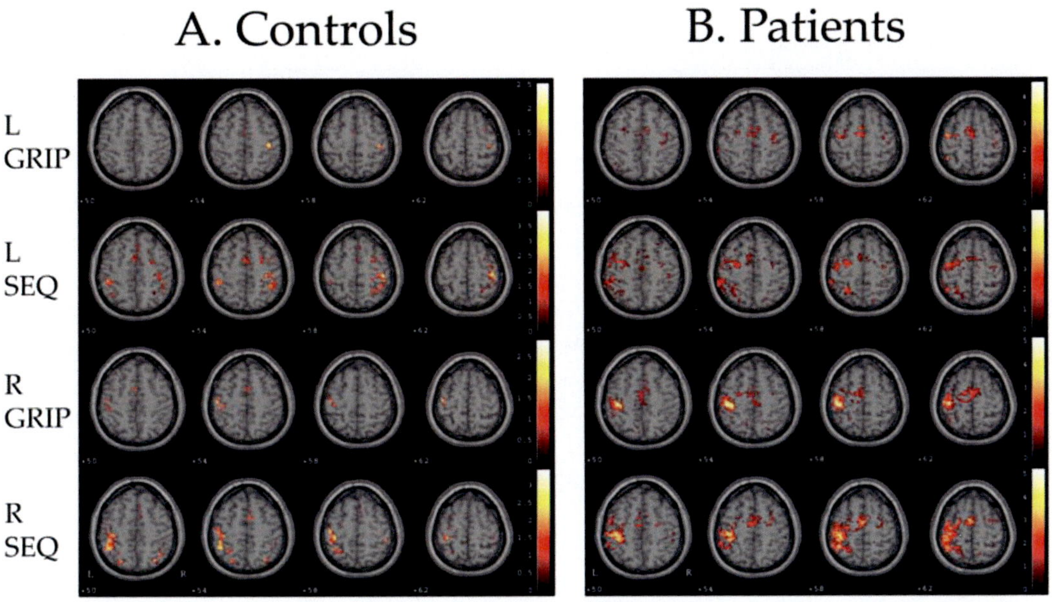


Figure 3. (Taken from Krakauer et al (2004).Group analyses on controls and patients with unilateral hemispheric hypoperfusion without stroke. Axial activation maps using a fixed-effects model with conjunction analysis ($p < 0.001$, uncorrected). Patients using the "affected" left hand predominantly activated left (ipsilateral) areas, whereas controls predominantly activated right (contralateral) areas. Both patients and controls activated contralaterally when using the "unaffected" right hand. Color bars to the right of each condition indicate the range of activation $t$ – values.

## Longitudinal Studies

Longitudinal studies of motor recovery after stroke image patients serially over the time course of recovery. The advantages of a longitudinal approach are that it allows study of patients who have not fully recovered and better captures a process that is known to change over time. A longitudinal study is a potentially powerful way to show reorganization if a *positive* correlation can be shown between an area of activation not seen in controls and longitudinal recovery on a behavioral measure. Such a result would be compelling because impaired motor performance would be expected to show the opposite correlation, i.e. negative, with the time course of recovery.

The first longitudinal functional imaging study of motor recovery after stroke scanned 8 patients with subcortical infarcts within 48 hours of their stroke and then again 3-6 months later [28]. Activation was compared between patients and controls and at the two time points by computing a laterality index using primary sensorimotor, medial and lateral premotor ROIs. The main findings were that patients showed more contralesional motor area activation than controls and that the laterality index increased, i.e. the ratio of ipsilesional to contralesional motor area activation, from the acute to the chronic timepoint, in parallel with improvement in hand function. This study suggested that recovery is associated with a return to a contralateral pattern of motor activation, consistent with the cross-sectional study by Ward et al. described above, which showed best recovery in those patients with patterns of activation indistinguishable from those seen in controls [23]. A similar result, with a shift in the balance of activation back to ipsilesional motor areas over time and a correlation of this shift with recovery, has been obtained in subsequent longitudinal studies using PET [29-31] and fMRI [32-34]. A particularly well-conducted study imaged 8 patients with first-ever subcortical stroke at frequent post-stroke time points and obtained detailed outcome measures at each of these timepoints [34]. A principal strength of this study was that the investigators sought to identify areas that were a function of recovery rather than of time after stroke. The first scan was obtained 10-14 days post-stroke onset and then patients were scanned weekly for at least the next four weeks and then at 3, 6 and, for some, 12 months post-stroke. The main finding was that task-related brain activations decreased over sessions in primary and premotor regions as a function of recovery in all patients, independent of initial severity or rate of recovery. Notably, whereas there were consistent decreases in activation that correlated with recovery there were no areas that showed a consistent increase in activation as recovery proceeded. Thus, as with earlier longitudinal studies, there was no evidence for sustained cortical reorganization that mediated behavioral improvement. As argued above, negative correlation would be expected if performance differences themselves drive differences in activation. However, the authors went to considerable lengths to control for performance differences within the scanner. When they controlled for absolute force and rate, they still found a negative correlation between novel activation and recovery. Thus the interpretation of what the negatively- correlated activation represents is complex. The authors postulate that it may represent either task difficulty or reorganization. The same level of performance might be more difficult to maintain early after stroke and then becomes easier and so activation decreases. Task difficulty is hard to define formally or to quantify. In addition, even if it could be defined, the reason why the task becomes less difficult as recovery proceeds would need to be explained. Either additional activation is playing an active role in making the task easier, e.g. a learning role, or some other recovery process is taking place and makes the additional areas less necessary over time. The latter mechanism should be associated with areas that positively correlate with recovery.

One longitudinal study specifically tested this hypothesis [35], using a form of ROI analysis, that over the course of stroke recovery, brain activation would increase in ipsi- and contra-lesional M1, premotor areas and in the cerebellum. Twelve patients were scanned at 1, 2, 3 and 6 months post-stroke on a finger opposition and wrist flexion/extension task. Patients were dichotomized into those with better versus worse recovery. Recovery was assessed with an index finger tapping task, the nine-hole peg test, and grip dynamometry. The investigators found a significant interaction between degree of recovery, hemisphere, and region of activation; which indicated that better recovery was associated with a pattern of activation that differed from the pattern seen in patients with poor recovery. *Post-hoc* analysis showed that the three-way interaction was driven entirely by significantly more ipsilateral cerebellar activation in the patients with better recovery compared with those with worse recovery. Notably, although there was increased activation in contralateral M1 when moving the paretic hand, it did not differ between better and worse recoverers. The authors speculate that the observed increased ipsilateral cerebellar activation may reflect a learning process, which contributes to recovery. In addition to the interesting positive result, this study emphasizes the fact that increased activation cannot be assumed to be relevant to recovery unless correlation is found with good behavioral measures. The activation might instead relate temporally to the evolution of other variables such as hemodynamics or diaschisis or represent a general response to hemiparesis or injury that is not relevant to recovery.

A more recent study [36] tested the hypothesis, based on results in non-human primates [37], that a stroke limited to a portion of primary motor cortex is associated with reorganization within the surrounding motor cortex and that this leads to reacquisition of a motor skill. Four right-handed patients with ischemic strokes limited to M1 were imaged longitudinally over three sessions: <20 days, 4 months, and 2 years after stroke. Four age-matched controls were imaged at the same intervals. The basic finding was that skilled motor recovery was associated with a transition from contralesional activation to ipsilesional activation in a location in M1, which was more dorsal compared to controls. The observed dorso-medial shift is consistent with **AN** adjacent cortical reorganization mechanism as has been seem in non-human primates.

## Functional Imaging Correlates of Stroke Rehabilitation

The cross-sectional and longitudinal studies described above were conducted in patients with both acute and chronic stroke. The studies did not control for the modality of or time spent in rehabilitation and therefore results may reflect a combination of spontaneous recovery and responses to therapeutic intervention. There have, however, been a few small studies that have used functional imaging to assess responses to specific forms of rehabilitation. All these studies attempted to control for performance confounds and obtained scans before and after treatment. One small study recruited four patients who had a chronic stroke, either left or right, cortical or subcortical, and suffered loss of finger individuation [38]. The motor task was 4-finger flexion-extension movements at 0.5 hz. Subjects received two weeks of constraint-induced therapy (CIT) [39-41]. ROIs were drawn for primary motor cortex, premotor cortex and SMA. The extent of activation was determined by counting the number of activated voxels and then a laterality index was calculated. Patients showed an improvement on the Fugl-Meyer stroke scale and on the Wolf-Motor function test. In association with this motor improvement there was a decrease in the laterality index, i.e. a shift towards contralesional activation. This result is interesting in so much that it contradicts most of the longitudinal studies described in the previous section, which showed an increase in the laterality index as recovery proceeded. It is important to note, however, that this was very small study with a heterogeneous mix of patients and not much can be concluded from it. Indeed, three other studies have shown that activation increases in motor areas on the ipsilesional side in response to task-oriented training [42] and CIT [43, 44]. In the most careful of these studies [44] , a group analysis of 7 patients with chronic hemiparesis showed that therapy-related improvements in hand-function correlated with increases in fMRI activity in the premotor and secondary somatosensory cortex on the ipsilesional side and bilateral superior cerebellum. Again, infarct location and side was heterogeneous, although the authors state that the hand region of the pre-central gyrus was not involved. The task was a paced 4-finger flexion/extension task and performance did not appreciably differ across scans.

At best, with the assumption that performance in the scanner did not change before and after therapy, the aforementioned studies suggest that motor representation changes in response to therapy. Not much more can be said because of the low patient number and the heterogeneity of lesion locations. The question whether reorganization in patients with chronic stroke in response to therapy is qualitatively different from spontaneous reorganization in the acute and sub-acute post-stroke period, as seen in the longitudinal studies described in the previous section, will require further investigation.

## Experiments That Complement Functional Imaging Studies

Functional imaging can only show that an area of activation correlates with motor behavior but not that it is necessary for recovery. If an area of novel activation mediates recovery then there should be re-emergence of the original deficit when the area is inactivated. This test has been applied in animal models with ablation or muscimol infusion and in humans with transcranial magnetic stimulation (TMS). A lesion of the hand representation in primary sensorimotor cortex in adult macaques resulted in complete loss of dexterity in the hand for 1-2 months. At around 3-4 months, there was a return to about 30% of pre-lesion dexterity. This improvement was reversed with muscimol infusion into the ipsilesional dorsal and ventral premotor areas but not with muscimol infusion into perilesional cortex or contralesional M1 [45]. More recently, it was shown that an ischemic lesion in the forelimb region of M1 in squirrel monkeys led to expansion of the hand representation in ipsilesional ventral premotor cortex (PMv) [46]. Interestingly, the degree of map reorganization in PMv was proportional to the amount of hand representation destroyed in M1. This result in monkeys provides a clue as to why novel functional activation patterns are seen most in patients with the greatest deficit. Similar results have been obtained using TMS in patients with chronic stroke and good recovery [47]. Four patients with capsular infarcts and good recovery from moderate to severe hemiparesis underwent single pulse TMS to the ipsilesional dorsal premotor cortex (PMd), which caused a delay in reaction time for the contralateral hand in patients but not in controls. In these well-recovered patients, TMS applied to contralesional M1 or PMd had no effect on reaction time. The same approach was used in a group of patients with more variable degrees of recovery [48]. TMS applied to contralesional PMd led to an increase in reaction time in the patients but not in controls. Importantly, the magnitude of the effect of TMS on contralesional PMd was correlated with the degree of hand impairment, consistent with the studies in monkeys described above. Thus reorganization can occur in cortex adjacent to the infarct, in premotor regions in the ipsilesional hemisphere and in motor regions in the contralesional hemisphere. Recruitment of more remote regions may depend both on the extent and location of the infarct and on stroke severity. This conclusion is supported by a recent study in rats [49], which showed that recruitment of the undamaged hemisphere depended on the degree of functional integrity of the remaining ipsilesional sensorimotor system.

The idea that contralesional motor recruitment is a function of degree of damage to motor areas on the ipsilesional side is attractive and explains several results in animals and humans. However, it is clear that this is not the whole story. We have already encountered situations above in which additional activation is seen in patients with good recovery and even in patients with no symptoms but with hemodynamic or structural lesions. A further example of the likely ability of remote regions to contribute to good recovery comes from reports of re-emergence of stroke deficits in patients who suffer a second stroke on the opposite side. C. Miller-Fisher [50] described two patients with pure motor hemiparesis with substantial recovery who then had subsequent mirror lesions (proven at autopsy) on the opposite side, the capsule in one patient and the medulla in the other patient, and presented with quadraparesis. A similar case has been reported more recently [51]. Thus, the contradiction seen between cross-sectional and longitudinal functional imaging studies in humans is also to some extent seen in animal experiments and clinical observations. With the current state of knowledge, all that can be said is that additional brain regions might be contributing to behavior in a number of different ways, only some of which have been effectively probed.

## Conclusions

Functional imaging seeks to correlate areas and patterns of brain activation with behavior. Even in healthy subjects, the technique is faced by considerable technical, anatomical and conceptual difficulties. These difficulties are compounded in studies of neurological patients, especially in the acute and subacute phases of a disease, because of the lack of stable baseline as brain systems are likely to be dynamically changing. Stroke is a particularly challenging disease to study because it is heterogeneous with respect to lesion location, initial severity and individual idiosyncrasies in the time-course of recovery. The complexities of using functional imaging to study brain reorganization after stroke are exemplified by the apparent contradictory findings between cross-sectional and longitudinal studies of stroke recovery. Cross-sectional studies often show altered brain activation patterns in patients with good recovery whereas longitudinal studies suggest that altered activation patterns are associated with the worst recovery. Part of the explanation for such conflicting results is that different types of stroke patient were selected for the two types of study. For example, in the initial PET studies of stroke recovery, patients with alleged full recovery may in fact have had deficits that were not adequately measured. Future studies will need to select larger and more homogeneous groups of patients with respect to lesion side and location and make great efforts to quantitatively measure performance and control for performance confounds. A change in conceptual approach that emphasizes interactions between brain regions rather than correlations between behavior and mean activations in single regions will likely prove more promising.

The use of functional imaging to assess responses to pharmacological and rehabilitation is also fraught with difficulties. Showing activation changes as patients respond to treatment is trivial unless performance can be kept constant across time points. This seems counterintuitive because the hope is that the patients will show substantial improvements with therapy. As in all science, it is necessary to have a hypothesis before embarking on a study using functional imaging techniques. It is useful to ask what question will be answered by functional imaging that otherwise could not be answered. The demonstration of changes in the brain in the absence of an either/or hypothesis is not very interesting. True insights into brain mechanisms of recovery from stroke will only come from complementing functional imaging studies with other types of experimental investigation in human and non-human animals.

## References

[1] Wolfe CD. The impact of stroke. *Br. Med. Bull.* 2000; 56:275-86.

[2] Calautti C, Serrati C, Baron JC. Effects of age on brain activation during auditory-cued thumb-to-index opposition: A positron emission tomography study. *Stroke* 2001; 32:139-46.

[3] D'Esposito M, Zarahn E, Aguirre GK, et al. The effect of normal aging on the coupling of neural activity to the bold hemodynamic response. *Neuroimage* 1999; 10:6-14.

[4] Shimizu T, Hosaki A, Hino T, et al. Motor cortical disinhibition in the unaffected hemisphere after unilateral cortical stroke. *Brain* 2002; 125:1896-907.

[5] Singh LN, Higano S, Takahashi S, et al. Comparison of ipsilateral activation between right and left handers: a functional MR imaging study. *Neuroreport* 1998; 9:1861-6.

[6] Bilecen D, Radu EW, Schulte AC, et al. fMRI of the auditory cortex in patients with unilateral carotid artery steno-occlusive disease. *J. Magn. Reson. Imaging*. 2002; 15:621-7.

[7] Rother J, Knab R, Hamzei F, et al. Negative dip in BOLD fMRI is caused by blood flow--oxygen consumption uncoupling in humans. *Neuroimage* 2002; 15:98-102.

[8] Cirstea MC, Levin MF. Compensatory strategies for reaching in stroke. *Brain* 2000; 123 ( Pt 5):940-53.

[9] Reinkensmeyer DJ, McKenna Cole A, Kahn LE, et al. Directional control of reaching is preserved following mild/moderate stroke and stochastically constrained following severe stroke. *Exp. Brain Res*. 2002; 143:525-30.

[10] Krakauer JW. Arm function after stroke: from physiology to recovery. *Seminars in Neurology* 2005.

[11] Gladstone DJ, Danells CJ, Black SE. The fugl-meyer assessment of motor recovery after stroke: a critical review of its measurement properties. *Neurorehabil. Neural. Repair* 2002; 16:232-40.

[12] Uttal WR. *The Psychobiology of Mind*: Lawrence Erlbaum., 1978.

[13] Carey JR, Kimberley TJ, Lewis SM, et al. Analysis of fMRI and finger tracking training in subjects with chronic stroke. *Brain* 2002; 125:773-88.

[14] Nelles G, Cramer SC, Schaechter JD, et al. Quantitative assessment of mirror movements after stroke. *Stroke* 1998; 29:1182-7.

[15] Chollet F, DiPiero V, Wise RJ, et al. The functional anatomy of motor recovery after stroke in humans: a study with positron emission tomography. *Ann. Neurol.* 1991; 29:63-71.
[16] Weiller C, Chollet F, Friston KJ, et al. Functional reorganization of the brain in recovery from striatocapsular infarction in man. *Ann. Neurol.* 1992; 31:463-72.
[17] Weiller C, Ramsay SC, Wise RJ, et al. Individual patterns of functional reorganization in the human cerebral cortex after capsular infarction. *Ann. Neurol.* 1993; 33:181-9.
[18] Seto E, Sela G, McIlroy WE, et al. Quantifying head motion associated with motor tasks used in fMRI. *Neuroimage* 2001; 14:284-97.
[19] Rickard TC. Methodological issues in functional magnetic resonance imaging studies of plasticity following brain injury. In: Levin HS, Graftman J, eds. *Cerebral reorganization of function after brain damage*, 2000:304-317.
[20] Cramer SC, Nelles G, Benson RR, et al. A functional MRI study of subjects recovered from hemiparetic stroke. *Stroke* 1997; 28:2518-27.
[21] Butefisch CM, Kleiser R, Korber B, et al. Recruitment of contralesional motor cortex in stroke patients with recovery of hand function. *Neurology* 2005; 64:1067-9.
[22] Newton J, Sunderland A, Butterworth SE, et al. A pilot study of event-related functional magnetic resonance imaging of monitored wrist movements in patients with partial recovery. *Stroke* 2002; 33:2881-2887.
[23] Ward NS, Brown MM, Thompson AJ, et al. Neural correlates of outcome after stroke: a cross-sectional fMRI study. *Brain* 2003; 126:1430-48.
[24] Luft AR, Waller S, Forrester L, et al. Lesion location alters brain activation in chronically impaired stroke survivors. *Neuroimage* 2004; 21:924-935.
[25] Reddy H, Narayanan S, Arnoutelis R, et al. Evidence for adaptive functional changes in the cerebral cortex with axonal injury from multiple sclerosis. *Brain* 2000; 123:2314-20.
[26] Krakauer JW, Radoeva PD, Zarahn E, et al. Hypoperfusion without stroke alters motor activation in the opposite hemisphere. *Ann. Neurol.* 2004; 56:796-802.
[27] Hanlon CA, Buffington AL, McKeown MJ. New brain networks are active after right MCA stroke when moving the ipsilesional arm. *Neurology* 2005; 64:114-20.
[28] Marshall RS, Perera GM, Lazar RM, et al. Evolution of cortical activation during recovery from corticospinal tract infarction. *Stroke* 2000; 31:656-61.
[29] Nelles G, Spiekramann G, Jueptner M, et al. Evolution of functional reorganization in hemiplegic stroke: a serial positron emission tomographic activation study. *Ann. Neurol.* 1999; 46:901-9.
[30] Calautti C, Leroy F, Guincestre JY, et al. Dynamics of motor network overactivation after striatocapsular stroke: a longitudinal PET study using a fixed-performance paradigm. *Stroke* 2001; 32:2534-42.
[31] Calautti C, Leroy F, Guincestre JY, et al. Displacement of primary sensorimotor cortex activation after subcortical stroke: a longitudinal PET study with clinical correlation. *Neuroimage* 2003; 19:1650-4.
[32] Feydy A, Carlier R, Roby-Brami A, et al. Longitudinal study of motor recovery after stroke: recruitment and focusing of brain activation. *Stroke* 2002; 33:1610-7.

[33] Jang SH, Kim YH, Cho SH, et al. Cortical reorganization associated with motor recovery in hemiparetic stroke patients. *Neuroreport* 2003; 14:1305-10.
[34] Ward NS, Brown MM, Thompson AJ, et al. Neural correlates of motor recovery after stroke: a longitudinal fMRI study. *Brain* 2003; 126:2476-96.
[35] Small SL, Hlustik P, Noll DC, et al. Cerebellar hemispheric activation ipsilateral to the paretic hand correlates with functional recovery after stroke. *Brain* 2002; 125:1544-57.
[36] Jaillard A, Martin CD, Garambois K, et al. Vicarious function within the human primary motor cortex? A longitudinal fMRI stroke study. *Brain* 2005; 128:1122-38.
[37] Nudo RJ, Wise BM, SiFuentes F, et al. Neural substrates for the effects of rehabilitative training on motor recovery after ischemic infarct. *Science* 1996; 272:1791-1794.
[38] Schaechter JD, Kraft E, Hilliard TS, et al. Motor recovery and cortical reorganization after constraint-induced movement therapy in stroke patients: a preliminary study. *Neurorehabil. Neural. Repair* 2002; 16:326-38.
[39] Taub E, Miller NE, Novack TA, et al. Technique to improve chronic motor deficit after stroke. *Arch. Phys. Med. Rehabil.* 1993; 74:347-54.
[40] van der Lee JH, Wagenaar RC, Lankhorst GJ, et al. Forced use of the upper extremity in chronic stroke patients: results from a single-blind randomized clinical trial. *Stroke* 1999; 30:2369-75.
[41] Dromerick AW, Edwards DF, Hahn M. Does the application of constraint-induced movement therapy during acute rehabilitation reduce arm impairment after ischemic stroke? *Stroke* 2000; 31:2984-8.
[42] Jang SH, Kim YH, Cho SH, et al. Cortical reorganization induced by task-oriented training in chronic hemiplegic stroke patients. *Neuroreport* 2003; 14:137-41.
[43] Levy CE, Nichols DS, Schmalbrock PM, et al. Functional MRI evidence of cortical reorganization in upper-limb stroke hemiplegia treated with constraint-induced movement therapy. *Am. J. Phys. Med. Rehabil.* 2001; 80:4-12.
[44] Johansen-Berg H, Dawes H, Guy C, et al. Correlation between motor improvements and altered fMRI activity after rehabilitative therapy. *Brain* 2002; 125:2731-42.
[45] Liu Y, Rouiller EM. Mechanisms of recovery of dexterity following unilateral lesion of the sensorimotor cortex in adult monkeys. *Exp. Brain Res.* 1999; 128:149-59.
[46] Frost SB, Barbay S, Friel KM, et al. Reorganization of remote cortical regions after ischemic brain injury: a potential substrate for stroke recovery. *J. Neurophysiol.* 2003; 89:3205-14.
[47] Fridman EA, Hanakawa T, Chung M, et al. Reorganization of the human ipsilesional premotor cortex after stroke. *Brain* 2004; 127:747-58.
[48] Johansen-Berg H, Rushworth MF, Bogdanovic MD, et al. The role of ipsilateral premotor cortex in hand movement after stroke. *Proc. Natl. Acad. Sci. USA* 2002; 99:14518-23.
[49] Biernaskie J, Szymanska A, Windle V, et al. Bi-hemispheric contribution to functional motor recovery of the affected forelimb following focal ischemic brain injury in rats. *Eur. J. Neurosci.* 2005; 21:989-99.
[50] Fisher CM. Concerning the mechanism of recovery in stroke hemiphegia. Canadian *Journal of Neurological Sciences* 1992; 19:57-63.

[51] Ago T, Kitazono T, Ooboshi H, et al. Deterioration of pre-existing hemiparesis brought about by subsequent ipsilateral lacunar infarction. *J. Neurol. Neurosurg. Psychiatry* 2003; 74:1152-3.

In: State-of-the-Art Imaging in Stroke, Volume 2
Editor: Bernhard Schaller, pp. 347-357
ISBN 978-1-60021-499-8


*Chapter XII*

# Imaging in Acute Stroke: Prospects for the Future

***Bernhard Schaller[1], Hans-Christoph Ludwig[2] and Michael Buchfelder[2]***
[1]Department of Neuroscience, Karolinska Institute, Stockholm, Sweden
[2]Department of Clinical Neuroscience, University Hospital, University of Göttingen, Germany

## A. Introduction

Cerebral ischemia implies a mismatch between blood flow and the metabolic needs of brain tissue. Hence maintenance of cerebral blood flow (CBF) above the infarction threshold is critical in preventing irreversible brain damage. The phenomenon of autoregulation is largely due to changes in the diameter of cerebral resistance vessels. One goal of acute intervention in stroke is therefore to maintain CBF above the infarction threshold.

CBF thresholds have led to the concept of the ischemic "penumbra" – an area of brain surrounding a dead infracted core where blood flows are between 10 and 20 ml/100g/minutes [1]. Many treatment strategies are therefore aimed at preserving and expanding the penumbra zone. Positron emission tomography (PET) studies have identified certain patterns indicative of the penumbra zone. In addition to decreased CBF, jeopardized brain tissue may show increased blood volume related to compensatory vasodilatation, or an increased oxygen extraction fraction (OEF), which maintains cerebral metabolism of oxygen in the face of reduced flow [2]. Unfortunately, PET is not widely available and is not a practical tool for urgent or repeated monitoring of CBF and cerebral metabolism in patients with rapidly evolving infarction. In addition, magnetic resonance (MR) diffusion imaging and functional MR imaging, combined with MR angiography, hold great promise for the early characterization of brain ischemia and their complications.

# B. Emergency Vascular Surgery

Emergency carotid endarterectomy (CEA) represents a controversial issue; the indications are not yet well defined. CEA early after cerebral infarction carries a high risk of perioperative worsening or massive hemorrhage into the infarct due to the sudden increase of perfusion pressure after restoration of blood flow. However, in selected cases emergency CEA may be indicated, for example, in patients suffering an acute carotid occlusion during hospitalization, during angiography, or immediately after carotid surgery.

Emergency CEA should also be considered for patients with fluctuating or progressive neurological deficits and high-grade stenosis of the internal carotid artery [3]. This includes patients with progressive stroke, waxing and waning neurological deficits, and crescendo TIAs despite anticoagulation. Even for a progressive stroke patient with a floating intraluminal thrombus, delay of CEA is usually advocated since immediate carotid surgery carries a high risk of perioperative embolism. If anticoagulation does not stop the attacks, CEA can be justified to prevent massive arterial embolization or acute thrombotic occlusion of the carotid artery. If fluctuating symptoms are of hemodynamic origin, CEA can restore blood flow and promptly improve or stabilize neurological deficits. This rare clinical scenario can be confirmed by transcranial ultrasound with estimation of the vasomotor reserve using $CO_2$ or diamox stimulation. In the future, angiography may be the treatment of choice in such cases, provided that the carotid stenosis is smooth and without ulceration. In rare cases with bilateral severe ICA stenoses, or occlusion on the symptomatic side with contralateral flow to the hemisphere producing clinical sigs of ischemia of hemodynamic origin. MCA embolectomy attempts to restore blood flow immediately, and there are some reports of favorable results if the operation is performed within six hours after the embolic event [4]. The operation is associated with the risk of large hematoma due to recirculation injury. Since local and systemic thrombolysis is now feasible, MCA embolectomy will be only of historical interest in the near future. As in thrombolysis, the extent of collateral blood flow documented during pre-treatment angiography is the best predictor of outcome.

## Cerebral Reperfusion Hemorrhage after Carotid Stenting or Carotid Endarterectomy

In 1981, Sundt et al. [5] used the term "hyperperfusion syndrome" to describe a triad of complications that included atypical migrainous phenomena, transient focal seizure activity, and intracerebral hemorrhage (ICH) after CEA. Symptoms usually developed five to seven days postoperatively and were often preceded by unilateral headaches; the triad was not complete in all patients. The features were attributed to elevated ipsilateral CBF without a significant change in systemic arterial blood pressure. Breen et al. [6] reported that the frequency of the hyperperfusion syndrome was 2.7% in their series, and in a recent review of the literature the frequency of ICH after CEA ranged from 0.3% to 1.2%. However, these authors noted that the blood pressure was elevated in the majority of patients at the time of presentation with the hyperperfusion syndrome. Percutaneous transluminal angioplasty (PTA) and angioplasty with stenting are increasingly being used as an alternative to carotid artery surgery in patients with carotid artery stenosis, but as experience with this relatively novel technique accrues, the true complication rate has not yet been established.

Cerebral hyperperfusion represents a rarer cause of stroke after these revascularization procedures. Clinical symptoms are thought to result from a sudden, rapid increase in CBF after reperfusion of a circulatory territory exposed to long-standing decreased perfusion pressure, although the pathophysiological characteristics of hyperperfusion syndrome remains poorly understood. Hemodynamic changes may not depend on degree of carotid artery stenosis alone [7, 8] but on a combination of factors contributing to cerebral circulation. The degree of carotid artery stenosis has been associated with impaired cerebral autoregulation [9] and the presence of collateral supply [10]. Other associated risk factors for hyperperfusion include hypertension [11], prior infarct [12, 13], severe ipsilateral and contralateral carotid artery stenosis [14, 15], clotting abnormalities [16], poor collateral circulation [17, 18], and decreased cerebrovascular reserve [19].

Despite the increasing use of PTA and stenting for the treatment of extracranial carotid artery stenosis, there are only four reports of "hyperperfusion injury" following PTA/stenting in the literature to date [20-22]. Two of these patients had ICA PTA [21, 22], one patient had common carotid artery stenting for recurrent stenosis after CEA [20], and one patient had PTA of the ICA and both vertebral arteries and stenting of the right subclavian artery [22]. Headache, seizures, ICH, and hypertension were noted in two patients (one of them developed diffuse basal subarachnoid hemorrhage) [22], headache and ICH (without reference to the blood pressure or seizures), in one patient [21], but the clinical details were not specified for the fourth patient [20]. Cerebral hyperperfusion injury may occur in the presence of normal or elevated arterial blood pressure after CEA [5, 6], but it has been associated with severe hypertension (240/100 mm Hg) after carotid angioplasty in the two cases in which it has been documented to date [22]. Because fatal hyperperfusion ICH has now been described after ICA stenting, in addition to PTA without primary stenting, one must be aware of this potential complication in both treatment groups.

## C. Pathophysiological Background of Hyperperfusion Syndrome

In patients with severe carotid artery stenosis, cerebral autoregulation may be impaired, as evidenced by decreased cerebrovascular reactivity [9]. One might assume that impaired autoregulation is most likely to occur in vascular territories distal to a marked stenosis [23]. However, Ko et al. did not find that the degree of vascular stenosis was predictive of CBF increases after treatment [23]. At least two possible explanations may account for this observation. First, the severity of carotid artery stenosis may not adequately reflect the extent of collateral perfusion pressure, which is available to the distal circulation (24). In particular, the development of a vascular stenosis due to atheromatous disease might be expected to stimulate the development or enlargement of collateral pathways. Future studies should assess the presence of collateral flow pathways and vasomotor reserve and their effect on CBF increases after endovascular stent placement [19, 25, 26]. Given the evidence gleaned from CEA, extent of collateral flow and vasomotor reserve seem likely to have an association in the setting of endovascular treatments. Second, the presence of hyperperfusion may be unrelated to hemodynamic factors and may involve other neuroeffectors. The autonomic nervous system is perturbed in the postoperative period after endovascular stent placement [27], and it may contribute, through some mechanism, to the observed changes in cerebral hemodynamics [18]. Such changes could involve the release of vasoactive neuropeptides involved in autoregulation.

### Carotid Artery Endarterectomy and Intracerebral Hemorrhagic Stroke

Hyperperfusion after CEA has been proposed as the main mechanism of intracerebral hemorrhage, which is a disastrous complication and contains a situation in which long-standing hypoperfusion results in chronic dilatation and loss of the normal compensatory autoregulation and vasoconstriction of cerebral vasculature. With restored blood flow, these dilated vessels then experience supranormal flow rates resulting in rupture and hemorrhage. The rate of intracerebral hemorrhagic stroke has been documented ranging from 0.4 to 2% [28-31]. Intracerebral hemorrhagic stroke generally occurred between 1 and 24 days postoperatively. In addition to prior recent stroke, factors identified with intracerebral hemorrhagic stroke are hypertension, headache, and increased flow velocities noted on transcranial Doppler [31, 32]. Ouriel et al. [28] added that younger age and severe cerebrovascular occlusive disease appeared to increase the risk of postoperative intracerebral hemorrhagic stroke. They further postulated that improved preoperative and postoperative management of cardiac disease and operative techniques resulting in decreased morbidity would cause the traditionally stable incidence of intracerebral hemorrhagic stroke to become a relatively more common complication.

The best treatment for hemorrhagic stroke would appear to be prevention. Control of arterial blood pressure and avoidance of anticoagulation and antiplatelet medication are important. Once intracerebral hemorrhagic stroke is documented, neurosurgical consultation is mandatory; however, the outlook is often poor. Clearly, further study is needed regarding the avoidance of this frequently fatal complication in the future.

## D. Intracerebral Hemorrhage and Imaging

Acute treatment options generally not differ according to intracerebral hemorrhage (ICH) etiologies, but the different pathophysiological origin of nontraumatic ICH may require different treatments. The vascular lesions underlying ICH often remain unrecognized; particularly the microvasculopathies that are often associated with hypertensive vasculopathy and CAA. It is possible to detect other small vasculopathic changes such as Charcot–Bouchard aneurysms in hypertensive vasculopathy or microaneurysms and vessel splitting associated with CAA by the current state-of-the-art-imaging modalities such as MRI and CT [33]. Another very promising approach to diagnosis of CAA lies in the molecular imaging with labeling the components of vascular amyloid, as for example the ß-amyloid peptide itself [34, 35].

In the near future, detection of old microhemorrages in ICH by gradient-echo MRI may be a promising imaging modalities that sheeds further light in the (pathophysiological) mechanism of ICH [36-38]. A potentially important advance in this regard is the development of very-high-field MRI technologies [39, 40], such as 8 Tesla. It is expected to receive more detailed knowledge on hemorrhages and individual blood products by these improvements in MRI technologies. Future imaging approaches to hematoma expansion should also allow fine differentiation of the age of clot that might be separated by minutes or hours rather than the current MRI classification of acute, subacute, and chronic. Finally, the ability to image the distribution of specific blood and cellular components such as thrombin, plasmin, plasminogen activators, inflammatory cells, platelet aggregation, and clot dissolution would be a major step toward elucidating the balance of thrombosis and thrombolysis in the process of clot expansion.

## Imaging of Vascular Properties: Perihematoma Perfusion and Hypoperfusion

Compromised cerebral perfusion, either as a direct consequence of ICH or as an unintended effect of candidate treatments such as blood pressure reduction for preventing expansion or rebleeding [41], represents a potential source of tissue injury in ICH and an important target for neuroimaging.

At some relatively large clot volume (depending on the extent of atrophy), there should be an elevation of intracranial pressure and a decrease of global cerebral perfusion, particularly in subjects treated with artrial blood pressure reduction. This effect would be global, perhaps with a gradient from the immediate perihematoma region to adjacent intracranial compartments [42]. An ideal modality for monitoring this effect would be a rapidly accessible, quantitative blood flow study. This information might be acquired by measure of a blood flow-related variable such as tissue oxygen availability. A matrix of tissue oxygen monitors using near-infrared spectroscopy [43] placed over both hemispheres (technology currently available) could provide access to continuous flow-related information that could help guide the question of global harm caused by hypoperfusion.

The safety of aggressive arterial blood pressure reduction for a smaller ICH demands monitoring of local flow changes. Flow information would be needed for this application, because it would not be desirable to reduce the pressure to the point of causing an elevation of lactate or glutamate or the depletion of ATP, steps that mark permanent damage to the surrounding tissues. Measurement of cerebral blood flow by MR spectroscopy and PET is an example of an emerging real-time, high-resolution technique also potentially available for bedside use with increasing availability.

A specific mechanism of compromised perfusion to be investigated by tomographic high-resolution flow imaging is the remote effects of ICH caused by compression of the anterior or posterior cerebral arteries. A similar set of questions pertains to the possible effects on perfusion of delayed perihematoma edema, which may cause compression of local perforating vessels as well as remote major cerebral vessels. Studies of perfusion at baseline or after manipulation of arterial blood pressure or $CO_2$, ideally coupled with measurements of metabolism and oxygen extraction, could provide insight as to whether such alterations in perfusion are a cause (rather than an effect) of perihematoma tissue injury.

Some caution will be required in determining whether post-ICH levels of perfusion decrease below ischemic thresholds, which are undoubtedly reduced by decreases in metabolic activity in the region of the hematoma [43]. Interpretation of the information will also be complicated by the fact that the greatest effect of subcortical ICH is on the white matter, for which we do not have a defined ischemic threshold. Diffusion-weighted imaging including apparent diffusion coefficient mapping offers an alternative approach for identifying perihematoma regions with bioenergetic compromise potentially caused by ischemia. Several small-scale studies suggest there may be a subgroup of patients with decreased perihematoma apparent diffusion coefficient values in the hyperacute phase [44]. Additional large-scale, prospective studies are needed to confirm this. Magnetic resonance spectroscopic studies acquired at the same scanning session can provide complementary information regarding the time course and frequency of changes in lactate and *N*-acetyl aspartate [45].

## E. Neuroimaging of Tissue Properties: Perihematoma Injury, Edema

An important target for imaging is the location and mechanism of neuronal cell death in ICH. Necrosis and apoptosis, related mechanisms of cell death, are candidates for imaging after ICH. Methodical approaches, as already used in the myocardium, adapted to brain cell death would be a major step toward understanding toxic mechanisms in ICH. A second set of targets for molecular probes are the inflammatory pathways induced by ICH. Metabolic markers such as deoxyglucose uptake [46] can image the high-energy requirements of various types of inflammatory cells. More specific identification of inflammatory cells has been approached through use of radiolabeled cytokines, lymphokines, and growth factors, which avidly bind to receptors on cells of specific classes and states of activation [47]. Further molecular probes for the intracellular and intercellular signaling pathways activated in response to ICH are likely to emerge with our growing understanding of these signal transduction pathways.

Another major goal in studying the tissue response to ICH is to understand the formation of perihematoma edema. Serial studies using MRI fluid-attenuated inversion recovery (FLAIR) sequences should be undertaken to document the evolution of edema and correlate it with hemorrhage size and location. Neuroimaging can also serve as a bridge between human ICH and experimental models, which have implicated thrombin and other blood breakdown products as contributors to perihematoma edema through effects on the blood–brain barrier and direct tissue injury [47]. Post-gadolinium FLAIR studies of the HARM (hyperintense acute reperfusion marker) phenomenon observed in ischemic stroke, for example, may provide insight into the nature and time course of blood–brain barrier disruption [48]. A potentially powerful method for defining molecular mechanisms active in the perihematoma tissue is analysis of the association between neuroimaging and gene expression data. Specimens for human studies could be derived from tissue obtained at surgical evacuation or biopsy. This would allow correlation of events occurring in the perihematoma molecular cascade of injury with radiological progression of ICH, edema, and clinical outcome.

These molecular approaches to tissue injury and inflammation can be supplemented by functional assessments of neuronal and neural circuit integrity. Functional neuroimaging provides the possibility of mapping not only deficits expected from the initial hemorrhage but also those functions potentially altered by further clot expansion or edema. Performing functional studies in acutely ill ICH patients will require new functional paradigms that can be applied to aphasic or patients with alteration in consciousness. Another emerging approach for detecting the integrity of neural circuits is through imaging of water diffusion along white matter tracts, including the sensitive techniques of diffusion-tensor and diffusion-spectrum imaging [49]. Both techniques allow characterization of the direction as well as the diffusibility of water in the brain; diffusion-tensor imaging assumes water mobility can be described by a Gaussian function or tensor, whereas diffusion-spectrum imaging does not make such simplifying (and time-saving) assumptions.

## F. New Imaging Agents

There are several important challenges in applying molecular imaging approaches to ICH. Probes will need to be modified to cross the blood–brain barrier. Studies aimed at delivery of drugs to the central nervous system have developed several promising approaches to this problem, such as use of drug-carrying nanoparticles coated with nonionic substances to reduce uptake by reticuloendothelial cells [50]. To minimize nonspecific backgrounds, the molecular probes will ideally exit the central nervous system rapidly as well. Finally, it will be important to develop agents detectable by MRI (for example, by conjugation to superparamagnetic iron oxide nanoparticles [51]) to take advantage of the high spatial resolution and widespread availability of this imaging modality.

## G. Imaging and Clinical Studies

The wide diversity of imaging protocols and software/hardware configurations has complicated attempts to pool data across collaborating sites. Creation of standardized parameters for imaging and a multicenter repository for clinical and radiographic data would be an important step toward assessing the clinical significance of novel radiographic markers and allowing them to be used in large-scale studies of ICH.

Further neuroimaging studies are needed to characterize radiographic markers of response to putative therapies such as hematoma drainage and neuroprotection, and of neurological outcome. In the case of ICH evacuation, serial imaging will likely provide a means to assess the effect of evacuation techniques and monitor for early hemorrhage recurrence. Additional studies are needed to identify baseline characteristics of patients likely to have good or bad outcome without intervention, as well as characteristics of patients most likely to experience ongoing injury or to respond to acute therapies.

# H. Take-Home-Message

These findings also offer support for use of hemorrhages detected by MRI as a surrogate outcome marker in studies of ICA. The cumulative number or incident appearance of hemorrhages predicts the likelihood of symptomatic ICH, suggesting that microhemorrhages reflect essentially the same underlying pathological process as symptomatic ICH. Although it remains unclear whether acute neurosurgical intervention improves the overall long-term outcome in intracerebral haemorrhage, it may reduce early mortality [52]. At experienced centres, aggressive interventional care shows promise in improving both morbidity and mortality [53]. One surrogate for neurosurgical availability is teaching hospital status. Observational evidence that differences in mortality exist by hospital type, after adjustment for case mix, is worth exploring.

# References

[1] Heiss WD, Thiel A, Grond M, et al. Contribution of immediate and delayed ischaemic damage to the volume of final infarcts. *Lancet* 1999; 353:1677-8.

[2] Heiss WD, Thiel A, Grond M, et al. Which targets are relevant for therapy of acute ischemic stroke? *Stroke* 2000; 30:1486-9.

[3] Heros RC. Carotid endarterectomy in patients with intraluminal thrombus. *Stroke* 19:667-668.

[4] Meyer FD, Piepgras TG, Sundt TM, et al. Emergency embolectomy for acute occlusion of the middle cerebral artery. *J. Neurosurg.* 1985; 62:639-47.

[5] Sundt TM, Sharbrough FW, Piepgras DG, et al. Correlation of cerebral blood flow and electroencephalographic changes during carotid endarterectomy. *Mayo. Clin. Proc.* 1981;56:533–543.

[6] Breen JC, Caplan LR, DeWitt LD, et al. Brain edema after carotid surgery. *Neurology.* 1996;46:175–181.

[7] Powers WJ, Press GA, Grubb RL Jr, et al. The effect of hemodynamically significant carotid artery disease on the hemodynamic status of the cerebral circulation. *Ann. Intern. Med.* 1987;106:27–34.

[8] Boysen G. Cerebral hemodynamics in carotid surgery. *Acta. Neurol. Scand. Suppl.* 1973;52:3–86.

[9] Reinhard M, Roth M, Muller T, et al. Cerebral autoregulation in carotid artery occlusive disease assessed from spontaneous blood pressure fluctuations by the correlation coefficient index. *Stroke* 2003;34:2138–2144.

[10] Henderson RD, Eliasziw M, Fox AJ, et al. Angiographically defined collateral circulation and risk of stroke in patients with severe carotid artery stenosis. North American Symptomatic Carotid Endarterectomy Trial (NASCET) Group. *Stroke* 2000;31:128–132.

[11] Sbarigia E, Speziale F, Giannoni MF, et al. Post-carotid endarterectomy hyperperfusion syndrome: preliminary observations for identifying at risk patients by transcranial Doppler sonography and the acetazolamide test. *Eur. J. Vasc. Surg.* 1993;7:252–256.

[12] Schroeder T, Sillesen H, Sorensen O, et al. Cerebral hyperperfusion following carotid endarterectomy. *J. Neurosurg.* 1987;66:824–829.
[13] Bernstein M, Fleming JFR, Deck JHN. Cerebral hyperperfusion after carotid endarterectomy: a cause of cerebral hemorrhage. *Neurosurgery* 1984;15:50–56.
[14] Reigel MM, Hollier LH, Sundt TM Jr, et al. Cerebral hyperperfusion syndrome: a cause of neurologic dysfunction after carotid endarterectomy. *J. Vasc. Surg.* 1987;5:628–634.
[15] Schroeder T, Holstein PE, Engell HC. Hyperperfusion following endarterectomy [letter]. *Stroke* 1984;15:758.
[16] Piepgras DG, Morgan MK, Sundt TM Jr, et al. Intracerebral hemorrhage after carotid endarterectomy. *J. Neurosurg.* 1988;68:532–536.
[17] Schroeder T, Engell HC, Sillesen H. Cerebral blood flow and cerebral perfusion reserve after carotid endarterectomy [Suppl]. *J. Cereb. Blood Flow Metab.* 1987;7:36.
[18] Macfarlane R, Moskowitz MA, Sakas DE, et al. The role of neuroeffector mechanisms in cerebral hyperperfusion syndromes. *J. Neurosurg.* 1991;75:845–855.
[19] Ogasawara K, Yukawa H, Kobayashi M, et al. Prediction and monitoring of cerebral hyperperfusion after carotid endarterectomy by using single-photon emission computerized tomography scanning. *J. Neurosurg.* 2003;99:504–510.
[20] Bergeron P, Chambran P, Benichou H, Alessandri C. Recurrent carotid disease: will stents be an alternative to surgery? *J. Endovasc. Surg.* 1996;3:76–79.
[21] Benichou H, Bergeron P. Carotid angioplasty and stenting: will periprocedural transcranial Doppler monitoring be important? *J. Endovasc. Surg.* 1996;3:217–223.
[22] Schoser BGH, Heesen C, Eckert B, et al. Cerebral hyperperfusion injury after percutaneous transluminal angioplasty of extracranial arteries. *J. Neurol.* 1997;244:101–104.
[23] Ko NU, Achrol AS, Chopra M, et al. Cerebral blood flow changes after endovascular treatment of cerebrovascular stenoses. *AJNR* 2005; 26:538-42.
[24] Derdeyn CP. Cerebral hemodynamics in carotid occlusive disease. *AJNR Am. J. Neuroradiol.* 2003;24:1497–1499.
[25] Schroeder T. Hemodynamic significance of internal carotid artery disease. *Acta Neurol. Scand.* 1988;77:353–372.
[26] Hosoda K, Kawaguchi T, Ishii K, et al. Prediction of hyperperfusion after carotid endarterectomy by brain SPECT analysis with semiquantitative statistical mapping method. *Stroke* 2003;34:1187–1193.
[27] Qureshi AI, Luft AR, Sharma M, et al. Frequency and determinants of postprocedural hemodynamic instability after carotid angioplasty and stenting. *Stroke* 1999;30:2086–2093.
[28] Ouriel K, Shortell CK, Illig KA, et al. Intracerebral hemorrhage after carotid endarterectomy: incidence, contribution to neurologic morbidity, and predictive factors. *J. Vasc. Surg.* 1999;29:82-89.
[29] Solomon RA, Loftus CM, Quest DO, et al. Incidence and etiology of intracerebral hemorrhage following carotid endarterectomy. *J. Neurosurg.* 1986;64:29-34.
[30] Reith HB, Edelmann M, Reith C. Spontaneous intracerebral hemorrhage following carotid endarterectomy. Experience of 328 operations from 1983-1988. *Int. Surg.* 1992;77:224-225.

[31] Jansen C, Sprengers AM, Moll FL, et al. Prediction of intracerebral hemorrhage after carotid endarterectomy by clinical criteria and intraoperative transcranial Doppler monitoring. *Eur. J. Vasc. Surg.* 1994;8:303-308.
[32] Mansoor GA, White WB, Grunnet M, et al. Intracerebral hemorrhage after carotid endarterectomy associated with ipsilateral fibrinoid necrosis: a consequence of the hyperperfusion syndrome? *J. Vasc. Surg.* 1996;23:147-151.
[33] Mandybur TI. Cerebral amyloid angiopathy: the vascular pathology and complications. *J. Exp. Neurol.* 1986; 45: 79-80.
[34] Schaller B, Tolnay M, Kleindienst A. State-of-the-art-imaging-methods to investigate the neurovascular mechanism in the origin of Alzheimer`s Disease. Differential diagnostic evaluations to other types of dementia. *Prog. Neurobiol.* 2005; in press.
[35] Klunk WE, Bacskai BJ, Mathis CA, et al. Imaging abeta plaques in living transgenic mice with microscopy and methoxy-x04, a systemically administered Congo red derivative. *J. Neuropathol. Exp. Neurol.* 2002; 61: 797-805.
[36] Kidwell CS, Saver JL, Villablanca JP, et al. Magnetic resonance imaging detection of microhemorrhages before thrombolysis: an emerging application. *Stroke.* 2002; 33: 95–98.
[37] Greenberg SM, Finklestein SP, Schaefer PW. Petechial hemorrhages accompanying lobar hemorrhage: detection by gradient-echo MRI. *Neurology.* 1996; 46: 1751–1754.
[38] Rosand J. Hypertens and the brain: stroke is just the tip of the iceberg. *Neurology.* 2004; 63: 6–7.
[39] Abduljalil AM, Schmalbrock P, Novak V, et al. Enhanced gray and white matter contrast of phase susceptibility-weighted images in ultra-high-field magnetic resonance imaging. *J. Magn. Reson. Imaging.* 2003; 18: 284–290.
[40] Kangarlu A, Burgess RE, Zhu H, et al. Cognitive, cardiac, and physiological safety studies in ultra high field magnetic resonance imaging. *Magn. Reson. Imaging.* 1999; 17: 1407–1416.
[41] Morgenstern LB, Yonas H. Lowering blood pressure in acute intracerebral hemorrhage: safe, but will it help? *Neurology.* 2001; 57: 5–6.
[42] Schaller B, Graf R. Different compartment of intracranial pressure and its relationship to cerebral blood flow. *J. Trauma* 2005; in press.
[43] Owen-Reece H, Smith M, Elwell CE, et al. Near infrared spectroscopy. *Br. J. Anaesth.* 1999; 82: 418–426.
[44] Carhuapoma JR, Wang PY, Beauchamp NJ, et al. Diffusion-weighted MRI and proton MR spectroscopic imaging in the study of secondary neuronal injury after intracerebral hemorrhage. *Stroke.* 2000; 31: 726–732.
[45] Flotats A, Carrio I. Non-invasive in vivo imaging of myocardial apoptosis and necrosis. *Eur. J. Nucl. Med. Mol. Imaging.* 2003; 30: 615–630.
[46] Hofstra L, Liem IH, Dumont EA, et al. Visualization of cell death in vivo in patients with acute myocardial infarction. *Lancet.* 2000; 356: 209–212.
[47] Hua Y, Bhasin RR, Ennis SR, et al. Mechanisms of edema formation after intracerebral hemorrhage: effects of extravasated red blood cells on blood flow and blood–brain barrier integrity. *Stroke.* 2001; 32: 2932–2938.

[48] Warach S, Latour LL. Evidence of reperfusion injury, exacerbated by thrombolytic therapy, in human focal brain ischemia using a novel imaging marker of early blood–brain barrier disruption. *Stroke*. 2004; in press.

[49] Kunimatsu A, Aoki S, Masutani Y, et al. Three-dimensional white matter tractography by diffusion tensor imaging in ischaemic stroke involving the corticospinal tract. *Neuroradiology*. 2003; 45: 532–535.

[50] Schroeder U, Sommerfeld P, Ulrich S, et al. Nanoparticle technology for delivery of drugs across the blood–brain barrier. *J. Pharm. Sci.* 1998; 87: 1305–1307.

[51] Signore A, Chianelli M, Bei R, et al. Targeting cytokine/chemokine receptors: a challenge for molecular nuclear medicine. *Eur. J. Nucl. Med. Mol. Imaging*. 2003; 30: 801–802.

[52] Qureshi AI, Tuhrim S, Broderick J, et al. Spontaneous intracerebral hemorrhage. N. Engl. J. Med. 2001;344: 1450-60.

[53] Naff NJ, Carhuapoma JR, Williams MA, et al. Treatment of intraventricular hemorrhage with urokinase: effects on 30-day survival. *Stroke* 2000:31: 841-7.

# Index

## D

## E

## F

## G



## H

## I

## J



## K



## L

## M

## N

## O

## P

## Q



## R

## S

## U



## V

## W



## X



## Y